Axonal Transport in Neuronal Growth and Regeneration

Advances in Neurochemistry

SERIES EDITORS

B. W. Agranoff, *University of Michigan, Ann Arbor*
M. H. Aprison, *Indiana University School of Medicine, Indianapolis*

ADVISORY EDITORS

J. Axelrod	F. Margolis	P. Morell	J. S. O'Brien
F. Fonnum	B. S. McEwen	W. T. Norton	E. Roberts

Volumes 1-4   Edited by B. W. Agranoff and M. H. Aprison

Volume 5   OLIGODENDROGLIA
Edited by William T. Norton

Volume 6   AXONAL TRANSPORT IN NEURONAL GROWTH
AND REGENERATION
Edited by John S. Elam and Paul Cancalon

A Continuation Order Plan is available for this series. A continuation order will bring delivery of each new volume immediately upon publication. Volumes are billed only upon actual shipment. For further information please contact the publisher.

Axonal Transport in Neuronal Growth and Regeneration

Edited by
John S. Elam
and
Paul Cancalon
Florida State University
Tallahassee, Florida

PLENUM PRESS • NEW YORK AND LONDON

Library of Congress Cataloging in Publication Data

Main entry under title:

Axonal transport in neuronal growth and regeneration.

(Advances in neurochemistry; v. 6)
Includes bibliographies and index.
1. Nervous system — Regeneration. 2. Axonal transport. 3. Nerves — growth.
I. Elam, John S., 1941–   . II. Cancalon, Paul. III. Series.
QP356.3.A37   vol. 6   [QP363.5]   599'.0188 s   84-16006
ISBN 0-306-41699-9   [599'.0188]

© 1984 Plenum Press, New York
A Division of Plenum Publishing Corporation
233 Spring Street, New York, N.Y. 10013

Printed in the United States of America

CONTRIBUTORS

BERNARD W. AGRANOFF • *Department of Biological Chemistry and Mental Health Research Institute, University of Michigan, Ann Arbor, Michigan 48109*

LARRY I. BENOWITZ • *Department of Psychiatry, Harvard Medical School and Mailman Research Center, McLean Hospital, Belmont, Massachusetts 02178*

MARK A. BISBY • *Department of Medical Physiology, Faculty of Medicine, University of Calgary, Calgary, Alberta, Canada T2N 4N1*

SCOTT T. BRADY • *Department of Developmental Genetics and Anatomy, Case Western Reserve University, Cleveland, Ohio 44106*

PAUL CANCALON • *Department of Biological Science, Florida State University, Tallahassee, Florida 32306*

G. CHAKRABORTY • *Department of Physiology, University of Medicine and Dentistry of New Jersey, New Jersey Medical School, Newark, New Jersey 07103*

JOHN S. ELAM • *Department of Biological Science, Florida State University, Tallahassee, Florida 32306*

THOMAS S. FORD-HOLEVINSKI • *Department of Biological Chemistry and Mental Health Research Institute, University of Michigan, Ann Arbor, Michigan 48109*

MARCIE GLICKSMAN • *Department of Anatomy and Neurobiology, Washington University School of Medicine, St. Louis, Missouri 63110*

JOHN W. GRIFFIN • *Departments of Neurology and Neuroscience, The Johns Hopkins University School of Medicine, Baltimore, Maryland 21205*

NOBUTAKA HIROKAWA • *Department of Anatomy, Faculty of Medicine, University of Tokyo, Hongo, Tokyo, 113 Japan*

PAUL N. HOFFMAN • *Department of Opthalmology, The Johns Hopkins University School of Medicine, Baltimore, Maryland 21205*

N. A. INGOGLIA • *Department of Physiology, University of Medicine and Dentistry of New Jersey, New Jersey Medical School, Newark, New Jersey 07103*

KRISTER KRISTENSSON • *Department of Pathology, Karolinska Institute, Huddinge University Hospital S-141 86, Huddinge, Sweden*

DAVID B. MCDOUGAL, JR. • *Department of Pharmacology, Washington University School of Medicine, St. Louis, Missouri 63110*

IRVINE G. MCQUARRIE • *Veterans Administration Medical Center and Department of Anatomy and Developmental Genetics, Case Western Reserve University, Cleveland, Ohio 44106*

KARINA MEIRI • *Department of Anatomy and Neurobiology, Washington University School of Medicine, St. Louis, Missouri 63110*

SIDNEY OCHS • *Department of Physiology and Biophysics, Indiana University School of Medicine, Indianapolis, Indiana 46223*

DONALD L. PRICE • *Departments of Pathology, Neurology, and Neuroscience, The Johns Hopkins University School of Medicine, Baltimore, Maryland 21205*

WILLIAM W. SCHLAEPFER • *Division of Neuropathology, Department of Pathology and Lab Medicine, University of Pennsylvania Medical School, Philadelphia, Pennsylvania 19104*

CAROLYN SIMON • *Department of Anatomy and Neurobiology, Washington University School of Medicine, St. Louis Missouri 63110*

J. H. PATE SKENE • *Department of Neurobiology, Stanford University, Palo Alto, California 94305*

MARK WILLARD • *Department of Anatomy and Neurobiology, Washington University School of Medicine, St. Louis, Missouri 63110*

DAVID L. WILSON • *Department of Physiology and Biophysics, University of Miami School of Medicine, Miami, Florida 33101*

M. F. ZANAKIS • *Department of Physiology, University of Medicine and Dentistry of New Jersey, New Jersey Medical School, Newark, New Jersey 07103*

UN-JIN P. ZIMMERMAN • *Division of Neuropathology, Department of Pathology and Lab Medicine, University of Pennsylvania Medical School, Philadelphia, Pennsylvania 19104*

PREFACE

Over the past several years, the pace of research on the control of axonal growth has increased at a remarkable rate, and this activity is reflected in a growing literature dealing with various aspects of axonal growth and regeneration. It appears timely to review the role played by axonal transport in the intrinsic responses of neurons in the growth and regrowth processes. Through the cooperation of the senior editors of this series, we have been given the opportunity to bring such a focus to the current volume.

We wish to acknowledge that the contributing authors attended a conference on "The Role of Axonal Transport in Neuronal Growth and Regeneration" held in Tallahassee, Florida in March, 1983, sponsored by the Psychobiology Research Center of the Florida State University. It is our hope that many of the perceptions and insights expressed in these chapters resulted from our interactions.

The chapters are arranged in an order that ranges from basic properties of axonal transport underlying growth to specific mechanisms by which transport may regulate growth. The reader will note that changes in axonal transport accompanying neuronal injury and growth include such diverse events as alterations in cell body synthesis, increases in transport rates, changes in the molecular composition of transported molecules, and posttranslational modification of molecules having undergone transport. Although the specific roles of each of these processes in regulating axonal growth are not known, it is inferred either that they signal the status of the axon to the cell body and surrounding tissues or that they contribute to the molecular environment necessary for the extension, connection (or reconnection), and maturation of neurites.

Where authors have conflicting opinions, we have encouraged them to sharpen their points of view, so that the reader may better appreciate controversy as well as established facts.

John S. Elam
Paul Cancalon

CONTENTS

CHAPTER 3

RETROGRADE SIGNALING AFTER NERVE INJURY

KRISTER KRISTENSSON

CHAPTER 4

*RETROGRADE AXONAL TRANSPORT AND NERVE
REGENERATION*

M. A. BISBY

CHAPTER 5

BIOCHEMICAL ASPECTS OF THE REGENERATING GOLDFISH VISUAL SYSTEM

BERNARD W. AGRANOFF AND THOMAS S. FORD-HOLEVINSKI

CHAPTER 6

AXONAL TRANSPORT OF GLYCOPROTEINS IN REGENERATING NERVE

JOHN S. ELAM

CHAPTER 9

*MOLECULAR EVENTS ASSOCIATED WITH PERIPHERAL NERVE
REGENERATION*

DAVID L. WILSON

CHAPTER 10

*TARGET-DEPENDENT AND TARGET-INDEPENDENT CHANGES IN
RAPID AXONAL TRANSPORT DURING REGENERATION OF THE
GOLDFISH RETINOTECTAL PATHWAY*

LARRY I. BENOWITZ

CHAPTER 11

REGULATION OF AXON GROWTH AND CYTOSKELETAL DEVELOPMENT

MARK WILLARD, J. H. PATE SKENE, CAROLYN SIMON, KARINA MEIRI, NOBUTAKA HIROKAWA, AND MARCIE GLICKSMAN

CHAPTER 12

EFFECT OF A CONDITIONING LESION ON AXONAL TRANS-PORT DURING REGENERATION: THE ROLE OF SLOW TRANSPORT

IRVINE G. MCQUARRIE

CHAPTER 15

*CALCIUM-ACTIVATED PROTEASE AND THE REGULATION OF
THE AXONAL CYTOSKELETON*

WILLIAM W. SCHLAEPFER AND UN-JIN P. ZIMMERMAN

CHAPTER 1

AXOPLASMIC TRANSPORT IN RELATION TO NERVE FIBER REGENERATION

SIDNEY OCHS

1. INTRODUCTION

This chapter represents a general review of the relationship of transport to regeneration. Views of how nerves regenerate have for some time been connected with the concept that transport supplies the materials required by the growing fibers. At first, when only slow transport was known, the similarity of the rates of transport and of regeneration at approximately several millimeters per day appeared to indicate their direct association. The more recent recognition of a faster rate of axoplasmic transport raised the question of how rapid transport might be related to regeneration. Currently, two general views are held: (1) that there is more than one transport system present in nerve fibers, one for slow transport, which is mainly responsible for the outgrowth of the major structural elements of the fiber, and another system mainly responsible for the rapid transport of membranous constituents of the axon and nerve terminal processes, and (2) that both rapid and slow transport are accomplished by one transport mechanism, a concept termed the "unitary hypothesis." In

SIDNEY OCHS ● Department of Physiology and Biophysics, Indiana University School of Medicine, Indianapolis, Indiana 46223 this chapter, I present an analysis of how the components needed for regeneration can be supplied on the basis of the unitary hypothesis. Another aspect of regeneration that is related to the transport mechanism is how a supply of materials can be provided to one subset of neurites growing or regenerating from a single neuron rather than to all the neurite branches supplied by the cell body. As is discussed below, this is entailed in the phenomenon of "routing," which can be accounted for by the same transport mechanism.

2. MODELS PROPOSED FOR REGENERATION

Ramon y Cajal (1928) saw fine regenerating fibers in and below partially constricted regions of sciatic nerves and a series of bulges and constrictions in the nerve fibers just above them, which he interpreted as representing a starting and stopping of nerve regeneration. In analogous experiments, Weiss and Hiscoe (1948) found similar irregular bulgings and swellings in the fibers above partial constrictions, which they viewed as a piling up or "damming" of the axoplasm continually "flowing" or "growing" down within the fibers, the damming being caused by a narrowing of the nerve fibers at the constrictions (Weiss, 1961, 1972). The rate of such flow was estimated at 1–3 mm/day, which corresponded to clinical estimates of nerve regeneration rates (Biondi *et al.,* 1972; Weiss and Mayr, 1971).

However, partial compression does not readily reduce the diameter of nerve fibers but rather causes fiber degeneration, especially of larger myelinated fibers which have a greater susceptibility to mechanical damage than the smaller fibers (Aguayo *et al.,* 1971; Gasser and Erlanger, 1929). The smaller-diameter fibers left remaining along with the regenerating fibers in the compressed region account for the observed shift toward a smaller-diameter population following this maneuver (Weiss, 1961). As originally observed by Perroncito (1905), a large number of regenerating neurites are seen to sprout from the fibers over a length of several millimeters above a transection of nerve fibers, and this could give rise to the bulging and tortuosities seen with the usual silver stains. Friede and Bischausen (1980) showed such sprouts in the reconstruction of fibers made from serial EM sections taken above a nerve transection, and in an earlier EM study, Spencer (1972) failed to find the kind of swellings in fibers above a constriction to be expected from a bulk flow.

Instead of a constant movement of the entire axoplasm down within the nerve fibers, Hoffman and Lasek (1975) proposed a slow outgrowth of some components of the axoplasm, mostly of the microtubules and neurofilaments. Using SDS-polyacrylamide gel electrophoresios (PAGE) they found in rat motor fibers injected with [^{3}H]leucine that the bulk of labeled activity in a wave moving at a rate of 1–1.2 mm/day consisted of tubulin and neurofilament polypeptides. These were proposed to be moving down within the nerve fibers in assembled form as microtubules and neurofilaments, these organelles undergoing a concomitant disassembly at the same rate in the nerve terminals (Lasek and Hoffman, 1976).

The rate of nerve regeneration in controlled studies in rats and other laboratory animals was determined to be 3.5–4.5 mm/day (Gutman et al., 1942; Bulger and Bisby, 1978; Griffin et al., 1976). This rate conflicts with an outgrowth of the microtubules and neurofilaments at a rate of 1.0 mm/day in that microtubules are seen in the base of the growth cones of regenerating nerve fibers (Bunge, 1973), and this would require that the microtubules also elongate at this rate. Otherwise the lengthening neurites would outdistance these organelles in the course of regeneration. Actually, the outflow of tubulin can be faster than 1 mm/day. In the rabbit vagus nerve, 54,000- and 56,000-molecular-weight polypeptides comigrating with tubulin were measured at a rate of 12–15 mm/day (McLean et al., 1983). This is much faster than the rate of regeneration of 3–4 mm/day found for this nerve (McLean and Sjöstrand, 1983). An outflow of polypeptide comigrating with tubulin at a rate close to this was also seen in rat sciatic nerve in our laboratory, along with a much smaller amount that was rapidly transported (Stromska et al., 1983).

The advance of tubulin ahead of the rate of regeneration of neurites is in accord with an alternative view, namely, that the tubulin and triplet subunits of microtubules and neurofilaments, rather than being added at the cell body, are carried down within the fibers as soluble proteins to enter a pool from which they then turn over in their respective organelles all along the length of the nerve fiber. The tubulin and neurofilament subunits from such a pool would also add onto the distal ends of the microtubules and neurofilaments in the course of nerve fiber regeneration. The means by which the soluble components are considered to be carried down within the nerve fiber are described in the following two sections.

3. THE TRANSPORT FILAMENT MODEL

In the transport filament model proposed for fast transport, the various materials carried down the nerve fibers are considered bound to carriers, the "transport filaments," which are moved axially in the fibers along the microtubules by means of side arms on the microtubules (Ochs, 1974). The energy needed to move the transport filaments is provided by ATP, which is utilized by a calmodulin-activated Ca^{2+}, Mg^{2+}-ATPase present on the side arms; the calmodulin is activated by Ca^{2+} in the micromolar range (Ochs and Iqbal, 1980), the level of Ca^{2+} likely to be present in the axoplasm (Baker, 1972, 1976). Calmodulin is present in nerve as shown by the blocking action of triflouperazine (TFP) on the calmodulin, Ca^{2+},Mg^{2+}-ATPase activity (Ochs and Iqbal, 1980). Additionally, axoplasmic transport *in vitro* is blocked by adding TFP to the incubation medium (Ochs and Iqbal, 1982; Ekström *et al.*, 1982). The addition of TFP only partially reduced $\sim$P levels in frog nerves (Ekström *et al.*, 1982), indicating that it is unlikely that the TFP block is acting in a nonspecific way by interfering with energy metabolism and production of ATP.

The necessity for Ca^{2+} to activate calmodulin could explain the dependence of axoplasmic transport on Ca^{2+}. A requirement for Ca^{2+} was shown in desheathed nerves by deletion of Ca^{2+} from the incubation medium (Ochs *et al.*, 1977; Lavoie *et al.*, 1979; Chan *et al.*, 1980). Agents interfering with Ca^{2+} influx, Co^{2+}, La^{3+}, verapamil, and Ni^{2+}, also cause a block of axoplasmic transport when added to the incubation medium (Ochs, 1982), most likely by a reduction in intraaxonal Ca^{2+}.

Strontium, which is closely similar in its chemical properties to Ca^{2+}, is able to maintain axoplasmic transport as well as Ca^{2+} (Ochs *et al.*, 1983). With an addition of higher levels of Sr^{2+}, the cation was found to be present along with Ca^{2+} in the same organelles that regulate Ca^{2+}, i.e., in the mitochondria and ER as well as along the axolemma and in the axoplasm. This suggests that Sr^{2+} might substitute for Ca^{2+} at storage sites, consequently releasing Ca^{2+} into the axoplasm and maintaining it at the level required to bind to calmodulin and in turn activate Ca^{2+},Mg^{2+}-ATPase. Alternatively, Sr^{2+}, which, like Ca^{2+}, binds to calmodulin, would enable the calmodulin to activate phosphodiesterase (Cox *et al.*, 1981) and Ca^{2+},Mg^{2+}-ATPase (Iqbal and Ochs, 1983).

4. SLOW TRANSPORT AS A DROP OFF AND TURNOVER OF COMPONENTS

Slow transport is typically seen as a declining exponential outflow of labeled protein in the nerve over a period of days and weeks after injection of [³H]leucine for uptake by the cells (Ochs, 1982); wavelike variations appear at later times. In rat motor nerves, waves that appeared to be slow moving were found by Lasek and Hoffman (1976). In rat and cat sensory nerves, however, the variations seen were so irregular as to obviate the identification of slow waves moving at definable rates (Stromska and Ochs, 1981). Similarly, little evidence of regularly moving slow waves was found in the sensory nerves and in dorsal roots of monkeys following L7 dorsal root ganglion injection with [³H]leucine (S. Ochs, unpublished observations). On the other hand, very regular slowly moving waves were found in the garfish olfactory nerve (Cancalon, 1979), most likely reflecting the uniformity of its population of unmyelinated fibers. These waves were seen to decrease in amplitude and broaden with time and distance, changes that can be accounted for by the "unitary hypothesis."

According to this hypothesis, differences in the binding of components to the transport filaments allow them to drop off more readily in the axon to constitute the slowly transported outflow (Figure 1). Those components carried all the way down to the nerve terminals by the carriers represent the rapidly transported components. Even the rapidly transported components, however, show some drop off down the length of the nerve, as indicated by the regular decrease in the amplitude of the fast transport crest with distance (Gross and Beidler, 1975; Ochs, 1975a; Muñoz-Martínez, 1981). This contributes both to the trailing behind the advancing crest and the increase in plateau height behind the crest seen in nerves ligated just behind the ganglion at different times after injection and outflow (Muñoz-Martínez, 1981; Ochs, 1975b).

Thus, in accordance with the unitary hypothesis, those components that are slowly transported are those that have a lower affinity for the transport mechanism and can drop off more rapidly in the axon. The amount remaining attached to the transport filaments is usually too small to be detected at a great distance. Although the bulk of the tubulins are slowly transported, a small amount of tubulin as well as actin (Stromska et al., 1983) and calmodulin (Iqbal and and Ochs, 1983) was seen to be rapidly transported. Rapid transport may be detected more readily if the nerve is sampled closer to the cell bodies, as was indicated for leucine (Schmid et al., 1983). In line with this view of a differential drop off, components that in earlier studies had been considered to be only slowly transported were subsequently found also to be carried in part at a fast rate (Brimijoin and Wiermaa, 1977).

Components that drop off locally in the fiber and/or their local turnover products may reattach to the transport mechanism for their redistribution in the anterograde and retrograde directions, as indicated in Figure 1. This process would account for the broadening of the slow transport wave. Retrograde

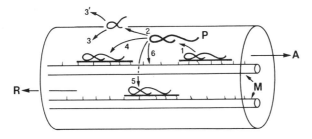

FIGURE 1. The unitary hypothesis is based on the transport filament hypothesis. Components that drop off from the transport mechanism enter an axonal pool (P). Their subsequent modes of redistribution contributing to slow transport are shown: (1) drop off, (2) insertion in membrane, (3 and 3') return or loss from membrane, (4) return to transport mechanisms for anterograde transport (A) or (5) retrograde transport (R); 6 represents components turning over in microtubules (M) (or in neurofilaments not shown).

transport of labeled proteins was shown by making a variety of distal ligations in nerves at different times after injecting [³H]leucine, allowing the labeled proteins to be transported to the ligation to collect there, and then, after their turnaround and retrograde transport, to collect below a proximally placed ligation made subsequently (Bulger and Bisby, 1978; Ochs, 1975*b*; Bisby, 1980; Bray *et al.*, 1971; Edstrom and Hanson, 1973; Lasek, 1968). A number of components are known to be carried retrogradely at approximately half the rate of fast anterograde transport (Ochs, 1982*a,b*). Additionally, a slow distal–proximal spread was also seen following the injection of nerve subperineurally with [³H]N-succinimidylproprionate ([³H]N-SP) by Fink and Gainer (1980). This agent enters the nerve fibers to label with proprionate various polypeptide species characterized by SDS-PAGE. By this method tubulin and neurofilament subunits were found to be transported anterogradely and a 68,000-dalton polypeptide retrogradely as slow waves, the latter identified as serum albumin (Gainer and Fink, 1982).

How the tubulin subunits might undergo turnover in the microtubules of the nerve fibers was clarified by recent evidence showing that the microtubules are present in nerve fibers as short segments ranging in length from several to several hundred micrometers staggered axially along the length of the fiber (Chalfie and Thomson, 1979; Bray and Bunge, 1981; Tsukita and Ishikawa, 1980). This finding caused a revision of the usual view that the microtubules are present in the fibers as a continuous organelle reaching from the cell body to the nerve terminals. *In vitro* studies had shown that tubulin is added at the ends of the microtubule segments, more readily at one than the other end (Allen and Borisy, 1974). The addition of subunits at one end and their ongoing disassembly at the other end of the segment results in a continuous "treadmill" (Wilson and Margolis, 1982) replacement of the tubulins in the microtubules. This process could take place at the ends of the microtubule segments all along the lengths of the mature nerve fibers and also at the microtubules at the distal ends of the regenerating neurites. Additionally, there is evidence that the neurofilaments also exist as short segments in nerve fibers (Tsukita and Ishikawa, 1980; Weiss and Mayr, 1971), and a similar process of turnover of their protein subunits could occur in them as well.

Among the components that drop off locally in the fibers to undergo turnovers are those incorporated into the axonal membrane (Ochs, 1982). Griffin *et al.* (1981) used autoradiographic EM to study the location of labeled glycoproteins transported down within the nerve fibers. They found the grains of labeled proteins to be distributed generally throughout the cross-sectional area of the axons at earlier times and then later to become localized peripherally at or in the axolemma. In regenerating fibers, even as early as a day after regeneration has started, a substantially greater amount of labeled material was seen localized at or in the axolemma, and after 7–14 days, almost all of the radioactivity was found in the axolemmal region. We would expect such a distribution in that the glycoproteins contribute to the newly formed axonal membrane.

The amount of labeled materials free to redistribute in the fibers declines with time (Ochs, 1975b). This was seen as a failure of the declining slope of outflow to level off when ligations were made below the ganglion several days after initiating downflow by injecting the ganglion with [³H]leucine, and it likely represents the incorporation of components into organelles in the course of turnover.

Another aspect of slow transport is the shift in the composition of labeled components leaving the cell body for export into the axon over a period of time. After only 15–20 min, the major portion if not all of the proteins have been synthesized. This was seen by the injection of puromycin or cycloheximide to block protein synthesis at different times after injecting [³H]leucine and finding no blocking effect after 15–20 min (Ochs *et al.,* 1970). The synthesized labeled proteins remain present in some pool in the cell bodies from which they can later move out into the fibers, with a shift toward the higher-molecular-weight proteins at the later times (Ochs, 1982a).

5. ROUTING IN RELATION TO TRANSPORT AND REGENERATION

A specialization of transport within the nerve fiber is shown by "routing," a phenomenon first described for the monkey (Ochs, 1972). This animal has exceptionally long L7 dorsal roots compared to the cat, allowing the rate of fast transport in the roots to be compared directly with that in the sensory nerves. These are supplied by one each of the two daughter fiber branches of the T-shaped dorsal root ganglion neurons. When the L7 dorsal root ganglia were injected with [³H]leucine, the fronts of labeled activity were seen to extend up to the same distance in the dorsal roots as in the descending sensory nerves, showing that the rate of rapid transport was the same in the branches. However, three to five times more labeled material was present in the crests in the sensory nerve fibers than in the dorsal roots. Similar asymmetries in the amounts of labeled activity fast-transported into the two nerve fiber branches of the dorsal root ganglion neurons were subsequently reported for the cat (Anderson and McClure, 1973), the rat (Komiya and Kurokawa, 1978), and for the superior and distal portions of the vagus nerve, after the nodose ganglion was injected with labeled precursor (Watson *et al.,* 1975).

Such large asymmetries in the amount of outflow could not be accounted for by morphological features of the fiber branches of the dorsal root ganglion neurons in the cat and monkey, neither by a greater diameter of the sensory fibers compared to those in the dorsal roots nor by a greater density of micro-tubules or neurofilaments in the sensory branch as compared to the roots (Ochs *et al.,* 1978). To account for the asymmetry in outflow, the transport filament model was invoked; more transport filaments carrying labeled materials and/ or more labeled materials bound to the transport filaments moved down into the sensory nerve fiber branch than into the dorsal root branch. This concept, called "routing," could also include the differential transport of components expected to be specific for the two branches of the dorsal root ganglion neurons, e.g., of those components required to support sensory transduction carried in the peripheral sensory nerve fibers to their terminals and of neurotransmitter and neurotransmitter-related materials transported via the dorsal root fibers to the presynaptic terminals in the CNS.

On the basis of the unitary hypothesis, we would expect to see an asymmetry of slow transport in the two branches of the dorsal root ganglia neurons as well as of fast transport. On this hypothesis, as a result of the greater amount of labeled materials carried by fast transport in the sensory fiber branch, we would expect a greater amount to drop off locally there compared to the dorsal roots. The slopes of outflow in the sensory nerves and dorsal roots seen after a period of days after injection of the dorsal root ganglia do in fact show such an asymmetry, with more labeled material present in the sensory nerves than in the dorsal roots (Lasek, 1968). Integration of the labeled radioactivity present under the curves of outflow in the dorsal root and sensory nerve taken at comparable lengths from the injected ganglia in our studies of slow transport showed that approximately two to three times more radioactivity was contained in the sensory nerves as in the dorsal roots (S. Ochs and D. Stromska, unpublished observations). An asymmetry of slowly transported labeled material in the two branches of the L7 dorsal root ganglion neurons of a group of six monkeys was also found, with some two times more labeled material present in the sensory nerves than in the dorsal roots (S. Ochs, unpublished observations).

Mori *et al.* (1979), using SDS-PAGE, found waves of triplet proteins, tubulins, and actin moving in the peripheral sensory nerve fiber branches at rates, respectively, of 2–3 mm/day, 9–13 mm/day, and 19 mm/day. In the dorsal root branch, the corresponding rates given were 1–2 mm/day, 3–4 mm/ day, and 4 mm/day. Rather than invoking six different rates and transport mechanisms to account for them, one can explain these variations by the unitary hypothesis as resulting from differences in the amount and rate of drop off of the various components transported in the fiber branches of the sensory neuron. Komiya and Kurokawa (1978) also found an asymmetry of slowly transported materials in the two branches of the dorsal roots and peripheral nerve fibers and interpreted their findings in terms of different rates of slow transport. Again, in accord with the unitary hypothesis, this could result from differences in the amounts of the different components dropped off.

6. A HYPOTHESIS FOR SELECTIVE NEURITE GROWTH ON THE BASIS OF ROUTING

Neurites in organ cultures (Harrison, 1910) and those visualized in the tadpole tail fin (Speidel, 1964) show growth in several directions, with some neurites advancing toward their ultimate targets and aberrant ones undergoing involution. A similar phenomenon is seen in regenerating peripheral nerve. At first a large number of neurites are seen to grow from the nerve fiber above a site of transection; later, the number becomes much diminished (Shawe, 1955), presumably when the pioneer neurites make contact with their targets and a trophic substance is supplied by the target cell to the neurite. The successful neurite then undergoes maturation, with an increase in its diameter toward the adult size of the nerve fiber.

Routing could underlie the selective supply of components to the growth of the neurites that succeed in establishing contact with their targets and provide for their maturation and the involution of aberrant neurites. We can consider a "signal" substance arising from the target cells taken up by the growth cones of those neurites growing in the right direction and then ascending by retrograde transport along the subset of microtubules supplying those neurites. On reaching the cell body, the signal substance induces an increased synthesis of components, which are then routed anterogradely down an allied subset of microtubules to supply the further growth of those same neurites. Thus, by the selective routing of the supply of the signal substances to the cell and subsequently of needed materials properly directed to those neurites, they will eventually outstrip the other neurites, which then undergo regression, either by default of supply or by the effect of some suppressor influence.

7. REFERENCES

Aguayo, A., Nair, C. P., and Midgley, R., 1971, Experimental progressive compression neuropathy in the rabbit: Histologic and electrophysiologic studies, *Arch. Neurol.* **24:**358–364.

Allen, C. C., and Borisy, G. G., 1974, Structural polarity and directional growth of *Chlamydomonas* flagella, *J. Mol. Biol.* **90:**381–402.

Anderson, L. E., and McClure, W. O., 1973, Differential transport of protein in axons: Comparison between the sciatic nerve and dorsal columns of cats, *Proc. Natl. Acad. Sci. U.S.A.* **70:**1521–1525.

Baker, P. F., 1972, Transport and metabolism of calcium ions in nerve, *Prog. Biophys. Mol. Biol.* **24:**177–223.

Baker, P. F., 1976, The regulation of intracellular calcium, *Symp. Soc., Exp. Biol.* **30:**67–88.

Biondi, R. J., Levy, M. J., and Weiss, P. A., 1972, An engineering study of the peristaltic drive of axonal flow, *Proc. Natl. Acad. Sci. U.S.A.* **69:**1732–1736.

Bisby, M.A., 1980, Retrograde axonal transport, *Adv. Cell. Neurobiol.* **1**:69–117.

Bray, D., and Bunge, M. B., 1981, Serial analysis of microtubules in cultured rat sensory axons, *J. Neurocytol.* **10**:589–605.

Bray, J. J., Kon, C. M., and Breckenridge, B. M., 1971, Reversed polarity of rapid axonal transport in chicken motoneurons, *Brain Res.* **33**:560–564.

Brimijoin, S., and Wiermaa, M. J., 1977, Rapid axonal transport of tyrosine hydroxylase in rabbit sciatic nerves, *Brain Res.* **121**:77–96.

Bulger, V. T., and Bisby, M. A., 1978, Reversal of axonal transport in regenerating nerves, *J. Neurochem.* **31**:1411–1418.

Bunge, M. G., 1973, Fine structure of nerver fibers and growth cones of isolated sympathetic neurons in culture, *J. Cell Biol.* **56**:713–735.

Cancalon, P., 1979, Influence of temperature on the velocity and on the isotope profile of slowly transported labeled proteins, *J. Neurochem.* **32**:997–1007.

Chalfie, M., and Thomson, J. N., 1979, Organization of neuronal microtubules in the nematode, *Caenorhabditis elegans, J. Cell Biol.* **82**:278–289.

Chan, S. Y., Ochs, S., and Worth, R. M., 1980, The requirement for calcium ions and the effect of other ions on axoplasmic transport in mammalian nerve, *J. Physiol. (Lond.)* **301**:477–504.

Cox, J. A., Malnoe, A., and Stein, E. Z., 1981, Regulation of brain cyclic nucleotide phosphodiesterase by calmodulin. A quantitative analysis, *J. Biol. Chem.* **256**:3218–3222.

Edström, A., and Hanson, M., 1973, Retrograde axonal transport of proteins *in vitro* in frog sciatic nerves, *Brain Res.* **61**:311–320.

Ekström, P., Kanje, M., and Edström, A., 1982, Effects of phenothiazines and dibensasepines on axonal transport and microtubule assembly *in vitro, Acta Physiol. Scand.* **116**:121–125.

Fink, D. J., and Gainer, H., 1980, Retrograde axonal transport of endogenous proteins in sciatic nerve demonstrated by covalent labeling *in vivo, Science* **208**:303–305.

Friede, L., and Bischausen, R., 1980, The fine structure of stumps of transected nerve fibers in subserial sections, *J. Neurol. Sci.* **44**:181–203.

Gainer, H., and Fink, D. J., 1982, Evidence for slow retrograde transport of serum albumin in rat sciatic nerve, *Brain Res.* **233**:404–408.

Gasser, H. S., and Erlanger, J., 1929, The role of fiber size in the establishment of a nerve block by pressure or cocaine, *Am. J. Physiol.* **88**:581–591.

Griffin, J. W., Price, D. L., and Drachman, D. B., 1976, Impaired regeneration in acrylamide neuropathy: Role of axonal transport, *Neurology (Minneap.)* **26**:350.

Griffin, J. W., Price, D. L., Drachman, D. B., and Morris, J., 1981, Incorporation of axonally transported glycoprotein into axolemma during nerve regeneration, *J. Cell Biol.* **88**:205–214.

Gross, G. W., and Beidler, L. M., 1975, A quantitative analysis of isotope concentration profiles and rapid transport velocities in the C-fibers of the garfish olfactory nerve, *J. Neurobiol.* **6**:213–232.

Gutman, E., Gutman, L., Medawar, P. B., and Young, J. Z., 1942, The rate of regeneration of nerve, *J. Exp. Biol.* **19**:14–44.

Harrison, R. G., 1910, The outgrowth of the nerve fiber as a mode of protoplasmic movement, *J. Exp. Zool.* **9**:787–846.

Hoffman, P. N., and Lasek, R. J., 1975, The slow component of axonal transport. Identification of major structural polypeptides of the axon and their generality among mammalian neurons, *J. Cell Biol.* **66**:351–366.

Iqbal, Z., and Ochs, S., 1983, The role of calcium binding protein in axoplasmic transport, *J. Neurochem* **41**(Suppl.):S69.

Komiya, Y., and Kurokawa, M., 1978, Asymmetry of protein transport in two branches of bifurcating axons, *Brain Res.* **139**:354–358.

Lasek, R. J., 1968, Axoplasmic transport of labeled proteins in rat ventral montoneurons, *Exp. Neurol.* **21**:41–51.

Lasek, R. J., and Hoffman, P. M., 1976, The neuronal cytoskeleton, axonal transport and axonal growth, in: *Cell Motility, Book C. Microtubules and Related Proteins* (R. Goldman, T. Pollard, and J. Rosenbaum, eds.), pp. 1021–1049, Cold Spring Harbor Laboratory, Cold Spring Harbor, New York.

Lavoie, P.-A., Bolen, F., and Hammerschlag, R., 1979, Divalent cation specificity of the calcium requirement for fast transport of proteins in axons of desheathed nerves, *J. Neurochem.* **32**:1745–1751.

McLean, W. G., and Sjostrand, J., 1983, Slow axonal transport of structural proteins and regeneration rate in rabbit vagus nerve, *J. Neurochem.* **41**(Suppl.):S97.

McLean, W. G., McKay, A. L., and Sjostrand, J., 1983, Electrophoretic analysis of axonally transported proteins in rabbit vagus nerve, *J. Neurobiol.* **14**:227–236.

Mori, H., Komiya, Y., and Kurokawa, M., 1979, Slowly migrating axonal polypeptides: Inequalities in their rate and amount of transport between two branches of bifurcating axons, *J. Cell Biol.* **82**:174–184.

Muñoz-Martínez, E. J., Núñez, R., and Sanderson, A., 1981, Axonal transport: A quantitative study of retained and transformed protein fractions in the cat, *J. Neurobiol.* **12**:15–26.

Ochs, S., 1972, Rate of fast axoplasmic transport in mammalian nerve fibres, *J. Physiol. (Lond.)* **227**:627–645.

Ochs, S., 1974, Energy metabolism and supply of $\sim$P to the fast axoplasmic transport mechanism in nerve, *Fed. Proc.* **33**:1049–1058.

Ochs, S., 1975*a*, A unitary concept of axoplasmic transport based on the transport filament hypothesis, in: *Third International Congress on Muscle Diseases* (W. G. Bradley, D. Gardner-Medwin, and J. N. Walton, eds.), pp. 128–133, Excerpta Medica, Amsterdam.

Ochs, S., 1975*b*, Retention and redistribution of proteins in mammalian nerve fibers by axoplasmic transport, *J. Physiol. (Lond.)* **253**:459–475.

Ochs, S., 1982*a*, *Axoplasmic Transport and Its Relation to Other Nerve Functions*, Wiley-Interscience, New York.

Ochs, S., 1982*b*, Block of axoplasmic transport by agents interfering with calcium flux: Cobalt, nickel, lanthanum, verapamil; and the maintenance of transport in calcium-free media by strontium, *Soc. Neurosci. Abstr.* **8**:826.

Ochs, S., and Iqbal, Z., 1980, Calmodulin and calcium activation of tubulin associated Ca-ATPase, *Soc. Neurosci. Abstr.* **6**:501.

Ochs, S., and Iqbal, Z., 1982, The role of calcium in axoplasmic transport in nerve, in: *Calcium and Cell Function*, Volume 3 (W. Y. Cheung, ed.), pp. 325–354, Academic Press, New York.

Ochs, S., Sabri, M. I., and Ranish, N., 1970, Somal site of synthesis of fast transported materials in mammalian nerve fibers, *J. Neurobiol.* **1**:329–344.

Ochs, S., Worth, R. M., and Chan, S. Y., 1977, Calcium requirement for axoplasmic transport in mammalian nerve, *Nature* **270**:748–750.

Ochs, S., Erdman, J., Jersild, R. A., Jr., and McAdoo, V., 1978, Routing of transported materials in the dorsal root and nerve fiber branches of the dorsal root ganglion, *J. Neurobiol.* **9**:465–481.

Ochs, S., Jersild, R. A., Jr., Breen, T., and Peterson, R., 1983, Comparison of calcium and strontium sequestration in nerve axons in relation to axoplasmic transport, *Soc. Neurosci. Abstr.* **9**:149.

Perroncito, A., 1905, La rigenerazione delle fibre nervose, *Boll. Soc. Med. Chir. Pavia* **4**:434–444.

Ramon Y Cajal, S., 1928, *Studies on Degeneration and Regeneration of the Nervous System* (R. M. May, trans.), Oxford University Press, Oxford. Reprinted 1968, Hafner, New York.

Schmid, G., Wagner, L., and Weiss, D. G., 1983, Rapid axoplasmic transport of free leucine, *J. Neurobiol.* **14**:133–144.

Shawe, G. D. H., 1955, On the number of branches formed by regenerating nerve fibers, *Br. J. Surg.* **42**:474–488.

Speidel, C. C., 1964, *In vivo* studies of myelinated nerve fibers, *Int. Rev. Cytol.* **16**:173–231.

Spencer, P. S., 1972, Reappraisal of the model for "bulk axoplasmic flow," *Nature (New Biol.)* **240**:283–285.

Stromska, D., and Ochs, S., 1981, Patterns of slow transport in sensory nerves, *J. Neurobiol.* **12**:441–453.

Stromska, D. P., Iqbal, Z., and Ochs, S., 1983a, Evidence for the fast transport of tubulin and actin in mammalian sciatic nerve, *Soc. Neurosci.* **9**:1191. *Abstr.* (in press).

Tsukita, S., and Ishikawa, H., 1980, The movement of membranous organelles in axons. Electron microscopic identification of anterogradely and retrogradely transported organelles, *J. Cell Biol.* **84**:513–530.

Watson, D. F., Donoso, J. A., Illanes, J. P., and Samson, F. E., 1975, Comparison of transported proteins in the central and peripheral processes of unipolar neurons, *Trans. Am. Soc. Neurochem.* **6**:109.

Weiss, P., 1961, The concept of perpetual neuronal growth and proximodistal substance convection, in: *Regional Biochemistry* (S. S. Kehy and J. Elkes, eds.), pp. 220–242, Pergamon Press, Oxford.

Weiss, P., 1972, Neuronal dynamics and axonal flow: Axonal peristalsis, *Proc. Natl. Acad. Sci. U.S.A.* **69**:1309–1312.

Weiss, P., and Hiscoe, H. B., 1948, Experiments on the mechanism of nerve growth, *J. Exp. Zool.* **107**:315–395.

Weiss, P., and Mayr, R., 1971, Organelles in neuroplasmic ('axonal') flow: Neurofilaments, *Proc. Natl. Acad. Sci. U.S.A.* **68**:846–850.

Wilson, L., and Margolis, R. L., 1982, Microtubule treadmills and their possible cellular functions, *Cold Spring Harbor Symp. Quant. Biol.* **46**(Part 1):199–205.

CHAPTER 2

BASIC PROPERTIES OF FAST AXONAL TRANSPORT AND THE ROLE OF FAST TRANSPORT IN AXONAL GROWTH

SCOTT T. BRADY

1. INTRODUCTION

In many respects, the extension of axons by neurons during development and regeneration reflects the aggregate effects of axonal transport processes that underlie this growth. For membranous organelles and structures in the axon, this means fast axonal transport. A number of functions have been suggested for fast transport during growth and regeneration, including the supply of

SCOTT T. BRADY ● Department of Developmental Genetics and Anatomy, Case Western Reserve University, Cleveland, Ohio 44106 plasma membrane components, regulation of growth cone activity, and delivery of trophic substances. Some of these are described in other chapters of this volume. However, new insights into the basic properties of fast axonal transport are beginning to illuminate the roles that it may play during axonal growth.

Although fast axonal transport is often used to refer solely to the movement of materials at the fastest orthograde rate, there is good reason for including in fast axonal transport the translocation of membranous organelles of all types in both directions (Lasek and Brady, 1982). The original descriptions of fast axonal transport (for example, see Lasek, 1967; Dahlstrom and Haggendahl, 1967; Grafstein, 1967) focused on the fastest moving elements leaving the cell bodies and defined this as fast axonal transport. More detailed studies demonstrated the existence of at least six rate components of axonal transport (see Grafstein and Forman, 1980, for review). Descriptions of axonal transport became more complex, but it was apparent that the slower moving components corresponded to the cytoplast, cytoskeletal elements and easily solubilized proteins, whereas faster moving materials were associated with membranous structures (Lasek and Brady, 1982; Tytell *et al.,* 1981; Baitinger *et al.,* 1982). In addition to containing membranes, the faster moving rate components share several important properties that suggest that they may be related processes (Brady *et al.,* 1982). This chapter is intended to summarize some of the similarities and differences in transport of specific membranous organelles and relate these observations to the roles each of these organelles may play in the growth of axons.

2. STRUCTURES IN FAST AXONAL TRANSPORT

The demonstration that fast axonal transport is movement of membrane-associated materials led to an obvious question: which membranous structures were moving? The prime candidates included agranular reticulum, mitochondria, synaptic vesicles, and lysosomal structures. All of these organelles had been observed in axonal or terminal regions of the neuron (Peters *et al.,* 1976), but the dynamics of these organelles were unknown. The possibility that some or all of the material in fast transport might be moving laterally within the plasma membrane can be excluded. Autoradiographic studies at the electron microscopic level clearly indicate that the fastest moving material in axonal transport was located within the axon, not in association with the plasmalemma (Droz and Leblond, 1963; Droz *et al.,* 1973). High-resolution autoradiography suggested that there might be an enrichment of fast transported material in the regions of the axon subjacent to the axolemma, but the data were most consistent with a location inside the plasma membrane (Tessler *et al.,* 1980).

Histochemical and immunohistochemical studies showed that proteins known to be moving at a fast rate tended to be associated with smooth membranous structures (Dahlstrom, 1971; Kasa, 1968), but analysis of the accumulation of enzyme activities at a lesion consistently indicated the presence of both a moving fraction and a stationary fraction for all enzymes studied (Brimijoin, 1975). It could not be stated with certitude whether the histochemical procedures were staining the moving structures, the stationary ones, or both fractions. There was also difficulty in identifying a specific organelle in thin-section electron micrographs as agranular reticulum or a discrete vesicle.

The agranular reticulum was found to be located near the plasma membrane and to extend for long distances within the axon (Tsukita and Ishikawa, 1976), so it became an early candidate for the fast transport vector (Droz *et al.*, 1975; Droz and Rambourg, 1982). Experiments designed to show that fast transport occurred in the lumen of the agranular reticulum or as migration within the membrane were equivocal, and the demonstration of discontinuities in the agranular reticulum at nodes of Ranvier (Berthold, 1982; Ellisman and Lindsey, 1982) effectively rules out this possibility. Most of the agranular reticulum also fails to be cleared from regions of axoplasm depleted of moving membranous organelles (Ellisman and Lindsey, 1982). It now appears that little, if any, of the material moving in fast transport is part of the agranular reticulum system of the axon, although it remains likely that fast moving materials may exchange with the reticulum.

Direct observation of membranous particles in neurites and teased frog sciatic nerves by light microscopy provided indications that the structures moving in the orthograde direction are not the same as those moving in the retrograde direction. Many of the membranous structures of the axon are too small to be seen with conventional light microscopic methods, but of the moving particles that were visible, most were moving in the retrograde direction (Forman *et al.*, 1977; Smith, 1972, 1980). This suggests that retrograde particles tend to be larger. The only structure that could easily be identified by direct observation using conventional light microscopy was the mitochondrion, which was distinguished by its characteristic size and shape. Many mitochondria were stationary, but the moving mitochondria moved in either direction and could be seen to reverse direction on occasion (Smith, 1972; Smith and Koles, 1976). Most of the retrograde particles were smaller than mitochondria and were spherical. When one of these retrograde moving particles was fixed and examined in the electron microscope, it was found to be a large vesicular structure of the type often considered to be lysosomal or prelysosomal (Breuer *et al.*, 1975).

The recent development of methods for video enhancement of contrast of light microscopic images, particularly the approaches pioneered by R. D. Allen and his associates (1981, 1983), has greatly extended the sensitivity of light microscopy. With these methods it is possible to detect structures as small as individual microtubules (25 nm) under appropriate conditions (Allen *et al.*, 1981). In collaboration with Dr. Allen, we have used these methods to study axonal transport of membranous organelles in the squid giant axon (Allen *et al.*, 1982) and isolated axoplasm (Brady *et al.*, 1982). Figure 1 illustrates the type of video records obtained using these methods on isolated axoplasm from the squid giant axon. The most striking feature in the video enhanced-contrast differential interference contrast (AVEC DIC) images is the presence of large numbers of low-contrast particles moving in the orthograde direction. These low-contrast particles have optical properties expected of organelles less than 100 nm in diameter and would not be detectable without video enhancement techniques. Direct observations of the movement of membranous organelles in axons thus suggest that orthograde transport represents movement of structures less than 100 nm in diameter and includes the bulk of the moving membranous elements. Particles moving in the retrograde direction tend to be larger and less numerous.

Zelena *et al.* (1968) showed that a local lesion of the axon produced a dramatic accumulation of membranous organelles on both the proximal and distal sides of the lesion. Several different laboratories have employed this method to characterize the vectors moving in both orthograde and retrograde fast transport. Smith (1980) examined individual teased myelinated axons from frog sciatic nerve and examined the nature and organization of membranous organelles accumulating on the proximal and distal sides of a single focal crush of the axon. At the same time, Tsukita and Ishikawa (1980) studied the accumulation of membranous organelles following focal cooling of mouse saphenous nerve. More recently, our laboratory (Fahim *et al.*, 1982) analyzed accumulations on either side of a cooled segment of the squid giant axon. All three studies found that the population of membranous organelles on the proximal side of the lesion was quite different from that of organelles on the distal side.

Mitochondria are found on both sides of a lesion, which is consistent with the observations of light microscopy, but may be more common on the proximal side of the lesion (Fahim *et al.*, 1982). This would indicate that mitochondria can move in both retrograde and orthograde transport, although the numbers moving in each direction may be different. It is not clear whether the mitochondria moving retrogradely differ from those moving orthogradely (i.e., older, metabolic differences, etc.). The movements of mitochondria, more often than that of the smaller organelles, involve stoppages and reversals of direction (Brady *et al.*, 1982). Such movements have historically been called saltatory, but this term is commonly used to describe rapid jumping movements. Real-time video records of mitochondrial movements are more suggestive of crawling or creeping than of leaping (Brady *et al.*, 1982). The term discontinuous

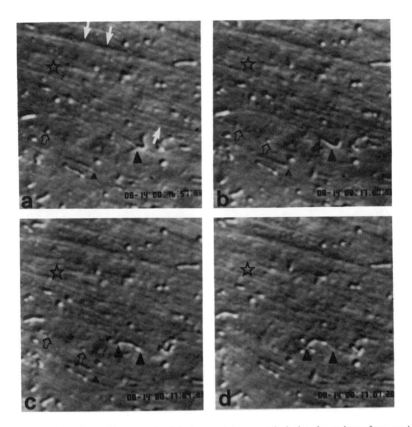

FIGURE 1. Stills from video records of fast axonal transport in isolated axoplasm from squid giant axon. The direction of the cell bodies was towards the lower right. Field of view in these stills is approximately 20 μm, and the images were recorded in real time [timing (day, hour, min, sec, ¹⁄₁₀₀ sec) is given by the numbers in the lower right-hand corner]. The large elongated structures (filled triangles in a) are mitochondria. Medium-sized particles (open arrow in a) most often move in the retrograde direction. Most of the particles, however, are small faint disks moving in the orthograde direction. (The region just above the star in part a contains several small particles.) The roughly parallel striations in the pictures (white arrows in a) are linear elements reflecting the cytoskeletal organization of the axoplasm. Most movement is parallel to these linear elements, but exceptions occur, as seen in the mitochondrion indicated by the large triangles in a–d. Panels b–d show positions of the various particles at subsequent times. (From Brady *et al,* 1982.)

may be more appropriate than saltatory for these movements because of the stoppages or changes of direction commonly seen. The reasons for this behavior are uncertain, but the large size and the role of mitochondria in generation of ATP make them unique among axonal organelles. Structural and metabolic properties may in general be responsible for the differences in the behaviors of the different-sized particles.

On the proximal side of the lesions in all three systems (Smith, 1980; Tsukita and Ishikawa, 1980; Fahim *et al.,* 1982), corresponding to orthograde transport, are large numbers of small, tubulovesicular structures (Figure 2a). Vesicles, approximately 50 nm in diameter, and tubular structures, 50 nm in

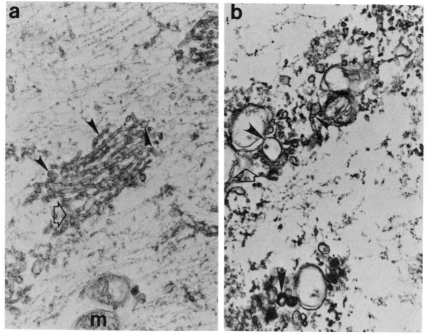

FIGURE 2. Transmission electron micrographs of membranous organelles moving in fast axonal transport after accumulation at a cold block in the squid giant axon. (a) Orthograde transport. Small 40- to 60-nm tubules and vesicles (arrowheads) are the most common structures found to accumulate on the proximal side of a lesion. An oblique section of a mitochondrion (m) is also seen in the micrograph. Although mitochondria can be found on both sides of a lesion, they are more frequently seen on the proximal side. (b) Retrograde transport. Larger, complex vesicles and multivesicular bodies are most often seen on the distal side of a lesion. Retrograde particles (arrowheads) are more heterogeneous in appearance, often ranging to 100–400 nm in diameter, and many have double membranes. Both orthograde and retrograde organelles are associated with an electron-dense granular matrix (open arrows). Micrograph taken by Dr. Mohammed Fahim. Bar, 0.5 μm.

diameter and several hundreds of nanometers in length, are both common. They can be very densely packed after prolonged accumulations, to the extent that the axon may become swollen from the numbers of organelles accumulated (Tsukita and Ishikawa, 1980). The overall appearance of the organelles on the proximal side tends to be relatively uniform, with smooth, single membrane boundaries and a moderately electron-dense interior (see Figure 2a), although dense-core vesicles may be seen. They are more uniform in diameter than agranular reticulum and appear to form discrete organelles without interconnections.

Organelles accumulating on the distal sides of lesions (Figure 2b) are fewer in number, producing sparser accumulations after similar incubation periods (Fahim et al., 1982; Tsukita and Ishikawa, 1980). The average diameter of distal organelles is greater, with many being 150 nm or more. The vertebrate preparations have a somewhat greater size range than the squid. Retrograde structures are more heterogeneous than orthograde structures, and many have double membranes (Figure 2a,b). Multilamellar and multivesicular bodies are common, particularly in vertebrate neurons.

Tubules or vesicles of only 50 nm, such as those in orthograde transport, would not be detectable by conventional light microscopy, but the size of the retrograde structures is above the resolution limit of conventional light microscopy. The multiple membranes on many retrograde organelles would also be highly refractile, making them easily detectable with either dark-field or differential interference contrast light microscopy. This would explain why most particles detected with conventional microscopic methods are moving in the retrograde direction. The accumulation studies also correlate well with the AVEC DIC microscopic studies. In the case of the squid giant axon, the same axon has been examined in AVEC DIC and electron microscopy after accumulation of organelles at a cold block (Fahim et al., 1982). Results show an enrichment of low-contrast small particles (in AVEC) and 50-nm vesicles (in EM) on the proximal side and an increase of larger, higher-contrast medium particles (in AVEC) and large double-membrane vesicles (in EM) on the distal side. The AVEC DIC microscopy thus indicates that the accumulated particles were moving prior to accumulation, and the electron microscopy confirms that the AVEC DIC methods are capable of detecting the full size range of membranous organelles moving in fast axonal transport.

3. ORGANIZATION OF FAST AXONAL TRANSPORT

Looking at the distribution of membranous organelles during and after accumulation at a lesion can also provide information on the distribution and associations of moving elements. For example, even after 6 hr or more of accumulation, when the axon is swollen from the amount of membranous organelles and associated materials, the neurofilament domains continue to exclude other axonal structures (see Figure 7 in Tsukita and Ishikawa, 1980). A neurofilament domain is a bundle of neurofilaments packed so that the distance between neurofilaments is minimized and cross bridges can be seen between neighboring filaments. It is presumed that the links between neurofilaments within domains are sufficiently stable to preclude entry of membranous organelles. Thus, neurofilament bundles may be displaced by accumulation of other axonal structures but remain as discrete domains.

If shorter accumulation periods are used, it becomes possible to extrapolate the distribution of membranous organelles back to the situation present in the undisturbed axon. In both the frog myelinated axon (Smith, 1980) and the squid giant axon (Fahim *et al.*, 1982), organelles accumulate in lines parallel to the long axis of the axon (Figure 3). These lines or files of particles are isolated columns of accumulated materials that may extend for some distance in the axon (the column in Figure 3 extends several micrometers in the plane of section). Files of particles are separated by neurofilament domains. In addition to the membranous organelles, two features are characteristic of the regions in which membranous organelles accumulate. If microtubules are preserved [as in the Smith study with frog sciatic nerve (1980)], then microtubules are often seen in association with the columns of membranous organelles. Microtubules do not, however, seem always to be present. In the cold-block studies with the squid giant axon, the number of microtubules is greatly reduced by the cold incubation, but the accumulated files of membranous organelles may extend for micrometers without evidence of microtubules (Fahim *et al.*, 1982). This suggests that the columns of accumulated elements can be maintained and perhaps be generated without continued interaction with microtubules.

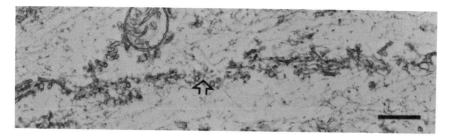

FIGURE 3. Columns of organelles in longitudinal sections at a cold block in the squid giant axon. Organelles accumulate in files or columns on both sides of a lesion, a feature that becomes apparent in longitudinal sections. Note the presence of the electron-dense granulofilamentous material (open arrow) along with membranous organelles. Micrograph taken by Dr. Mohammed Fahim. Bar, 0.5 μm.

A more consistent observation is the presence of a granular electron-dense material surrounding the membranous organelles accumulated on both proximal and distal sides of the lesion (see Figures 2a and 2b). Suggestions of this material can be seen not only in the three studies of accumulation at a lesion (Smith, 1980; Tsukita and Ishikawa, 1980; Fahim *et al.*, 1982) but also in micrographs of intact axons. Figure 4 is an electron micrograph of toad peripheral nerve axon at a Schmidt–Lantermann cleft taken by Dr. Allan Hodge at

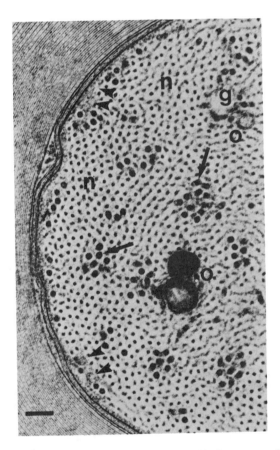

FIGURE 4. Cross section of toad peripheral nerve at a Schmidt–Lantermann cleft. The constriction of the axon associated with the Schmidt–Lantermann cleft emphasizes the fundamental order of axoplasm. Neurofilaments (n) form almost crystalline arrays interrupted by groups of microtubules (arrows). Electron-dense granular material (g) and on occasion membranous organelles (o) are found preferentially in these microtubule-associated interruptions of the neurofilament domains. Similar regions containing granular material and membranous organelles are located adjacent to the plasmalemma of the axon (arrowheads). Micrograph taken by Dr. Alan Hodge. Bar, 0.1 μm. (Adapted from Hodge and Adelman, 1983.)

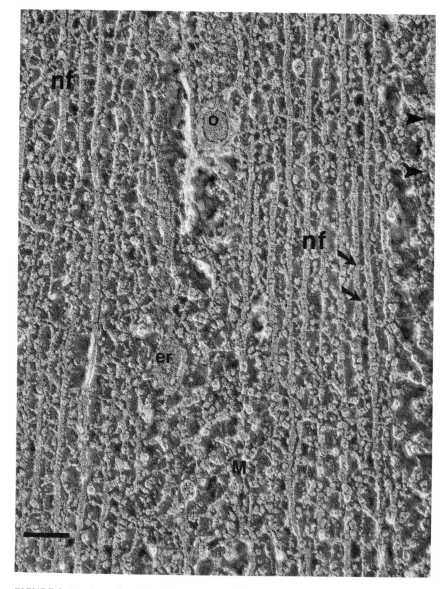

FIGURE 5. Axoplasm of turtle optic axon prepared by rapid freezing, freeze fracture, and minimal etching. The axoplasm was rotary shadowed to reveal the complex structure of the axoplasm with several discrete domains. The neurofilament domains (nf) contain longitudinally arranged, parallel neurofilaments connected by an extensive set of cross bridges (arrows). The relative homogeneity of this region is in contrast to the regions of the axoplasm that contain the granulofilamentous matrix (M) that is characteristic of the regions Schnapp and Reese (1982) call

the Marine Biological Laboratory in Woods Hole, Massachusetts. The axon is slightly compressed at Schmidt–Lantermann clefts, which results in an enhancement of the order already seen in the rest of the internodal axon. The neurofilament domains are readily apparent in this micrograph. Membranous organelles are present only in "islands" of granular electron-dense material very similar to those seen in Figures 2a and 2b. Cross sections of squid giant axons such as the one seen in longitudinal section in Figure 3 look very similar to the micrograph in Figure 4: islands of membranous organelles and electron-dense granular material separated by neurofilament domains. Figure 4 also shows that a similar granular electron-dense material is often seen in the axoplasm just beneath the plasma membrane. Again, microtubules and membranous organelles are often found in association with this granular matrix. Understanding of the mechanisms of fast axonal transport seems likely to be dependent on an understanding of the nature of these regions of the axon.

4. MOLECULAR BASES OF MOVEMENT

The precise composition and nature of the granular matrices are not well understood at present, but several inferences may be drawn from the cell biology literature. We have previously suggested (Brady and Lasek, 1981, 1982a) that such granulofilamentous matrices in the axon represent the morphological correlate of slow component b (SCb), which includes actin (Black and Lasek, 1979; Willard *et al.*, 1979), glycolytic enzymes (Brady and Lasek, 1981; Brady, 1982), calmodulin (Brady *et al.*, 1981), and several hundred other polypeptides (see Brady and Lasek, 1982a, for review). Using freeze–etch and freeze–substitution methods for maximum preservation of structural detail (Figure 5), Schnapp and Reese (1982) have shown complex globular and filamentous material in regions they refer to as microtubule domains because these structures are generally associated with microtubules but never with neurofilaments. The distribution and complexity of these structures correspond closely to the predicted properties of the SCb structure.

Much of the literature on the molecular basis of the movement of organ-

---

microtubule-associated domains (no microtubules are apparent in this region). It is in these matrix regions that membranous organelles (o) are located, the primary exception being the elements of the smooth endoplasmic reticulum (er), which may be found in either matrix regions or neurofilament domains. The appearance of the matrix (M) is similar in many respects to the subplasmalemmal cortex of the axoplasm (arrowheads). For more detailed descriptions of the technique and images, see Schnapp and Reese (1982). Micrograph provided by Dr. Bruce Schnapp. Bar, 0.1 μm.

elles in fast axonal transport has focused on the role of the axonal microtubules (see Grafstein and Forman, 1980; Hanson and Edstrom, 1978, for reviews), but it has always been noted that microfilaments were also candidates for the structures underlying the mechanisms of motility (Grafstein and Forman, 1980). Unfortunately, very little has been known about the organization and distribution of microfilaments within the axon. Schnapp and Reese (1982) find structures similar in appearance to their microtubule domains adjacent to the plasma membrane, but near the plasma membrane, microfilaments can be identified as well. The presence of microfilaments adjacent to the plasma membrane has been reported by several different laboratories (Hirokawa, 1982; Metuzals and Tasaki, 1978; Lebeux and Willemot, 1975), but relatively little was known about the organization of actin in other areas of the axoplasm. Several recent studies indicate that microfilaments may play a fundamental role in the movement of membranous organelles.

Fast axonal transport in isolated axoplasm was found to be effectively independent of the concentrations of Ca^{2+} that range from effectively zero to 10–100 μm (Brady and Lasek, 1982b). As a result, it becomes possible to introduce agents into the axoplasm that are sensitive to calcium concentration and determine the effect on transport. Gelsolin is a 90,000-dalton protein that can produce rapid depolymerization of actin microfilaments in the presence of micromolar concentrations of Ca^{2+} but that has no effect on microfilaments at lower concentrations of Ca^{2+} (Yin *et al.,* 1980). If gelsolin is perfused into isolated axoplasm in the presence of micromolar levels of Ca^{2+}, it blocks the movements of all membranous organelles. Gelsolin has no effect on fast axonal transport at lower levels of Ca^{2+} (Brady *et al.,* 1984). The effects of gelsolin confirm and extend earlier studies by Goldberg *et al.* (1980) and by Isenberg *et al.* (1980) using deoxyribonuclease I and other agents that disrupt microfilament organization. All these studies are consistent with the hypothesis that microfilaments are present in regions of the axoplasm well away from the plasma membrane and that these microfilaments are important elements in the mechanisms of fast axonal transport.

A detailed model for the molecular mechanisms of fast axonal transport is still not practical. Too many pieces are missing from the puzzle at this time. However, certain properties of fast transport must be explained by any model. First, the absence of regulation by Ca^{2+} makes fast axonal transport unique among types of cell motility studied to date. It can be argued that the traffic of membranous organelles in the axon is always "on" and that it would be disadvantageous to have these processes subject to interruption by the normal regulatory events of cellular metabolism, many of which involve changes in Ca^{2+} levels. However, this fails to explain the observation that the maximal rates of fast axonal transport differ in central and peripheral neurons (Grafstein and Forman, 1980). The actions of treatments that disrupt cytoskeletal organization *in situ* must be better understood. Treatments that disrupt cyto-skeletal elements *in vitro* generally also inhibit transport, but not always (see Brady *et al.,* 1980; Byers, 1974; Papasozomenos *et al.,* 1982, for exceptions on the microtubules; see Goldberg *et al.,* 1980; Isenberg *et al.,* 1980, for excep-tions on the microfilaments).

Finally, any model must explain how different classes of particles differ in direction of movement and characteristic types of movement, i.e., why some particles are retrograde and others orthograde in the axon, and still others may move in either direction. We now know that the orthograde organelles are mor-phologically distinct from the retrograde organelles, but it is not clear how this structural difference is translated into differences in net direction. This ques-tion becomes particularly interesting in light of the report by Adams and Bray (1983) that polystyrene beads of appropriate dimensions and surfaces injected into axons will move in a manner essentially indistinguishable from endogenous organelles. These artificial organelles have so far been found to move only in the orthograde direction. Many other properties of fast axonal transport must also be explained before a satisfactory model is defined. These represent only a few key features that are not adequately explained by available models.

5. ROLE OF FAST AXONAL TRANSPORT IN AXONAL GROWTH AND REGENERATION

Axonal transport is now being defined in terms of the organelles and struc-tures that move within the axon. The function of each rate component can be discussed with regard to identified proteins and cellular structures. Thus, Slow Component a provides for the continual renewal of the neurofilament–micro-tubule network of the axon (Lasek and Brady, 1982). Any discussion of the morphology of neurons, particularly of the dynamics of neuronal form, rapidly becomes concerned with the properties of Slow Component a for that neuron. In the same manner, fast axonal transport, as defined in this review, involves the movement of membranous organelles in the axon and must be considered when the role of the neuronal surface in growth or the supply of membrane-associated enzymatic activities is important for the development of the axon.

One of the important steps in understanding fast axonal transport has been the determination of which axonal organelles are moving and which are not. Identification of the moving structure and the direction of movement is an essential part of understanding the metabolic function of an axonal structure. Development of new approaches and new preparations for the study of fast axonal transport processes has been necessary to achieve this goal, but we now have a better understanding of the classes of membranous organelles within the axon and the organization of the interior of the axon.

The three classes of membranous organelles moving within the axon have been identified both in living preparations with light microscopic methods and in fixed preparations with the electron microscope: tubulovesicular structures 40–60 nm in diameter move in the orthograde direction; larger complex vesicles move mainly in the retrograde direction; and mitochondria move in both directions. The result is a more complete picture of the dynamics for all the membranous structures within the axon. If the smooth endoplasmic reticulum and plasma membrane are not being actively translocated in fast axonal transport, then turnover of proteins associated with these structures must be mediated by the processes of fast orthograde and retrograde transport. Thus, changes in axonal length or diameter that require an increase in membrane surface area would be expected to result from changes in the amount, composition, or destination of materials moving in fast axonal transport. Such alterations in fast axonal transport have, in fact, been reported during growth and regeneration of axonal processes (Grafstein and McQuarrie, 1978; Skene and Willard, 1981*a,b*).

Having progressed this far in our understanding of axonal growth and fast axonal transport, we can see several directions for future research that look particularly promising. Now that the structures corresponding to the different subcategories of fast axonal transport have been identified, it becomes possible and desirable to isolate and characterize the different structures and organelles in transport. We still know little or nothing about why a class of organelles moves preferentially in one direction. Are there receptors of orthograde and retrograde polarities on the organelles, or do retrograde and orthograde organelles follow different pathways in the axon? The video records suggest that there are no directed pathways, but even this may be deceptive. Many other questions remain about regulation of the movement of membranous organelles in the axon and the role this dynamic process plays in the growth and maintenance of axons. For example, how is a specific mitochondrion targeted for a specific destination, and what determines the direction of movement? What is the function of the proteins that change markedly in amount during growth or regeneration of axons (Skene and Willard, 1981*a,b*)? Many proteins appear to be present in both orthograde and retrograde transport, but what are the steps that convert a membranous element from an orthograde to a retrograde moving particle? Some of these questions have eluded explanation for many years, but it has now become possible to consider the answers.

ACKNOWLEDGMENTS

The author wishes to thank Dr. Raymond Lasek for his continuing support and many stimulating collaborations in the laboratory and discussions. The author is also grateful to Alison Hall for commenting on the manuscript. The original research described in this chapter received support from the following grants made by the National Institutes of Health: NS18361, AG00795, NS14900, and NS15731.

6. REFERENCES

Adams, R. J., and Bray, D., 1983, Rapid transport of foreign particles microinjected into crab axons, *Nature* **303**:718–720.

Allen, R. D., and Allen, N. S., 1983, Video-enhanced microscopy with a computer frame memory, *J. Micros.* **129**(Part I):3–17.

Allen, R. D., Allen, N. S., and Travis, J. L., 1981, Video-enhanced contrast, differential interference contrast (AVEC-DIC): A new method capable of analyzing microtubule related motility in the reticulopodial network of *Allogromia laticollaris, Cell Motil.* **1**:291–302.

Allen, R. D., Metuzals, J., Tasaki, I., Brady, S. T., and Gilbert, S., 1982, Fast axonal transport in squid giant axon, *Science* **218**:1127–1129.

Baitinger, C., Levine, J., Lorenz, T., Simon, C., Skene, P., and Willard, M., 1982, Characteristics of axonally transported proteins, in: *Axoplasmic Transport* (D. G. Weiss, ed.), pp. 110–120, Springer-Verlag, Berlin, Heidelberg, New York.

Berthold, C.-H., 1982, Some aspects of the ultrastructural organization of peripheral myelinated axons in the cat, in: *Axoplasmic Transport* (D. G. Weiss, ed.), pp. 40–54, Springer-Verlag, Berlin, Heidelberg, New York.

Black, M., and Lasek, R. J., 1979, Axonal transport of actin: Slow component b is the principle source of actin for the axon, *Brain Res.* **171**:401–413.

Brady, S. T., 1982, Axonal transport of glycolytic enzymes: Aldolase and pyruvate kinase, *Trans. Am. Soc. Neurochem.* **13**:226.

Brady, S. T., and Lasek, R. J., 1981, Nerve specific enolase and creatine phosphokinase in axonal transport: Soluble proteins and the axoplasmic matrix, *Cell* **23**:523–531.

Brady, S. T., and Lasek, R. J., 1982a, The slow components of axonal transport: Movements, compositions, and organization, in: *Axoplasmic Transport* (D. G. Weiss, ed.), pp. 206–217, Springer-Verlag, Berlin, Heidelberg, New York.

Brady, S. T., and Lasek, R. J., 1982b, Fast axonal transport in isolated axoplasm: Roles of neurofilaments and microtubules, *J. Cell Biol.* **95**:330a.

Brady, S. T., and Lasek, R. J., 1983, Axonal transport in isolated axoplasm: Gelsolin as a probe for actin, *Trans. Am. Soc. Neurochem.* **14**:21.

Brady, S. T., Crothers, S., Nosal, C., and McClure, W. O., 1980, Fast axonal transport in the presence of high Ca^{2+}: Evidence that microtubules are not required, *Proc. Natl. Acad. Sci. U.S.A.* **77**:5909–5913.

Brady, S. T., Tytell, M., Heriot, K., and Lasek, R. J., 1981, Axonal transport of calmodulin: A physiological approach to identification of longterm associations between proteins, *J. Cell Biol.* **89**:607–614.

Brady, S. T., Lasek, R. J., and Allen, R. D., 1982, Fast axonal transport in extruded axoplasm from squid giant axon, *Science* **218**:1129–1131.

Brady, S. T., Lasek, R., Allen, R., Yin, H., and Stossell, T., 1984, Gelsolin inhibition of fast axonal transport indicates a requirement for actin microfilaments, *Nature* (in press).

Breuer, A. C., Christian, C. M., Henkart, M., and Nelson, P. G., 1975, Computer analysis of organelle translocation in primary neuronal cultures and continuous cell lines, *J. Cell Biol.* **65**:562–576.

Brimijoin, S., 1975, Stop flow: A new technique for measuring axonal transport and its application to the transport of dopamine-β-hydroxylase, *J. Neurobiol.* **6**:379–394.

Byers, M., 1974, Structural correlates of rapid axonal transport: Evidence that microtubules may not be directly involved, *Brain Res.* **75**:97–113.

Dahlstrom, A., 1971, Axoplasmic transport (with particular respect to adrenergic neurons), *Phil. Trans. R. Soc. Lond. [Biol.]* **261**:325–358.

Dahlstrom, A., and Haggendal, J., 1967, Studies on the transport and lifespan of amine storage granules in the adrenergic neuron system of the rabbit sciatic nerve, *Acta Physiol. Scand.* **69**:153–157.

Droz, B., and Leblond, C. P., 1963, Axonal migration of proteins in the central nervous system and peripheral nerves as shown by radioautography, *J. Comp. Neurol.* **121**:325–346.

Droz, B., and Rambourg, A., 1982, Axonal smooth endoplasmic reticulum and fast orthograde transport of membrane constituents, in: *Axoplasmic Transport* (D. G., Weiss, ed.), pp. 110–120, Springer-Verlag, Berlin, Heidelberg, New York.

Droz, B., Koenig, H. L., and DiGiamberardino, L., 1973, Axonal transport of protein and glycoprotein to nerve endings. I. Radioautographic analysis of the renewal of protein in nerve endings of chicken ciliary ganglion after intracerebral injection of [³H]-L-lysine, *Brain Res.* **60**:93–127.

Droz, B., Rambourg, A., and Koenig, H. L., 1975, The smooth endoplasmic reticulum: Structure and role in the renewal of axonal membrane and synaptic vesicles by fast axonal transport, *Brain Res.* **93**:1–13.

Ellisman, M. H., and Lindsey, J. D., 1982, Organization of axoplasm—membranous and fibrillar components possibly involved in fast neuroplasmic Transport, in: *Axoplasmic Transport* (D. G. Weiss, ed.), pp. 55–63, Springer-Verlag, Berlin, Heidelberg, New York.

Fahim, M., Brady, S. T., and Lasek, R. J., 1982, Axonal transport of membranous organelles in squid giant axons and axoplasm, *J. Cell Biol.* **95**:330a.

Forman, D., Padjen, A. L., and Siggins, G., 1977, Axonal transport of organelles visualized by light microscopy: cinemicrographic and computer analysis, *Brain Res.* **136**:197–213.

Goldberg, D. J., Harris, D. A., Lubit, B. W., and Schwartz, J. H., 1980, Analysis of the mechanism of fast axonal transport by intracellular injection of potentially inhibitory macromolecules: Evidence for a possible role of actin filaments, *Proc. Natl. Acad. U.S.A.* **77**:7448–7452.

Grafstein, B., 1967, Transport of protein by goldfish optic nerve fibers, *Science* **157**:196–198.

Grafstein, B., and Forman, D. S., 1980, Intracellular transport in neurons, *Physiol. Rev.* **60**:1167–1283.

Grafstein, B., and McQuarrie, I., 1978, Role of the nerve cell body in axonal regeneration, in: *Neuronal Plasticity* (C. Cotman, ed.), pp. 155–195, Raven Press, New York.

Hanson, M., and Edstrom, A., 1978, Mitosis inhibitors and axonal transport, *Int. Rev. Cytol.* [*Suppl.*] **7**:373–402.

Hirokawa, N., 1982, Cross-linker system between neurofilaments, microtubules, and membranous organelles in frog axons revealed by quick-freeze, deep-etching method, *J. Cell. Biol.* **94**:129–142.

Hodge, A., and Adelman, W., 1983, in: *Structure and Function in Excitable Cells* (D. Chang, I. Tasaki, W. Adelman, and H. Leuchtag, eds.), pp. 75–111, Plenum Press, New York.

Isenberg, G., Schubert, P., and Kreutzberg, G. W., 1980, Experimental approach to test the role of actin in axonal transport, *Brain Res.* **194**:588–593.

Kasa, P., 1968, Acetylcholinesterase transport in the central and peripheral nervous tissue: The role of tubules in the enzyme transport, *Nature* **218**:1265–1267.

Lasek, R. J., 1967, Bidirectional transport of radioactivity labeled axoplasmic components, *Nature* **216**:1212–1214.

Lasek, R. J., 1968, Axoplasmic transport in cat dorsal root ganglion cells as studied with [³H]-L-leucine, *Brain Res.* **7**:360–377.

Lasek, R. J., and Brady, S. T., 1982, The structural hypothesis of axonal transport: Two classes of moving elements, in: *Axoplasmic Transport* (D. G. Weiss, ed.), pp. 397–405, Springer-Verlag, Berlin, Heidelberg, New York.

Lebeux, Y. J., and Willemot, J., 1975, An ultrastructural study of the microfilaments in rat brain by heavy meromyosin labelling: The perikaryon, dendrites, and the axon, *Cell Tissue Res.* **160:**1–36.

Metuzals, J., and Tasaki, I., 1978, Subaxolemmal filamentous network in the giant nerve fiber of the squid (*Loligo pealei* L.) and its possible role in excitability, *J. Cell Biol.* **78:**597–621.

Papasozomenos, S., Yoon, M., Crane, R., Autillio-Gambetti, L., and Gambetti, P., 1982, Redistribution of proteins of fast axonal transport following administration of β,β-iminodiproprionitrile: A quantitative autoradiographic study, *J. Cell Biol.* **95:**672–675.

Peters, A., Palay, S. L., and Webster, H., 1976, *The Fine Structure of the Nervous System,* W. B. Saunders, Philadelphia.

Schnapp, B., and Reese, T., 1982, Cytoplasmic structure in rapid-frozen axons, *J. Cell Biol.* **94:**667–679.

Skene, P., and Willard, M., 1981*a*, Changes in axonally transported proteins during axon regeneration in toad retinal ganglion cells, *J. Cell Biol.* **89:**86–95.

Skene, P., and Willard, M., 1981*b*, Axonally transported proteins associated with axon growth in rabbit central and peripheral nervous systems, *J. Cell Biol.* **89:**96–103.

Smith, R. S., 1972, Detection of organelles in myelinated nerve fibers by dark field microscopy, *Can. J. Physiol. Pharmacol.* **50:**467–469.

Smith, R. S., 1980, The short term accumulation of axonally transported organelles in the region of localized lesions of single myelinated axons, *J. Neurocytol.* **9:**39–65.

Smith, R. S., and Koles, Z. J., 1976, Mean velocity of optically detected intraaxonal particles measured by a cross correlation method, *Can. J. Physiol. Pharmacol.* **54:**859–869.

Tessler, A., Autillio-Gambetti, L., and Gambetti, P., 1980, Axonal growth during regeneration: A quantitative autoradiographic study, *J. Cell Biol.* **87:**197–203.

Tsukita, S., and Ishikawa, H., 1976, Three-dimensional distribution of smooth endoplasmic reticulum in mylenated axons. *J. Electron Micros*, **25:**141–149.

Tsukita, S., and Ishikawa, H., 1979, Morphological evidence for the involvement of the smooth endoplasmic reticulum in axonal transport, *Brain Res.* **174:**315–318.

Tsukita, S., and Ishikawa, H., 1980, The movement of membranous organelles in axons: Electron microscopic identification of anterogradely and retrogradely transported organelles, *J. Cell Biol.* **84:**513–530.

Tytell, M., Black, M. M., Garner, J., and Lasek, R. J., 1981, Axonal transport: Each of the major rate components consists of distinct macromolecular complexes, *Science* **214:**179–181.

Willard, M., Wiserman, M., Levine, J., and Skene, P., 1979, Axonal transport of actin in rabbit retinal ganglion cells, *J. Cell Biol.* **81:**581–591.

Yin, H., Zaner, K. S., and Stossel, T. P., 1980, Ca^{2+} control of actin gelation: Interaction of gelsolin with actin filaments and regulation of actin gelation, *J. Biol. Chem.* **255:**9494–9500.

Zelena, J., Lubinska, L., and Gutmann, E., 1968, Accumulation of organelles at the ends of interrupted axons, *Z. Zellforsch. Mikrosk. Anat.* **91:**200–219.

CHAPTER 3

RETROGRADE SIGNALING AFTER NERVE INJURY

KRISTER KRISTENSSON

1. NERVE CELL BODY RESPONSE TO AXOTOMY

The nerve cell body's reaction after an axonal lesion was first described in 1892 by Nissl. This reaction, later to be termed chromatolysis, is characterized by dispersion of the Nissl bodies and decreased cytoplasmic basophilia. The functional meaning of chromatolysis is still not completely understood, and we do not know the mechanism by which the cell body is signaled from the injured axon to bring about such a reaction (Torvik, 1976).

There is biochemical evidence that after an axonal lesion the nerve cell body increases its synthesis of materials needed to reconstitute the axonal membranes and cytoskeletal elements necessary for regeneration and that the synthesis of enzymes involved in the neurotransmittor synthesis is diminished (Kreutzberg, 1982).

It has therefore generally been assumed that chromatolysis in some way reflects such metabolic adjustments. However, Torvik (1976) has reported that after a crush to the facial nerve in rabbits, classical chromatolysis develops,

KRISTER KRISTENSSON ● Department of Pathology, Karolinska Institute, Huddinge University Hospital S-141 86, Huddinge, Sweden

whereas in mice, an increased cytoplasmic basophilia occurs, and in rats no reaction is seen at all. In spite of these remarkable differences in the nerve cell bodies' morphological reactions, the nerves regenerate in a similar way in all three species. Therefore, the question of what in the nerve cell's response reflects alterations related to regeneration and what instead reflects degenerative or other changes induced by the injury remains to be answered. Another reaction, rapid nerve cell death, may also occur during defined periods of time in the early postnatal development of the different neuronal populations. In certain neurons of mature animals, for instance, the dorsal motor vagal neurons in rats and rabbits, nerve transection also causes a rapid death of the cell bodies (Aldskogius *et al.*, 1980). Since the nerve cell body's responses to an axonal injury vary, the signal(s) by which these are mediated may also vary.

In his classical review article, "What is the signal for chromatolysis?" Cragg in 1970 considered ten hypotheses. These include signaling by blood-borne substances, depolarization of the cell by the cut end of the axon, loss of axon potentials, proliferation of neurofilaments and of Schwann cells, breakdown of a blood-nerve barrier, increased loss of axoplasm or axoplasmic constituents from the injured axon, loss of a trophic substance coming from the periphery, and loss of a repressor substance from the cell body. None of these hypothetical signal mechanisms was considered to account perfectly for all experimental findings known at that time, but the last hypothesis, which implies that the neuron produces a substance that represses neuronal RNA production and loses some of these repressors when the axon is injured or when it sprouts, appeared to come nearest to explaining these findings. That a loss of a trophic substance coming from the peripheral target organ should induce chromatolysis seemed less likely. That hypothesis failed to explain the observations that nucleolar RNA production returns to near normal levels at the same time whether the axons reinnervate a muscle or form a neuroma and that the nucleolar reaction can be induced again by cutting off a neuroma. Also, at that time there was no definite proof for a retrograde transport in axons *in vivo*.

Since many studies during the last decade have shown that in fact transport of substances in axons from the periphery to the nerve cell body does exist, the possibility that the signal(s) are transferred by retrograde transport is reconsidered in this chapter. Such signals may include, in addition to a loss of trophic substances coming from the periphery, alterations in the transport induced by factors at the site of the lesion. If the signal(s) in fact are transferred by retrograde transport, this may have practical application, since ways may be offered to selectively alter the nerve cell bodies' response after an axonal injury. For example, in certain circumstances, factors may be introduced to prevent a rapid nerve cell death; in others, a weak and insufficient regenerative response may be enhanced; and in still others, improper reinnervation or neuroma formation may be eliminated.

2. RETROGRADE AXONAL TRANSPORT: PHYSIOLOGICAL SIGNIFICANCE

At axon terminals, macromolecular substances can be incorporated either by so-called fluid-phase endocytosis or by adsorptive endocytosis (Kristensson, 1978). In fluid-phase endocytosis, a substance does not interact with the axonal surface, and the incorporation is in direct proportion to the concentration of the substance in the surrounding medium. The second mechanism implies that the substance is adsorbed to the surface, a process that may be facilitated by nonspecific electrostatic factors; e.g., cationized ferritin is readily adsorbed and incorporated at axon terminals, whereas anionic ferritin is not. Certain lectins are also incorporated into neurons as a result of the high degree of affinity they have for defined sugar groups at the cell surface. Other substances of particular molecular composition can be selectively adsorbed at low concentrations by so-called receptor-mediated endocytosis. This is the means by which different polypeptide hormones can be incorporated into different cell types (Pastan and Willingham, 1981). The hormone (ligand), after binding to receptors, causes the latter to aggregate into clusters, which move into coated pits. These are invaginations of the plasma membrane undercoated by a radially striated material containing clathrin. From such coated pits, vesicles move into the cytoplasm and fuse with prelysosomal organelles, which then move into the region of the Golgi apparatus. The fate of the receptors has not, because of technical difficulties, been followed. The ligand may in some cases be recirculated to the cell surface and in others be transferred to lysosomes for degradation.

Most hormones appear to elicit their primary metabolic alterations in the cell from the cell surface via a second messenger released during the ligand–receptor binding and receptor aggregation. It has been debated whether ligands incorporated into intracellular vesicles also can stimulate some type of metabolic response. The incorporation may simply be a pathway for inactivation of ligand–receptor complexes, but the possibility still exists that some type of effect can be elicited at the level of prelysosomal organelles moving into the Golgi region by release of either a second messenger or an activated ligand.

It has never convincingly been demonstrated that a ligand or a product of it can be transferred to the nucleus. However, from virologic experiments it is well known that DNA viruses such as herpes viruses can be taken up at nerve endings and travel retrogradely in axons, and from the perikaryon the virus nucleic acid must be transferred to the nucleus, where the virus replicates (Wildy *et al.,* 1982). Since viruses in many other instances use a cell's normal mechanism for their transport and assembly, it therefore seems likely that there are pathways in neurons by which exogenous macromolecular substances can reach the cell nucleus after somatopetal axonal transport.

At axon terminals, tracer substances have been localized to coated vesicles and to larger vacuoles that lack a coat. It is well known that the uptake of substances by fluid-phase endocytosis can be increased by synaptic activity, which apparently reflects a recirculation of synaptic vesicle membranes (Holtzman *et al.*, 1971). Less is known about the relationship between synaptic vesicles and high-affinity uptake involving ligand–receptor binding, and it is unclear how substances taken up by adsorptive endocytosis relate to recycling of synaptic vesicles. For the economy of the cell, it would seem likely that vesicles incorporated by this mechanism would recycle back to the surface membrane after the ligand and/or the receptor has been delivered to some sort of transport vacuole. The transport in axons also occurs in large elongated vacuolar structures and does not seem to involve vesicles of the size of a synaptic vesicle to any larger extent (Figure 1).

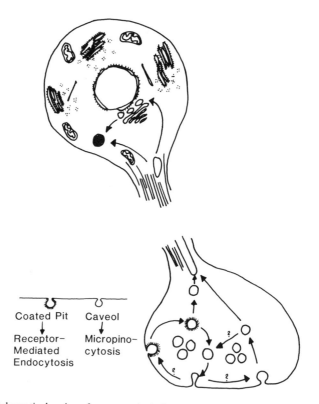

FIGURE 1. Schematic drawing of a neuron depicting principles for endocytotic uptake of macromolecules at axon terminal. The retrograde transport occurs in larger elongated vacuoles and terminates in lysosomal organelles or passes through the Golgi region in the cell body, depending on the properties of the macromolecule.

In order to examine if the amount of retrogradely transported materials also varies with synaptic activity, quantitative cytofluorometric determinations of neuronal accumulation of a fluorochrome were performed during different physiological states of the neuron (Enerbäck *et al.,* 1980). Botulinus toxin, which inhibits the release of synaptic vesicle content, caused only a slight reduction in the amount of tracer substances transported retrogradely in the áxons, whereas stimulation after exposure to tetanus toxin caused an increase. Since sensory neurons, which do not have any synaptic activity at their peripheral nerve endings, also incorporate tracers from the periphery, it is suggested that neurons, like other cells, have a basal rate of endocytosis delivering membranes and exogenous materials to the perikaryon and that this rate can be somewhat modulated by the synaptic activity.

The physiological significance of retrograde axonal transport could then include bulk turnover of membranes from the axon terminal surface and from the synaptic vesicles (Holtzman and Mercurio, 1980), regulation or modulation of the number of receptor molecules at the axon surface, and incorporation of biologically active ligands via receptor-mediated endocytosis either for their inactivation in lysosomal organelles or, possibly, as a pathway for them to elicit effects directly at the level of the cell body (Thoenen and Schwab, 1978).

3. CHROMATOLYSIS AND RETROGRADE AXONAL TRANSPORT: TIME RELATIONSHIP

By compiling data from the literature, Cragg (1970) estimated that the signal for chromatolysis should reach the nerve cell body with a velocity of about 1 mm/day, which is much slower than retrograde transport for tracer-containing organelles. However, there is a latent period of several hours between the time the signal has reached the perikaryon and the time the chromatolytic reaction develops. Chromatolysis develops after DNA-dependent RNA synthesis, and from experiments with intracerebral injections of actinomycin D at various time intervals in relation to the axonal injury, it is known that this synthesis precedes chromatolysis by several hours (Torvik and Heding, 1969). Horseradish peroxidase (HRP) applied topically to a nerve at the site of a lesion will be incorporated into the injured axons and transported to the nerve cell body, where it also appears several hours prior to the earliest morphological signs of chromatolysis. By crushing the sciatic nerves at two different levels in different groups of rats and examining the appearance of spinal ganglion neurons at regular time intervals thereafter, we found that the velocity of the ascent of signal for chromatolysis must be much faster than previously estimated and within the same range as retrograde transport of HRP (Kristensson and Olsson, 1975). Thus, there is a time relationship between the two phenomena—appearance in the nerve cell body of materials transported retrogradely and the signal for chromatolysis. Whether there also is a causal relationship is discussed in the next section.

4. POSSIBLE SIGNAL MECHANISMS MEDIATED BY RETROGRADE TRANSPORT

4.1. Loss of Repressor Factors

One growth factor for neurons that has been studied extensively and characterized is the nerve growth factor (NGF) for sympathetic neurons (Thoenen and Schwab, 1978). A number of experiments have shown that NGF is transported retrogradely in sympathetic neurons and also in small neurons in the spinal ganglia. If a sympathetic nerve is cut in immature animals, the neurons will rapidly degenerate and disappear. This rapid nerve cell death can be prevented by topical application of nerve growth factor to the ganglion (Hendry *et al.,* 1974; Hendry and Campbell, 1976). In this case, it seems that the cause of cell death is the loss of NGF, or of a factor induced by it, coming from the periphery, unless the topical application of NGF counteracts noxious effects of other factors transported with the axons. In mature animals, axonal lesions generally induce a regenerative response instead of nerve cell death, but it is not known if NGF can act as a maintenance or repressor factor in adult neurons instead of as a growth-stimulating factor. Axotomy of frog spinal neurons at 15°C causes no signs of chromatolysis in cell bodies. This makes it less likely that the chromatolytic response seen after transection at 25°C can be solely caused by the elimination of a trophic agent coming from the periphery, since that agent should also be eliminated at 15°C (Carlsen *et al.,* 1982). Also, in long-term cultures of rat sympathetic neurons, neurites will regenerate after a neuritotomy in the virtual absence of nonneuronal cells around the neurites and when nerve growth factor has been withdrawn from the cultures, which again suggests that the induction of regenerative response of the neuron is not mediated by the loss of an exogeneous trophic factor coming from the periphery (Campenot, 1981).

4.2. Alterations at the Site of the Lesion

We have observed that HRP topically applied to a crushed nerve can diffuse into the area of the crush and into the injured axons. Later, HRP is found in vacuoles more proximally in the axons and then in the nerve cell bodies. This would imply that the exogenous molecule, after diffusion into the axon over the injured membrane, is sequestered into organelles prior to transport. This is a transient influx, since HRP applied 1 hr after the crush is no longer transported to any substantial degree (Kristensson and Olsson, 1976). In this way, exogenous factors can enter neurons. Such factors may include (1) factors from the serum leaking into the damaged nerve, (2) factors from the inflammatory response induced by the trauma, and (3) factors released by the nonneuronal cells surrounding the axons. However, this can also mean that damaged or altered axonal membranes (both from the axolemma and the endoplasmic reticulum) may be transferred back to the nerve cell bodies (Figure 2). There seem to be alterations in the transport of lectins to the nerve cell bodies from the site of axon injury as compared to that from intact axon terminals (Nennesmo, 1983), indicating such membrane and binding changes. The trauma to the axolemma and/or the permeability disturbances induced in it may also release factors from the membranes that may be transported back to the nerve cell body. Alterations in retrograde transport of endogenous axonal materials and their relation to the signal for chromatolysis are further discussed by Bisby in this volume (Chapter 4).

The hypothesis that factors released at the site of the lesion can signal the response of the nerve cell body is compatible with experiments showing that the type of the lesion can influence the type of the nerve cell body response. For instance, if the facial nerve of the rat is evulsed, a dramatic degeneration with cell death occurs; if the nerve is crushed, no histological changes are visible at the light microscopic level; if the nerve is cut, the reaction is intermediate (Søreide, 1981) (Figure 3). Conceivably, different types of trauma may cause different changes of the axonal membranes and constituents or expose the axons differently to nonneuronal factors. This hypothesis is further supported by the observations that a chromatolytic response may ensue after a

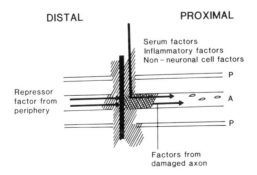

FIGURE 2. Possible signaling mechanisms for chromatolysis following an axonal crush. These include exogenous or endogenous materials transported from the site of the lesion and loss of a hypothetical repressor factor coming from the periphery. A, axon; P, perineurium.

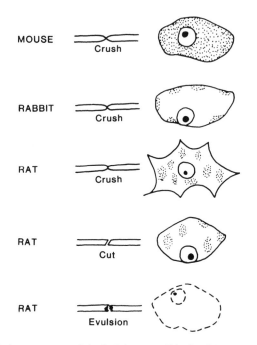

FIGURE 3. Various responses of the facial nerve cell bodies following different types of axonal injuries in different animal species.

neuronma formation is cut (Watson, 1974) and that peripheral nerve transplantations into the CNS may induce a regenerative response in otherwise nonregenerating CNS neurons, showing that extrinsic factors in the axon's environment are of importance for regeneration (Aguayo *et al.,* 1982).

Biochemical changes in the nerve cell body occur after the injection of botulinum toxin into the area of neuromuscular junction. Watson (1974) suggested that since botulinum toxin causes a block of synaptic vesicle release, endocytosis associated with recycling of membranes should also be inhibited, and, consequently, a block of uptake of a trophic substance from the periphery could cause the cell body changes. However, as an argument against this hypothesis, we have observed that botulinum toxin, although it induces a complete paralysis, only causes a minor reduction in retrograde axonal transport in the facial nerves of the mouse and no light microscopic changes in the nerve cell bodies (Enerbäck *et al.,* 1980). Therefore, it is possible that the previous biochemical alterations described may either be a toxic effect on the neuron induced by botulinum toxin transported up to the nerve cell bodies or reflect some minor metabolic adjustments to the altered function in the neuron and not the dramatic picture of chromatolysis.

Further evidence that retrograde axonal transport and factors from the site of the axonal lesion mediate the signal for the nerve cell body's response is suggested by experiments on the rat hypoglossal nerve, where an axotomy causes an increased glucose consumption in the hypoglossal nucleus as assayed by an increased $[^{14}C]$2-deoxyglucose uptake. This increased glucose uptake can be blocked by injections of colchicine into the nerve proximal to the lesion, a treatment that also effectively blocks retrograde transport of HRP (Fernandez *et al.,* 1981).

Since the nerve cell body's response can vary markedly from species to species, with the age of the animal, and with the type of axonal injury, it is difficult to conceive how such different reactions can be induced by a single factor that at one extreme causes the neuron to regenerate with no light microscopic perikaryal changes and at the other extreme causes a rapid cell death. The factors leading to rapid cell death may therefore be different from those inducing the regenerative response. Apparently, regeneration does not follow as a consequence to chromatolysis, since the initial response to axotomy is the same whether the nerve cell will die or not (Aldskogius *et al.,* 1980), and rat facial neurons regenerate without any visible degenerative alterations in the cell.

In general cell pathology, it has not yet been determined what factors cause an irreversible cell damage. The early hypothesis that the leakage of lysosomal enzyme should be the cause of damage is less likely to be valid, since such leakages are generally late events and probably just a consequence of cell damage. In immature neurons, which die rapidly after axotomy, we found no signs of any early leakage of tracer substances from lysosomes (Olsson and Kristensson, 1979). Another hypothesis involves activation of Ca^{2+}-dependent phospholipases, which, in ischemic liver and myocardial cells, degrade plasma membranes and endoplasmic reticulum membranes (Farber *et al.,* 1981), thereby possibly causing the irreversible damage. Activation of such enzymes may well also occur after damage to axon membranes, and more severe axonal damages could cause more extensive activation. There have been no experiments performed to test such a hypothesis; however, an interesting observation is that in dorsal vagal motor neurons, which in adult rats and rabbits rapidly die after axotomy, numerous cytoplasmic lipid droplets occur in the perikaryon, often in connection with degenerated endoplasmic reticulum membranes (Aldskogius, 1978).

New information on the signaling mechanism for chromatolysis may also be obtained from basic studies of neurovirulent viruses. A classic chromatolysis develops in motor neurons after infection with poliomyelitis virus, which travels retrogradely in the axons to the nerve cell bodies following injection in the periphery (Bodian, 1948). In other cell types, poliovirus causes a disaggregation and reaggregation of polyribosomes, which reflect a cut-off of the host cell's protein synthesis and an induction of virus protein synthesis (Martin and Kerr, 1968). The disaggregation of polyribosomes can be prevented by actinomycin D, which is reminiscent of the observation that the dispersion of Nissl bodies after axonal lesion can be prevented by the same treatment. In addition, transection of a nerve root or trauma to the peripheral field of innervation of a ganglion can reactivate herpes simplex virus infections in spinal or cranial ganglia. During latency, the viral DNA is probably in some way integrated in the nerve cell nucleus (Wildý *et al.*, 1982), and the mechanisms by which the virus is activated may be similar to those for eliciting the chromatolytic response after an axonal trauma.

5. RETROGRADE TRANSPORT DURING REGENERATION

After a nerve crush, the perineurium is damaged, and serum proteins and other macromolecular substances diffuse into the endoneurium. Such molecules will also leak into the distal stump of the nerve (Olsson and Kristensson, 1973), and the outgrowing nerve fibers will consequently be exposed to a milieu rich in serum factors that may well promote regeneration similar to the situation *in vitro* in which introduction of NGF causes a more extensive and long-term regeneration of sympathetic neurons following neuritotomy; in the absence of NGF, regeneration is limited to a few days (Campenot, 1981).

Another alteration in the metabolism of the nerve cell occurs when the regenerating axons have reached their target area and established functioning connections. By using quantitative cytofluorometric methods, we have observed that there is an increased accumulation of tracer substances, both those incorporated by fluid-phase endocytosis and those taken up by adsorptive endocytosis, from the periphery when a nerve is reinnervating its muscle (Enerbäck *et al.*, 1980; Nennesmo, 1983). Such an increased accumulation probably represents an increased uptake area, each axon giving rise to several branches with an early polyneuronal innervation of reinnervated muscles. This polyneuronal innervation is subsequently eliminated, and during the same time period, the increased incorporation of tracer substances from the periphery is normalized. Such alterations in the amount of materials transported may be of significance for an understanding of how the cell body interacts with its peripheral field of innervation and how it returns to its normal metabolic state after an axonal injury.

6. CONCLUDING REMARKS

Axotomy may induce alterations in both the metabolism and structure of the nerve cell body. The morphological changes include classical chromatolysis in many nerve cell populations, although in certain populations no changes at all are displayed despite the fact that the nerve regenerates. It is therefore not clear what the chromatolytic reactions signify. Probably, they are not necessary for the initiation of regeneration but may reflect long-term changes in nerve cell metabolism required for a proper outgrowth of axons. In the very young animal and in some nerve cell populations of mature animals, a rapid nerve cell death may follow axotomy. Since the responses of neurons vary, the signals that induce such responses may also vary. The signals may be mediated by retrograde axonal transport, as the estimated velocity for the ascent of signal for chromatolysis is within the same range as that for retrograde transport. Since the cell body's response also varies with the type of lesion, an elimination of trophic factors coming from the peripheral target organ cannot be solely involved. Directly from the site of the lesion there is a transient influx of exogenous materials into the cell body. Such exogenous materials may include factors from the serum, the inflammatory response, or the nonneuronal cells. Also, damaged axonal constituents or endogenous factors released from such damaged structures may be involved. Since retrograde axonal transport offers a selective way of introducing factors into a nerve cell body and thus manipulating its metabolism during regeneration, it is important to define clearly what factors after a nerve lesion stimulate axonal growth and what factors cause neuronal death.

ACKNOWLEDGMENTS

The author wishes to thank Marie Gustafsson for excellent technical assistance. This work was supported by a grant from The Swedish Medical Research Council, project No. B81-12X-04480-07A.

7. REFERENCES

Aguayo, A. J., Richardson, P. M., David, S., and Beufey, M., 1982, Transplantation of neurons and sheath cells—a tool for the study of regeneration, in: *Repair and Regeneration of the Nervous System* (J. G. Nicholls, ed.), pp. 91–105, Springer-Verlag, Berlin, Heidelberg, New York.

Aldskogius, H., 1978, Lipid accumulation in axotomized adult rabbit vagal neurons. Electron microscopical observations, *Brain Res.* **140**:349–353.

Aldskogius, H., Barron, K. D., and Regal, R., 1980, Axon reaction in dorsal motor vagal and hypoglossal neurons of the adult rat. Light microscopy and RNA-cytochemistry, *J. Comp. Neurol.* **193**:165–177.

Bodian, D., 1948, The virus, the nerve cell and paralysis. A study of experimental poliomyelitis in the spinal cord, *Bull. Johns Hopkins Hosp.* **83**:1–108.

Campenot, R. B., 1981, Regeneration of neurites in long-term cultures of sympathetic neurons deprived of nerve growth factor, *Science* **214**:579–581.

Carlsen, R. C., Kiff, J., and Ryugo, K., 1982, Suppression of the cell body response in axotomized frog spinal neurons does not prevent initiation of nerve regeneration, *Brain Res.* **234**:11–25.

Cragg, B. G., 1970, What is the signal for chromatolysis? *Brain Res.* **23**:1–21.

Enerbäck, L., Kristensson, K., and Olsson, T., 1980, Cytophotometric quantification of retrograde axonal transport of a fluorescent tracer (Primuline) in mouse facial neurons, *Brain Res.* **186**:21–32.

Farber, J. I., Chien, K. R., and Mittnacht, S., 1981, The pathogenesis of irreversible cell injury in ischemia, *Am. J. Pathol.* **102**:271–281.

Fernandez, H. L., Singer, P. A., and Mehler, S., 1981, Retrograde axonal transport mediates the onset of regenerative changes in the hypoglossal nucleus, *Neurosci. Lett.* **25**:7–11.

Gonatas, J., Stieber, A., Olsnes, S., and Gonatas, N. K., 1980, Pathways involved in fluid phase and adsorptive endocytosis in neuroblastoma, *J. Cell Biol.* **87**:579–588.

Hendry, I. A., and Campbell, J., 1976, Morphometric analysis of rat superior cervical ganglion after axotomy and nerve growth factor treatment, *J. Neurocytol.* **5**:351–360.

Hendry, I. A., Stoeckel, K., Thoenen, H., and Iversen, L. L., 1974, The retrograde axonal transport of nerve growth factor, *Brain Res.* **68**:103–121.

Holtzman, E., Freeman, A. R., and Kashner, Z. A., 1971, Stimulation-dependent alterations in peroxidase uptake at lobster neuromuscular junctions, *Science* **173**:733–736.

Holtzman, F., and Mercurio, A. M., 1980, Membrane circulation in neurons and photoreceptors: Some unresolved issues, *Int. Rev. Cytol.* **67**:1–67.

Kreutzberg, G. W., 1982, Acute neural reaction to injury, in: *Repair and Regeneration of the Nervous System* (J. G. Nicholls, ed.), pp. 57–69, Springer-Verlag, Berlin, Heidelberg, New York.

Kristensson, K., 1978, Retrograde transport of macromolecules in axons, *Annu. Rev. Pharmacol. Toxicol.* **18**:97–110.

Kristensson, K., and Olsson, Y., 1975, Retrograde transport of horseradish peroxidase in transected axons. II. Relations between rate of transfer from the site of injury to the perikaryon and onset of chromatolysis, *J. Neurocytol.* **4**:653–661.

Kristensson, K., and Olsson, Y., 1976, Retrograde transport of horseradish in transected axons. 3. Entry into injured axons and subsequent localization in perikaryon, *Brain Res.* **115**:201–213.

Martin, E. M., and Kerr, I. M., 1968, Virus-induced changes in host-cell macromolecular synthesis, in: *The Molecular Biology of Viruses* (L. V. Crawford and M. G. P. Stoker, eds.), pp. 15–46, Cambridge University Press, Cambridge.

Nennesmo, I., 1983, Cytofluorometric quantitation of somatopetally transported FITC-labelled lectins: Enhanced uptake of concanavalin A and wheat germ agglutinin from the periphery in regenerating facial nerve, *J. Neurocytol.* **12**:1007–1016.

Nissl, F., 1982, Uber die Veranderungen der Ganglienzellen um Facialiskern des Kannuncheng nach Ansreissung der Nerve, *Allq. Z. Psychiatrie* **48**:197–206.

Olsson, Y., and Kristensson, K., 1973, The perineurium as a diffusion barrier to protein tracers following trauma to nerves, *Acta Neuropathol. (Berl.)* **23**:105–111.

Olsson, T., and Kristensson, K., 1979, Uptake and retrograde axonal transport of horseradish peroxidase in normal and axotomized motor during postnatal development, *Neuropathol. Appl. Neurobiol.* **5**:377–387.

Pastan, I. H., and Willingham, M. C., 1981, Receptor-mediated endocytosis of hormones in cultured cells, *Annu. Rev. Physiol.* **43:**239–250.
Søreide, A. J., 1981, Variations in the axon reaction after different types of nerve lesion, *Acta Anat.* **110:**173–188.
Thoenen, H., and Schwab, M., 1978, Physiological and pathophysiological implications of retrograde axonal transport of macromolecules, *Adv. Pharm. Ther.* **5:**37–59.
Torvik, A., 1976, Central chromatolysis and the axon reaction: A reappraisal, *Neuropathol. Appl. Neurobiol.* **2:**423–432.
Torvik, A., and Heding, A., 1969, Effect of actinomycin D on retrograde nerve cell reaction, *Acta Neuropathol. (Berl.)* **14:**62–71.
Watson, W. E., 1974, Cellular responses to axotomy and to related procedures, *Br. Med. Bull.* **30:**112–115.
Wildy, P., Field, H. J., and Nash, A. A., 1982, Classical herpes latency revisited, in: *Virus Persistence* (B. W. J. Mahy, A. C. Minson, and G. K. Darby, eds.), pp. 133–167, Cambridge University Press, Cambridge.

CHAPTER 4

RETROGRADE AXONAL TRANSPORT AND NERVE REGENERATION

M. A. BISBY

1. INTRODUCTION

The ability of neurons to take up exogenous protein molecules and to transport them in a retrograde direction (i.e., from axon to cell body) enables neuroanatomists to trace neuronal pathways (LaVail, 1978). Toxins (Mellanby and Green, 1981) and certain viruses (K. Kristensson, Chapter 3, this volume) use this route to enter the CNS. The retrograde transport of lectins (e.g., Borges and Sidman, 1982) and neurotransmitters (Streit, 1980) shows that specific components of the neuronal membrane, that is, the receptors for these ligands, are returned to the cell body where they were synthesized originally (Laduron, 1980; Laduron and Janssen, 1982). With the exception of nerve growth factor (NGF) (Schwab et al., 1981), the physiological significance of the retrograde transport of these exogenous molecules remains to be determined, but it is widely believed that the sampling of the axonal environment provided to the cell body by this process has informational significance.

M. A. BISBY ● Department of Medical Physiology, Faculty of Medicine, University of Calgary, Calgary, Alberta, Canada T2N 4N1

These exogenous molecules are passengers on a transport system that also recycles to the cell body the endogenous components of the axon that were previously conveyed into the axon by anterograde transport. The rationale for the recycling is unclear, but presumably it is energetically advantageous to return materials to the cell body for reuse rather than to break them down and excrete them from the axon. The central issues in this chapter are: Does the cell body receive information about the status of its axon only through changes in amounts or types of exogenous materials reaching it through retrograde transport? Can alterations in the dynamics of transport of endogenous materials also signal to the cell body that metabolic adjustments are required to meet changes in the status of the axon?

2. RETROGRADE TRANSPORT FOLLOWING AXONAL INJURY

2.1. The Injury Signal

The cell body reaction to axonal injury demonstrates that the cell body does receive information about the status of its axon. A reaction can also be elicited by less traumatic stimuli such as axonal sprouting (Watson, 1973), so it seems likely that the cell body continually monitors changes in the axon and its environment.

The signal for the cell body reaction to axonal injury is probably conveyed from the site of injury by retrograde transport rather than by action potentials or diffusion (Cragg, 1970). The signal could be negative, for example, loss of target-derived trophic factor, or positive, for example, abnormal entry into the neuron of exogenous materials through regions of increased permeability at the site of injury, or some combination of signals. It is also likely that at different times in the development of the nervous system the relative importance of different signals varies. Neurons in the process of finding and securing their connections with target cells would be expected to be more sensitive to loss of signals emanating from those target cells. Thus, removal of the peripheral target or axotomy frequently results in the death of developing neurons (Oppenheim, 1981). Following axotomy, developing neurons sensitive to NGF can be rescued by direct administration of NGF (Hendry, 1975; Banks and Walter, 1977; Nja and Purves, 1978; Hamburger et al., 1981), suggesting that the primary signal in these neurons is absence of NGF derived from the target tissue.

In "adult" neurons, the response to axotomy, is, in most circumstances, chromatolysis rather than death (Lieberman, 1974), indicating that in those neurons that had achieved functional contact with target, there is reduced dependence on target-derived trophic factor. Three lines of evidence suggest that "positive" signals emanating from the site of injury are also important.

First, the onset of cell body reaction in cat hypoglossal motoneurons can be delayed if colchicine is applied proximal to the site of injury (Singer *et al.,* 1982). Since colchicine blocks axonal transport, then if the signal were loss of target-derived trophic factor, colchicine should do no more than the axotomy. If the signal were derived from the axotomy site, colchicine would prevent its arrival at the cell body. Axonal colchicine application alone causes a cell body reaction in parasympathetic and sympathetic neurons (Pilar and Landmesser, 1972; Purves, 1975), and if direct effects of colchicine on the cell body can be excluded, this result may mean that these autonomic neurons are more heavily dependent than somatic motoneurons on target-derived trophic factors.

Second, Hall and Wilson (1982) have examined the changes in protein synthesis that occur in superior cervical ganglion following axotomy and NGF administration, essentially repeating the procedures of Nja and Purves (1978), who found that NGF prevented the depression of ganglionic transmission that follows axotomy. Hall and Wilson (1982) found that NGF did not reverse the changes in protein synthesis produced by axotomy but did induce further changes. Together, these results imply that the reaction to injury is multidimensional; depression of ganglionic transmission may be a result of lack of NGF derived from the target [and so colchicine application to axons has the same effect as axotomy (Purves, 1975)], whereas many changes in cell body protein synthesis that are not sensitive to NGF may be a response to a direct axon injury or loss of axoplasm signal.

Third, neurons will react to an axonal injury even if the neurons are not in contact with their target. In rat hypoglossal nucleus, a second lesion, made as soon as 24 hr after the first, causes the death of a considerable proportion of neurons, whereas the first lesion provokes a marked cell body reaction but little if any cell death (Arvidsson and Aldskogius, 1982). The more severe reaction to the second injury cannot be the result of a further loss of trophic factor because the injured axons could not have reestablished contact with their targets in the 24 hr intervening between the first and second lesions.

Sumner (1979) found that if the cut proximal stump of the hypoglossal nerve was directed into the sternomastoid muscle (innervated by the spinal accessory nerve), then even after 84 days a second axotomy would provoke a cell body reaction. The diverted hypoglossal nerve had not formed functional synapses, and the cell body reaction to the first axotomy was only partially reversed (Sumner, 1976). In the absence of functional contact with the target, the motoneurons were abnormal, but a second axotomy could still provoke a cell body reaction. These results mean that motoneurons are dependent on a target-derived trophic factor for normal metabolism, but there is a separate and additional sensitivity to axonal injury.

The observation that the severity of the cell body reaction is roughly inversely proportional to the distance between cell body and lesion (Lieberman, 1974) is difficult to explain on the basis of loss of target-derived trophic factor (except in the situation where terminal branches leave the parent axon at regular intervals). The uptake of abnormal materials at the site of injury does not easily explain the phenomenon either, but it may be explained on the basis of an abnormality of retrograde transport of endogenous materials, with the proportion of abnormal to normal transport higher with axotomies closer to the cell body. This point is discussed further in Section 2.4.

The cell body reaction to injury is a response both to loss of contact with the target and to loss of axoplasm or axonal injury. The relative importance of these two factors varies during neuronal development and for different neuronal types, and the two factors regulate different aspects of neuronal metabolism. During regeneration as, first, axonal repair and, second, contact with the target occur, we would expect to see a return to normal neuronal structure and metabolism, with different aspects showing different time courses.

2.2.   Retrograde Transport of Endogenous Materials in Intact Axons

We have studied the retrograde of proteins and phospholipids by combining isotopic tracer techniques with ligature techniques in order to collect labeled material in transit. If a mixture of L-$[^{35}S]$methionine and $[^3H]$glycerol is injected into the lumbosacral spinal cord of rats, and at various time intervals a double ligature is applied to the sciatic nerve, $[^3H]$-labeled phospholipid (over 90% phosphatidylcholine) and $[^{35}S]$-labeled protein accumulate proximal to the proximal collection ligature and distal to the distal collection ligature (Figure 1). These accumulations, expressed relative to the total activity trapped in the isolated segment between the two ligatures, give a measure of the fraction of labeled material in the nerve that is mobile. In normal motor axons, anterograde transport of labeled material begins to decline within 3 hr after precursor injection, but retrograde transport peaks between 20 and 30 hr post-injection (Figure 2). Assuming that the material undergoing retrograde transport (i.e., accumulating at the distal side of the distal ligature) is returning to the cell body, the turnover time in the axons is about 1 day, in general agreement with values obtained by others (Droz, 1975; Goodrum and Morell, 1982).

The similar time course for retrograde transport of phospholipid and protein is consistent with previous observations of coordinated fast anterograde transport of lipid and proteins (Abe *et al.*, 1973; Grafstein *et al.*, 1976; Longo and Hammerschlag, 1980). The cotransport of proteins and lipid in both anterograde and retrograde directions involves intracellular membranes, with smooth endoplasmic reticulum as the most likely candidate for anterograde transport, as determined by ultrastructural studies on autoradiography of labeled protein (Rambourg and Droz, 1980) and lipid (Droz *et al.*, 1978) and on material accumulating adjacent to a crush (Smith, 1980) or cold block (Tsukita and Ishikawa, 1980). However, recent work questions whether the

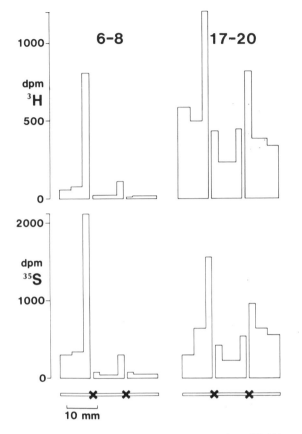

FIGURE 1. Anterograde and retrograde transport of labeled protein and lipid in rat sciatic nerve motor axons. A mixture of precursors ([³H]glycerol for phospholipid, upper two panels; [³⁵S] methionine for protein, lower two panels) was injected into the lumbosacral spinal cord, and 6 hr later (left-hand panels) or 17 hr later (right-hand panels) double collection crushes were placed on the sciatic nerve and left in place for a further 2–3 hr. The nerves were then removed, and activity of each segment determined. At 6 to 8 hr post-injection, there is only anterograde transport of the labeled [³H]phospholipid and [³⁵S]protein. By 17–20 hr post-injection, retrograde transport has begun, as shown by accumulations of activity distal to the collection crushes. Profiles from two individual experiments (M. A. Bisby, unpublished data).

smooth-membrane transport vectors and the axoplasmic reticulum are part of the same membrane system (Ellisman and Lindsey, 1983). Retrograde transported membranes take the form of "prelysosomal" structures such as multivesicular bodies, as determined by observation of organelles in retrograde motion (Breuer et al, 1975) or organelles accumulating on the distal side of a block (Smith, 1980; Tsukita and Ishikawa, 1980) and also by localization of

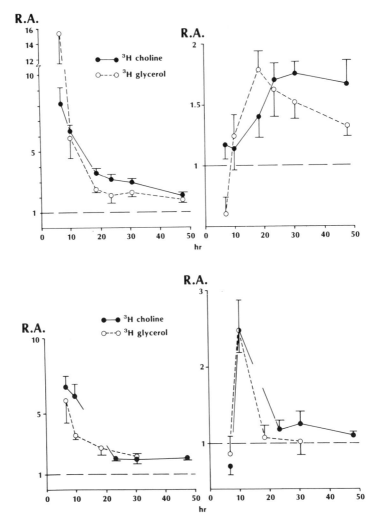

FIGURE 2. Time course of retrograde axonal transport of phospholipid. Precursors ([³H]glycerol or [³H]choline) were injected into lumbosacral spinal cord, and at various postinjection periods nerves were double-ligated for 2–3 hr. Vertical axis: accumulation proximal or distal to collection crushes relative to activity in the isolated nerve segment. Horizontal axis: elapsed time since precursor injection. Left-hand panels, anterograde transport; right-hand panels, retrograde transport. Upper two panels, intact axons; lower two panels, injured axons (i.e., sciatic nerve crushed far distally at the time of precursor injection). Means ± S.E., $n \geq 6$. Note that in the injured axons retrograde transport of the labeled phospholipid occurs earlier and more synchronously than in the intact axons. (M. A. Bisby, unpublished data.)

exogenous tracers undergoing retrograde transport (LaVail *et al,* 1980; Claude *et al.,* 1982).

The endogenous proteins undergoing retrograde transport (characterized according to molecular weights of their polypeptide chains on SDS-polyacrylamide gel electrophoresis) were similar to those undergoing anterograde transport in the same axons (Abe *et al.,* 1974; Bisby, 1981), even though only about half of the proteins anterogradely transported into motor axons are subsequently returned to the cell body (Bisby and Bulger, 1977). This raises the problem of how the same protein molecules can be transported in different directions at different times during their life cycle. The one-dimensional gel electrophoresis technique would not detect changes in tertiary structure attendant on retrograde transport. Posttranslational modification of a fast transported polypeptide in injured axons has been recently reported (Tedeschi and Wilson, 1983). The reduced enzymatic activity of dopamine-β-hydroxylase undergoing retrograde transport (Nagatsu *et al.,* 1976) and alterations in properties of receptors undergoing anterograde and retrograde transport (Zarbin *et al.,* 1982; Zarbin *et al.,* 1983) suggest that such changes do occur. Since the two types of organelles implicated in anterograde and retrograde transport differ, it is likely that some feature of their membranes gives them a distinctive "flavor" which determines the directionality of their interaction with the transport system. An alternative explanation based on the existence of two oppositely polarized transport systems for anterograde and retrograde transport, is becoming less tenable with the mounting evidence for involvement of microtubules in axonal transport (Allen *et al.,* 1981), microtubules which are uniformly polarized (Burton and Paige, 1981).

The site of transport reversal in intact axons is not known. Although the highest concentration of transported material may be at the axon terminals, in long axons most of the transported protein leaves the transport system within the axon. For rat sciatic nerve, it is estimated using the equations of Munoz-Martinez *et al.* (1981), that less than 10% of the transported protein leaving the cell body reaches the axon terminals directly. The ability to load expended axonal material onto the retrograde transport system at the initial site of offloading would seem more efficient, but it is also possible that material initially deposited along the axon has to be remobilized and transported to the terminal axon in order to undergo the transformations necessary for retrograde transport. Defects in the retrograde transport of endogenous material produced by acrylamide intoxication (Sahenk and Mendell, 1981; Jakobsen and Sidenius, 1983) lead to the accumulation of vesicular material in the distal axon (Souyri *et al.,* 1981; Chretien *et al.,* 1981), indicating that the terminal regions are the major site of transport reversal, as originally suggested by Bray *et al.* (1971).

2.3. Acute Effects of Injury on Retrograde Transport of Endogenous Materials

If the sciatic nerve is crushed distally at the same time as precursor is applied to the cell bodies, the retrograde transport of protein and phospholipid occurs earlier than in intact axons, with a peak at 9–11 hr post-injection (Figure 2). The major site of reversal in these injured axons was assumed to be immediately proximal to the injury, and this was demonstrated directly by Schmidt *et al.* (1980), who also showed that enzymes associated with three different subcellular organelles (smooth endoplasmic reticulum, lysosomes, and mitochondria) all reversed direction of transport at an injury. As in intact axons, reversal of transport occurs without proteolysis (Bisby, 1981).

The time taken for the development of the ability to reverse transport at an injury was determined by delaying the injury until just before the labeled transported protein reached the site of injury. Reversal was delayed by approximately 1 hr, showing that development of the reversal process takes less than 1 hr (Bisby and Bulger, 1977). Using position-sensitive detectors, O'Brien and Snyder (1982) estimated that reversal began within 0.4 hr of the arrival of labeled protein at a ligature.

The mechanism of reversal at an injury is just as obscure as the mechanism in intact axons. Influx of calcium ions through the distorted axolemma at the injury might activate enzymes that would alter the "flavor" of the transported membranes, allowing them to move in a retrograde direction. Such a calcium-activated process might also act in normal terminals and at the tips of regenerating axons where Ca^{2+} levels should also be high (Meiri *et al,* 1981). A number of calcium-activated enzyme systems exist in axons, including a Mg^{2+}/Ca^{2+}-activated ATPase (Shecket and Lasek, 1982), proteases which degrade neurofilaments (Schlaepfer and Hasler, 1979; Pant and Gainer, 1980), and modify them during their axonal transport (Nixon *et al,* 1983) and a vesicle-bound $Ca^{2+}/calmodulin$-dependent kinase which phosphorylates synaptic vesicle tubulin (Burke and De Lorenzo, 1982). This latter enzyme, since it affects a transported organelle rather than a cytoskeletal element, might be a candidate for altering the mobility of the organelle.

There has been little direct experimental work done on the mechanism of turnaround. In isolated axons, elevated extracellular Ca^{2+} concentrations initially stimulated but later depressed movement of visible organelles (Stearns, 1982). Retrograde transport of visible organelles was shown to be Mg^{2+} rather than Ca^{2+} dependent in *Xenopus* axons (Smith, 1982), but retrograde transport of acetylcholinesterase in *Rana* axons was Ca^{2+} dependent (Lavoie, 1982).

Koles *et al.* (1982) presented a model for the reversal process based on the behavior of visible particles at a nerve crush (Smith, 1980). Transported organelles bear sites for both anterograde and retrograde transport. Accumulation at an injury is followed by gradual conversion of anterograde to retrograde sites, leading to eventual retrograde movement away from the injury. During the transition period, organelles would bear approximately equal numbers of sites, leading to the oscillations exhibited by some organelles before they commenced retrograde transport.

2.4. Abnormal Reversal of Transport as a Putative Axotomy Signal

Could the abnormal reversal of transport at an injury provide the axonal component of the signal for the cell body reaction? In order for this process to be a candidate, it is necessary to show that the signal would arrive at the cell body before the first detectable response to injury. The time taken for protein to reverse direction of transport at the injury was estimated to be 1.4 hr, beginning 0.8 hr after the injury was sustained. The retrograde transport for [^{3}H]protein returning from an injury was measured as 8.6 mm·hr^{-1} using a reversible cold block (Bisby and Buchan, 1981). The time taken for a signal to reach the cell body was thus estimated as 8 hr for a lesion made 50 mm from the cell body. The earliest detectable cell body reaction was reported in sympathetic ganglia, 6 hr after an injury made 2 mm from the cell body (Matthews and Raisman, 1972). Applying our figures for turnaround time, etc. to this situation would give an arrival time of 2.4 hr.

Since the cell body does not count the ^{3}H label used to reveal the phenomenon of reversal at an injury, the exact nature of a putative injury signal is open to question. Relatively more of the anterogradely transported protein shipped into the axon is returned following injury, and for endogenous enzymes, retrograde transport, relative to anterograde transport, is also increased following axon injury (Schmidt and McDougal, 1978). Perhaps some sort of feedback control exists in the cell body so that an increased return of fast-transported protein following axotomy reduces synthesis of those proteins and also causes the altered patterns of structural protein synthesis characteristic of regenerating neurons (Hoffman and Lasek, 1980; Sinicropi and McIlwain, 1983).

For endogenous proteins undergoing steady-state transport in the axon, reversal at an injury would be expected to produce an increase in enzyme content at the cell body. This would be the "error signal" that would initiate the cell body reaction. Sinicropi *et al.* (1982) performed a quantitative analysis of the amount of AChE in cell body and axon following injury to frog motoneuron axons: reversal of transport of AChE at an injury has been well documented (Schmidt and McDougal, 1978; Couraud and Di Giamberardino, 1982). No increase in cell body AChE was found. However, a rapid reduction in amount of AChE accumulating at the injury showed that there was rapid reduction in cell body AChE synthesis. Thus, increased return of enzyme to the cell body could be a signal if it is assumed that the regulation of synthesis is so sensitive to variations in amounts of AChE returning from the axon that the "error signal" is hard to detect.

There are examples of transient increases of fast-transported materials in the cell body after axotomy followed by a later decline, as pointed out by Grafstein and McQuarrie (1978) and Sinicropi *et al.* (1982). In such instances, the axotomy was made very close to the cell body (Anden *et al.*, 1966; Reis and Ross, 1973; Ross *et al.*, 1975), or colchicine was applied directly to the cell body (Fonnum *et al.*, 1973). Both procedures would cause a sudden and rapid build-up of transported materials in the cell body, to which the regulatory system might not be able to respond sufficiently by decreased synthesis of transported materials.

An important challenge to the idea that reversal of transport at an injury has any informational significance has come from the recent study of Aletta and Goldberg (1982). In the giant cerebral neuron of *Aplysia,* rapid and precise reduction in axonal transport of serotonin occurred after section of one of the two main axon branches of the neuron. In this neuron, axotomy of one branch causes diversion of transported materials into the other branch. The reduction in transported serotonin meant that the remaining intact branch received an approximately normal supply of serotonin. There was no evidence for increased serotonin-containing vesicle content in the segment of axon proximal to the bifurcation; this suggests that there is no increase in return of vesicles to the cell body, and so increased return of serotonin vesicles to the cell body is unlikely to be the signal that depresses serotonin synthesis. The vesicles reversing direction at the site of axotomy are presumably diverted into the remaining intact axon. Aletta and Goldberg (1982) favor some signal derived from the synapses as the regulator of serotonin transport. In mammalian aminergic neurons, axotomy of one axon branch results in depression of amine content in all branches, suggesting that diversion of amine storage vesicles into intact axon branches does not occur (Reis and Ross, 1973), so the generality of these observations is questionable.

As an alternative to changes in amounts of proteins returning to the cell body, the characteristics of the material returning from an injury may differ from those returning from an intact axon, although a first attempt at detection of such differences was negative (Bisby, 1981) (however, see D. L. Wilson, Chapter 9, this volume).

Abnormal reversal of transport at an injury could provide information about the extent of axoplasmic loss: it is difficult to understand how loss of target-derived trophic materials or uptake of exogenous materials at the site of injury could do this. Fast-transported material is deposited in the axolemma all along the axon (Ochs, 1975; Gross and Beidler, 1975; Munoz-Martinez *et al.*, 1981). Following a far distal injury, the majority of transported proteins would be deposited normally along the axon, undergo a normal life-span, and be returned normally to the cell body. Only the fraction of transported proteins destined for regions of axon distal to the site of injury would be subject to abnormal reversal, so that the cell body receives a weak signal. If the injury is made more proximally, the proportion of transported protein undergoing abnormal reversal would be greater, and the cell body would receive a stronger signal, evoking a stronger reaction.

To conclude this section, it is clear that axonal injury provokes a reversal of axonal transport proximal to the site of injury, and the evidence is also good for an injury signal arising at the injury site. What is unclear is whether the abnormal reversal of endogenous material at the injury has any informational significance or whether this process serves to convey exogenous "wound substances," which enter the injured axon and ascend to the cell body.

3. CHANGES IN RETROGRADE TRANSPORT DURING REGENERATION

3.1. Time Course of Endogenous Protein Transport

We have studied the time course of retrograde transport of endogenous [^{3}H]protein in motor axons that were briefly crushed, resulting in regeneration at 4 mm·day^{-1} after an initial delay of 1½ days (Bulger and Bisby, 1978). Immediately after injury, the period of maximum retrograde transport is 9–11 hr after precursor injection (Figure 3).

During the first 5 days, retrograde transport maintains the time course characteristics of acutely injured axons but is increased in amount. As regeneration proceeds, the time course and amount of retrograde transport return to normal (Figure 3). In axons that were ligated to prevent regeneration, retrograde transport remained elevated in the 9- to 11-hr postinjection period (Bulger and Bisby, 1978).

Since the major destination of rapidly transported protein in regenerating axons is the growing axon (Bisby, 1979; Forman and Berenberg, 1979), where incorporation occurs adjacent to the growth cone (Tessler *et al.,* 1980; Feldman *et al.,* 1981; Griffin *et al.,* 1981; Pfenniger and Maylie-Pfenniger, 1981), the major site of transport reversal should be the growth cones, and the shift in time course as regeneration proceeds can be explained in part by axonal elongation and the increase in transit time between growth cones and the collection ligatures. An alternative explanation for the shift in time course might be that rapidly transported protein incorporated into existing axolemma has a different turnover time than protein incorporated into new membrane at the growing tip. As the axon elongates, relatively more rapidly transported protein will be

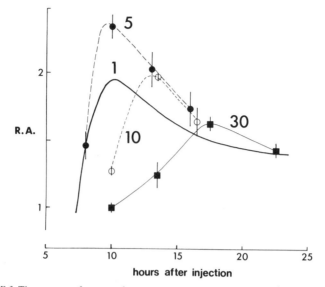

FIGURE 3. Time course of retrograde transport in regenerating axons. [³H]Leucine was injected into lumbosacral spinal cord of rats that had received sciatic nerve crush 1, 5, 10, or 30 days previously. Relative accumulations were determined at various postinjection intervals. The time course of retrograde transport shifts from a maximum at 9–11 hr post-injection to a later maximum as regeneration proceeds, following an initial period of at least 5 days when no shift in time course is detectable. (Redrawn from Bulger and Bisby, 1978.)

incorporated into existing axolemma rather than being incorporated into new membrane at the growing tip.

It is not known whether the change in dynamics of retrograde axonal transport during regeneration is accompanied by changes in amount or composition of materials returning to the cell body. We can speculate that in cases of abortive regeneration relatively more of the exported protein would return to the cell body than in the cases of successful regeneration, where optimal growth requires continued supply of rapidly transported materials and their incorporation into new membranes.

3.2. Retrograde Transport of Signals for Axon Elongation and for Reinnervation of Target

In peripheral nerves, the amount of many anterogradely transported material decreases rapidly following axotomy (e.g., labeled protein, Frizell and

Sjostrand, 1974; Bisby, 1978; Bulger and Bisby, 1978; acetylcholinesterase, Frizell and Sjostrand, 1974; O'Brien, 1978; Schmidt and McDougal, 1978; Heiwall *et al.,* 1979; DiGiamberardino *et al.,* 1982) but gradually increases during regeneration. If regeneration is frustrated, recovery does not occur (Bulger and Bisby, 1978; O'Brien, 1978; Heiwall *et al.,* 1979). Recovery toward normal values of transport of these materials begins soon after injury, at the time when axonal outgrowth begins, and long before contact with the target is restored. For example, in motor axons, recovery of protein transport begins on day 1–3 after crush injury to the sciatic nerve (Bulger and Bisby, 1978), and in sensory axons, on day 2–3 (Bisby, 1978). Approximately normal amounts of transported protein are restored by day 14, yet reinnervation of muscle as measured by EMG recordings or functional indices of locomotion does not occur until day 14–18. Similar results have been obtained in studies on acetylcholinesterase transport (DiGiamberardino *et al.,* 1982). Some axotomy-induced cell body changes also reverse prior to reinnervation but during the period of axonal elongation (e.g., cell body RNA synthesis, Scott and Foote, 1982). Other instances of changes in the cell body occurring prior to axonal reinnervation of target are cited by Grafstein and McQuarrie (1978).

Since the increase in transport during regeneration occurs gradually during the period of elongation, it is possible that the cell body has some way of sensing the length (or volume or surface area) of its axon and synthesizes and transports an amount of fast-transported material appropriate for the maintenance of its processes as well as for the formation of new membrane during regeneration. The elongation signal could be a change in the retrograde transport of endogenous materials or, alternatively, a trophic factor derived from Schwann cells or degenerating axons in the distal stump.

When the regenerating axons contact the target, other components of the cell body reaction to injury return to normal. For example, the changes in composition of fast-transported protein that occur following axotomy of the sciatic nerve reach a maximum 14 days after injury and thereafter decline, that is, with the same time course as reinnervation but later than axonal elongation (Bisby, 1980). If axons are prevented from regenerating, these changes do not reverse (Bisby, 1982). The existence of a specific reinnervation signal has been shown by the work of Watson (1970) and Sumner (1977). Reinnervation of muscle by the hypoglossal nerve was delayed by implantation of the proximal nerve stump into the sternomastoid muscle. If the spinal accessory nerve was then removed, the hypoglossal axons innervated the sternomastoid, and synaptic bouton relationships in the hypoglossal nucleus returned towards normal, even after a delay of 84 days. Similar results were reported by Purves (1975) in studies on superior cervical ganglion.

This reinnervation signal is probably target derived, and clues to the nature of the signal have been provided by Kuno and collaborators, who found that the degree of recovery of the physiological properties of motoneurons following axotomy was related to the degree of motor reinnervation (Kuno *et al.,* 1974). Subsequently, they discovered that muscle inactivity caused by tetrodotoxin block of the muscle nerve or spinal transection resulted in similar changes to those produced by axotomy, implicating absence of muscle activity rather than absence of motoneuron activity as the reason for the inactivity changes (Czeh *et al.,* 1978). When muscle was immobilized in a shortened position, atrophy occurred, and changes were seen in motoneurons. When muscles were immobilized in the lengthened position, neither atrophy nor motoneuron changes occurred (Gallego *et al.,* 1979). The conclusion was that the trophic factor is produced by the muscle, and production is related to overall metabolic activity in the muscle. If this hypothesis is correct, then only functional innervation of muscle would result in production of the trophic factor and return to normal of motoneuron cell body properties. Since the cell bodies of motor neurons whose axons are diverted into muscle already innervated by another nerve do not return to normal, it is further necessary that the regenerating axons establish neuromuscular transmission in order to receive the trophic factor.

To summarize this section, during axonal regeneration, there are two separate retrogradely transported signals that reach the cell body: one is related to the successful elongation of axons, cannot be target derived, but might be Schwann cell derived or might be associated with changes in retrograde transport. The second signal is associated with reinnervation of the target and might be caused by the renewed arrival at the cell body of a target-derived trophic factor. These dual signals for regeneration changes are related to the initial signals for cell body reaction. In Section 2.1 evidence was presented for both target- and axon-derived injury signals.

4. CONTROL OF REGENERATION RATE

The rate at which axons regenerate is not a constant for a particular type of neuron. Once growing axons *in vivo* have traversed the disrupted zone at the site of injury, their rate of elongation depends on the age of the animal (Black and Lasek, 1979; Pestronk *et al.,* 1980), the past history of the nerve, and the chemical environment, though this is an area of confused claims (e.g., Strand and Kung, 1980) and counterclaims (e.g., Verghese *et al.,* 1982) complicated by assessment of different parameters of regeneration. *In vitro,* it is more evident that nerve growth factor (Campenot, 1977; Campenot, 1981; Turner *et al.,* 1982) and less-well-characterized ingredients of conditioned media (Collins and Dawson, 1982; Dribin and Barrett, 1982; Muhlach and Pollack, 1982; Schwartz *et al.,* 1982; Smith and Appel, 1983) can influence growth rate.

The "conditioning lesion" phenomenon (Forman *et al.,* 1981; I. G.

McQuarrie, this volume) shows that the past history of the nerve can influence regeneration rate. The rate measured from a test lesion is greater if a conditioning lesion was made on the nerve several days previously. One explanation for this phenomenon is that the first (conditioning) lesion primes the neuron so that it is already in a metabolic state to sustain regeneration when the test lesion is made (Ducker *et al.*, 1969) and, in some cases, shows an enhanced and sustained reaction to the second (test) injury.

An alternative explanation, originally proposed by Lubinska (1952) and revived by Brown and Hopkins (1981), is that the conditioning lesion causes predegeneration of axons so that when the test lesion is made the regenerating axons can grow more rapidly through the distal nerve. This explanation could not account for the demonstration of the conditioning lesion effect in neurons *in vitro* (Feldman *et al.*, 1981; Landreth and Agranoff, 1979; Turner *et al.*, 1982) or for the modest 22% increase in regeneration rate found in rat sciatic sensory axons when the conditioning lesion was made at the ankle and the test lesion was made at the hip (McQuarrie *et al.*, 1977). In this situation, the axons regenerating from the test lesion were not in predegenerated regions of nerve. We have repeated these experiments, making the test and conditioning lesions at the same place on the sciatic nerve, so that axons regenerating from the test lesion enter predegenerated segments of nerve, and obtained an increase in regeneration rate of 67% (Bisby and Pollock, 1983). This result suggests that both enhanced cell body reaction and the axonal environment can influence regeneration rate. How might these two factors regulate the rate of axon outgrowth?

Lasek and colleagues (Black and Lasek, 1979; Hoffman and Lasek, 1980) have emphasized the similarity between regeneration rate and the velocity of slow axonal transport component b. This component contains proteins such as actin and clathrin associated with growth cones. A correlation between slow component b velocity and regeneration rate in the central and peripheral axon branches of dorsal root ganglia neurons strengthens the hypothesis that slow component b controls regeneration rate through the supply of the cytoskeletal elements necessary to advance the growth cones (Wujek and Lasek, 1983). If this is so, then it is necessary to explain the enhanced conditioning lesion effect observed by us as an effect at the cell body, most likely through the retrograde transport to the cell body of some trophic factors derived from degenerated nerve (Schwann cells or degenerating axons). In goldfish optic nerve, where a marked conditioning lesion effect is obtained, the increased regeneration rate is associated with an increased velocity of slow transport (McQuarrie and Grafstein, 1982).

The existence of trophic factors within distal nerve stumps has been demonstrated by the work of Lundborg and colleagues (Lundborg *et al.*, 1982; Longo *et al.*, 1983). Axon regeneration occurred through a silicone chamber into which the proximal nerve stump had been implanted only if the other end of the chamber contained a distal stump and only if the gap between stumps was 10 mm or less. The fluid collected from the chamber exerted a trophic effect on chick embryo sensory, spinal motor, and sympathetic neurons. It was concluded that the distal nerve stump secreted a proteinaceous trophic material.

Politis *et al.* (1982) showed that regenerating sciatic axons grew preferentially into the arm of a Y-tube containing a sciatic nerve graft. When an 0.2-μm-pore filter was placed between the proximal stump and the graft, preferential growth was noted so long as the distance between proximal stump and filter did not exceed 5 mm. Distal nerve stumps exert an attractive influence on regenerating axons, but this effect has a limited range.

The limited range of a putative trophic effect may account for differences in regeneration rate obtained by McQuarrie *et al.* (1977), Carlsen (1982), and Bisby and Pollock (1983). All three laboratories were studying the conditioning lesion effect on sensory axons in rat sciatic nerve, but McQuarrie separated conditioning and test lesions (made at the ankle and hip, respectively) by the greatest distance and obtained a 22% increase in regeneration rate. Carlsen (1982) made conditioning and test lesions at the knee and hip, respectively, and obtained a 40% increase in regeneration rate. Bisby and Pollock obtained a 42% increase when conditioning and test lesions were made at the knee and hip and a 67% increase when the two lesions were made at the same site. The closer together the two lesions were made, the greater the subsequent regeneration rate.

If degenerating axons or "denervated" Schwann cells can exert a growth-promoting effect on regenerating axons, it is strange that the rate of regeneration *in vivo* after a single lesion does not increase as regeneration proceeds and the axons enter more distal regions of nerve that have been denervated for longer times and should be producing trophic factors. If the rate of regeneration changes at all in long nerves, it decreases (Sunderland, 1978). The rate of regeneration seems to be set at the time the test lesion is made. Trophic factors taken up over a short period at the time of injury and retrogradely transported back to the cell body must set the subsequent rate of cytoskeletal protein synthesis.

5. CONCLUSION

We have followed the sequence of events from initial axon injury through axonal elongation to reinnervation of target. This sequence involves cell body regulation through a variety of "signals" derived from the axon and its environment and conveyed to the cell body by retrograde axonal transport. The initial cell body reaction to axonal injury is a response both to loss of target-derived trophic factors and to loss of axoplasm, with the exact nature of this latter signal unknown. Both uptake of "wound substances" at the site of injury and alterations in retrograde transport of endogenous materials could be involved. During regeneration, there is at least a partial reversal of the reaction to injury. The first phase of recovery is a response to axonal outgrowth and could be signaled either by exogenous trophic materials derived from the distal nerve stump that is invaded by the regenerating axons or by return to normal of the dynamics and/or composition of retrograde transport of endogenous materials. If functional contact with the target is achieved, a second phase of recovery occurs, probably signaled by the reappearance at the cell body of the target-derived trophic factor. Finally, the rate of regeneration may be regulated by factors derived from degenerating nerves taken up and retrogradely transported to the cell body that, on arrival at the cell body, regulate synthesis of cytoskeletal components carried in slow component b.

The original problems posed in this chapter were: Does the cell body receive information about the status of its axon only through changes in the types and amounts of exogenous molecules derived from other cell types reaching it? Can alterations in amounts or composition of endogenous material returned to the cell body provide this information?

I have failed to provide a clear answer to both questions but have, I hope, emphasized the issues. Although the definitive experiments have still to be planned, careful quantitative work along the lines of the studies of Aletta and Goldberg (1982) and Sinicropi *et al.* (1982) will soon lead to a refinement of our crude hypotheses.

ACKNOWLEDGMENT

The author's work has been funded by an operating grant from the Medical Research Council of Canada and by equipment grants and trainee support from the Alberta Heritage Foundation for Medical Research.

6. REFERENCES

Abe, T., Haga, T., and Kurokawa, M., 1973, Rapid transport of phosphatidyl-choline occurring simultaneously with protein transport in the frog sciatic nerve, *Biochem. J.* **136**:731–740.
Abe, T., Haga, T., and Kurokawa, M., 1974, Retrograde axoplasmic transport: Its continuation as anterograde transport FEBS *Lett.* **47**:272–275.
Aletta, J. M., and Goldberg, D. J., 1982, Rapid and precise down regulation of fast axonal transport of serotonin in an identified neuron, *Science* **218**:913–916.

Allen, R. D., Travis, J. L., Hayden, J. H., Allen, N. S., Breuer, A. C., and Lewis, I. J., 1981, Cytoplasmic transport: Moving ultrastructural elements common to any cell types revealed by video-enhanced microscopy, *Cold Spring Harbor Symp. Quant. Biol.* **46**:85–87.

Anden, N. E., Dahlstrom, A., Fuxe, K., Larsson, K., Olson, L., and Ungerstedt, O., 1966, Ascending monoamine neurons to the telencephalon and diencephalon, *Acta Physiol. Scand.* **67**:313–326.

Arvidsson, J., and Aldskogius, H., 1982, Effect of repeated hypoglossal nerve lesions on the number of neurons in the hypoglossal nucleus of adult rats, *Exp. Neurol.* **75**:520–524.

Banks, B. E. C., and Walter, S. J., 1977, The effects of postganglionic axotomy and nerve growth factor on the superior cervical ganglia of developing mice, *J. Neurocytol.* **6**:287–297.

Bisby, M. A., 1978, Fast axonal transport of labelled proteins in sensory axons during regeneration, *Exp. Neurol.* **61**:281–300.

Bisby, M. A., 1979, Differences in incorporation of axonally transported protein in regenerating motor and sensory axons, *Exp. Neurol.* **65**:680–684.

Bisby, M. A., 1980, Changes in the composition of labelled protein transported in motor axons during their regeneration, *J. Neurobiol.* **11**:435–445.

Bisby, M. A., 1981, Reversal of axonal transport: Similarity of proteins transported in anterograde and retrograde directions, *J. Neurochem.* **36**:741–745.

Bisby, M. A., 1982, Prolonged alterations in composition of fast-transported protein in axons prevented from regenerating after injury, *J. Neurobiol.* **13**:377–381.

Bisby, M. A., and Buchan, D. H., 1981, Velocity of labelled protein undergoing anterograde and retrograde transport, *Exp. Neurol.* **74**:11–20.

Bisby, M. A., and Bulger, V. T., 1977, Reversal of axonal transport at a nerve crush, *J. Neurochem.* **29**:313–320.

Bisby, M. A., and Pollock, B., 1983, Increased regeneration rate in peripheral nerve axons following double lesions: Enhancement of the conditioning lesion effect, *J. Neurobiol.* **14**:467–472.

Black, M. M., ad Lasek, R. J., 1979, Slowing of the rate of axonal regeneration during growth and maturation, *Exp. Neurol.* **63**:108–119.

Borges, L. F., and Sidman, R. L., 1982, Axonal transport of lectins in the peripheral nervous system, *J. Neurosci.* **2**:647–653.

Bray, J. J., Kon, C. M., and Breckenridge, B. McL. 1971, Reversed polarity of rapid axonal transport in chicken motoneurons, *Brain Res.* **33**:560–564.

Breuer, A. C., Christian, C. N., Henkart, M., and Nelson, P. G., 1975, Computer analysis of organelle translocation in primary neuronal cultures and continuous cell lines, *J. Cell Bio.* **65**:562–576.

Brown, M. C., and Hopkins, W. G., 1981, Role of degenerating axon pathways in regeneration of mouse soleus motor axons, *J. Physiol. (Lond.)* **318**:365–373.

Bulger, V. T., and Bisby, M. A., 1978, Reversal of axonal transport in regenerating nerves, *J. Neurochem.* **31**:1411–1418.

Burke, B. E., and De Lorenzo, R. J., 1982, Ca^{2+} and calmodulin-dependent phosphorylation of endogenous synaptic vesicle tubulin by a vesicle-bound calmodulin kinase system *J. Neurochem.* **38**:1205–1218.

Burton, P. R., and Paige, J. L., 1981, Polarity of axoplasmic microtubules in the olfactory nerve of the frog, *Proc. Natl. Acad. Sci. U.S.A.* **78**:3269–3273.

Campenot, R. B., 1977, Local control of neurite development by nerve growth factor, *Proc. Natl. Acad. Sci. U.S.A.* **74**:4516–4519.

Campenot, R. B., 1981, Regeneration of neurites in long-term cultures of sympathetic neurons deprived of nerve growth factor, *Science* **214**:579–581.

Carlsen, R. C., 1982, Comparison of adenylate cyclase activity in segments of rat sciatic nerve with a condition/test or test lesion, *Exp. Neurol.* **77**:254–265.

Chretien, M., Patey, G., Souyri, F., and Droz, B., 1981, Acrylamide-induced neuropathy and impairment of axonal transport of protein. II. Abnormal accumulations of smooth endoplasmic reticulum at sites of focal retention of fast transported proteins. Electron microscopic radioautographic study, *Brain Res.* **205:**15–28.

Claude, P., Hauroi, E., Dunis, D. A., and Campenot, R. B., 1982, Binding, internalization, and retrograde transport of ^{125}I-nerve growth factor in cultured rat sympathetic neurons, *J. Neurosci.* **2:**431–442.

Collins, F., and Dawson, A., 1982, Conditioned medium increases the rate of neurite elongation: Separation of this activity from the substratum-bound inducer of neurite outgrowth, *J. Neurosci.* **2:**1005–1010.

Couraud, J.-Y., and DiGiamberardino, L., 1982, Axonal transport of the molecular forms of acetylcholinesterase. Its reversal at a nerve transection, in: *Axoplasmic Transport* (D. G. Weiss, ed.), pp. 144–152, Springer-Verlag, Berlin, Heidelberg, New York.

Cragg, B. G., 1970, What is the signal for chromatolysis? *Brain Res.* **23:**1–21.

Czeh, G., Galego, R., Kudo, N., and Kuno, M., 1978, Evidence for the maintenance of motoneuron properties by muscle activity, *J. Physiol. (Lond.)* **281:**239–252.

DiGiamberardino, L., Couraud, J.-Y., Hassig, R., and Gorio, A., 1982, Recovery of axonal transport of acetylcholinesterase in regenerating sciatic nerve precedes muscle reinnervation, in: *Axoplasmic Transport in Physiology and Pathology* (D. G. Weiss and A. Gorio, eds.), pp. 77–80, Springer-Verlag, Berlin, Heidelberg, New York.

Dribin, L. B., and Barrett, J. N., 1982, Characterization of neuritic outgrowth-promoting activity of conditioned medium on spinal cord explants, *Devel. Brain Res.* **4:**435–441.

Droz, B., 1975, Synthetic machinery and axoplasmic transport: Maintenance of neuronal connectivity, in: *The Nervous System,* Vol. I (D. B. Tower, ed.), pp. 111–117, Raven Press, New York.

Droz, B., DeGiamberardino, L., Koenig, H. L., Boyenval, J., and Hassig, R., 1978, Axon–myelin transfer of phospholipid components in the course of their axonal transport as visualized by radioautography, *Brain Res.* **155:**347–353.

Ducker, T. B., Kempe, C. G., and Hayes, G. J., 1969, The metabolic background for peripheral nerve injury, *J. Neurosurg.* **30:**270–280.

Ellisman, M. H., and Lindsey, J. D., 1983, The axoplasmic reticulum within myelinated axons is not transported rapidly. *J. Neurocytol.* **12:**393–411.

Feldman, E. L., Axelrod, D., Schwartz. M. Heacock, A. M., and Agranoff, B. W., 1981, Studies on the localization of newly added membrane in growing neurites, *J. Neurobiol.* **12:**591–598.

Fonnum F., Frizell, M., and Sjostrand, J., 1973, Transport, turnover and distribution of choline acetyltransferase and acetylcholinesterase in the vagus and hypoglossal nerves of the rabbit, *J. Neurochem.* **21:**1109–1120.

Forman, D., and Berenberg, R. A., 1979, Regeneration of motor axons in the rat sciatic nerve studied by labelling with axonally transported radioactive proteins, *Brain Res.* **156:**213–225.

Forman, D. S., McQuarrie, I. G., Grafstein, B., and Edwards, D. L., 1981, Effect of a conditioning lesion on axonal regeneration and recovery of function, in: *Lesion-Induced Neuronal Plasticity in Sensorimotor Systems* (H. Flohr and W. Precht, eds.), pp. 103–113, Springer-Verlag, Berlin, Heidelberg, New York.

Frizell, M., and Sjostrand, J., 1974, Transport of protein, glycoproteins and cholinergic enzymes in regenerating hypoglossal nerves, *J. Neurochem.* **22:**845–880.

Gallego, R., Kuno, M., Nunez, R., and Snider, W. D., 1979, Dependence of motoneuron properties on the length of immobilized muscle, *J. Physiol. (Lond.)* **219:**179–189.

Goodrum J. F. and Morell, P., 1982, Axonal transport, deposition and metabolic turnover of glycoproteins in the rat optic pathway, *J. Neurochem.* **38:**696–704.

Grafstein, B., and McQuarrie, I. G., 1978, Role of the nerve cell body in axonal regeneration, in: *Neuronal Plasticity* (C. W. Cotman, ed.), pp. 155–195, Raven Press, New York.

Grafstein, B., Miller, J. A., Ledeen, R. W., Haley, J., and Specht, S. C., 1976, Axonal transport of phospholipid in goldfish optic system, *Exp. Neurol.* **46**:261–281.

Griffin, J. W., Price, D. L., Drachman, D. B., and Morris, J., 1981, Incorporation of axonally transported glycoproteins into axolemma during nerve regeneration, *J. Cell Biol.* **88**:205–214.

Gross, G. W., and Beidler, L. M., 1975, A quantitative analysis of isotope concentration profiles and rapid transport velocities in the C-fibres of the garfish olfactory nerve, *J. Neurobiol.* **6**:213–232.

Hall, M. E., and Wilson, D. L., 1982, Nerve growth factor effects on protein synthesis after nerve damage, *Exp. Neurol.* **77**:625–633.

Hamburger, V., Brunsobechtqld, J. K., and Yip, J. W., 1981, Neuronal death in the spinal ganglia of the chick embryo and its reduction by nerve growth factor, *J. Neurosci.* **1**:60–71.

Heiwall, P. O., Dahlstrom, A., Larson, P. A., and Booj, S., 1979, The intra-axonal transport of acetylcholine and cholinergic enzymes in rat sciatic nerve after various types of axonal trauma, *J. Neurobiol.* **10**:119–136.

Hendry, I. A., 1975, The response of adrenergic neurons to axotomy and nerve growth factor, *Brain Res.* **94**:87–97.

Hoffman, P. N., and Lasek, R. J., 1980, Axonal transport of the cytoskeleton in regenerating neurons: Constancy and change, *Brain Res.* **202**:317–333.

Jakobsen, J., and Sidenius, P., 1983, Early and dose-dependent decrease of retrograde axonal transport in acrylamide-intoxicated rats, *J. Neurochem.* **40**:447–454.

Koles, Z. J., McLeod, K. D., and Smith, R. S., 1982, A study of the motion of organelles which undergo retrograde and anterograde rapid axonal transport in *Xenopus, J. Physiol. (Lond.)* **328**:469–484.

Kuno, M., Miyata, Y., and Munoz-Martinez, E. J., 1974, Properties of slow and fast α-motoneurons following re-innervation, *J. Physiol. (Lond.)* **242**:273–288.

Laduron, P., 1980, Axoplasmic transport of muscarnic receptors, *Nature* **286**:287–288.

Laduron, P. M., and Janssen, P. F. M., 1982, Axoplasmic transport and possible recycling of opiate receptors labelled with ^{3}H-lofentanil, *Life Sci.* **31**:457–462.

Landreth, G. E., and Agranoff, B. W., 1979, Explant culture of goldfish retina: A model for the study of CNS regeneration, *Brain Res.* **151**:39–53.

LaVail, J. H., 1978, A review of the retrograde transport technique, in: *Neuroanatomical Research Techniques* (R. T. Robertson, ed.), pp. 356–384, Academic Press, New York.

LaVail, J. H., Rapisardi, S., and Sugino, I. K., 1980, Evidence against the smooth endoplasmic reticulum as a continuous channel for the retrograde axonal transport of horseradish peroxidase, *Brain Res.* **191**:3–20.

Lavoie, P. A., 1982, Ionic requirements for *in vitro* retrograde axonal transport of acetylcholinesterase, *Neurosci Lett.* **33**:213–216.

Lieberman, A. R., 1974, Some factors affecting retrograde neuronal responses to axonal lesions, in: *Essays on the Nervous System* (R. Bellairs and E. G. Gray, eds.), pp. 71–105, Clarendon Press, Oxford.

Longo, F. M., and Hammerschlag, R., 1980, Relation of somal lipid synthesis to the fast axonal transport of protein and lipid, *Brain Res.* **193**:471–485.

Longo, F. M., Manthorpe, M., Skaper, S. D., Lundborg, G., and Varon, S., 1983, Neuronotrophic activities accumulate *in vivo* within silicone nerve regeneration chambers, *Brain Res.* **261**:109–117.

Lubinska, L., 1952, The influence of the state of the peripheral stump on the early stages of nerve regeneration, *Acta Biol. Exp. (Warsaw)* **16**:55–63.

Lundborg, G., Dahlin, L. B., Danielson, N., Gelberman, R. H., Longo, F. M., Powell, H. C., and

Varon, S., 1982, Nerve regeneration in silicone chambers: Influence of gap length and of distal stump components, *Exp. Neurol.* **76**:361–375.

Matthews, M. R., and Raisman, G., 1972, A light and electron microscopic study of the cellular response to axonal injury in the superior cervical ganglion of the rat, *Proc. Roy. Soc. Lond. [Biol.]* **181**:43–79.

McQuarrie, I. G., and Grafstein, B., 1982, Protein synthesis and axonal transport in goldfish retinal ganglion cells during regeneration accelerated by a conditioning lesion, *Brain Res.* **251**:25–37.

McQuarrie, I. G., Grafstein, B., and Gershon, M. D., 1977, Axonal regeneration in the rat sciatic nerve: Effect of a conditioning lesion and of dbCAMP, *Brain Res.* **132**:443–453.

Meiri, H., Spira, M. E., and Parnas, I., 1981, Membrane conductance and action potential of a regenerating axonal tip, *Science* **211**:709–712.

Mellanby, J., and Green, J., 1981, How does tetanus toxin act? *Neuroscience* **6**:281–300.

Muhlach, W. L., and Pollack, E. D., 1982, Target tissue control of nerve fibre growth rate and periodicity *in vitro, Dev. Brain Res.* **4**:361–364.

Munoz-Martinez, E. J., Nunez, R., and Sanderson, A., 1981, Axonal transport: A quantitative study of retained and transported protein fraction in the cat, *J. Neurobiol.* **12**:15–26.

Nagatsu, I., Kondo, Y., and Nagatsu, T., 1976, Retrograde axoplasmic transport of inactive dopamine-β-hydroxylase in sciatic nerves, *Brain Res.* **116**:277–286.

Nixon, R. A., Brown, B. A. and Marotta, C. A., 1983, Limited proteolytic modification of a neurofilament protein involves a proteinase activated by endogenous levels of calcium, *Brain Res.* **275**:384–388.

Nja, A., and Purves, D., 1978, Effects of nerve growth factor and its antiserum on synapses in the superior cervical ganglion of the guinea pig, *J. Physiol.* **277**:53–75.

O'Brien, D. W., and Snyder, R. E., 1982, Position-sensitive detector studies of the axonal transport of a pulse of radioisotope, *J. Neurobiol.* **13**:435–445.

O'Brien, R. A. D., 1978, Axonal transport of acetylcholine, choline acetyltransferase and cholinesterase in regenerating peripheral nerve, *J. Physiol. (Lond.)* **282**:91–103.

Ochs, S., 1975, Retention and redistribution of proteins in mammalian nerve fibres by axoplasmic transport, *J. Physiol. (Lond.)* **253**:459–475.

Oppenheim, R. W., 1981, Neuronal cell death and some related regressive phenomena during neurogenesis: A selective historical review and progress report, in: *Studies in Developmental Neurobiology: Essays in Honor of Viktor Hamburger* (W. M. Cowan,. ed.), pp. 74–133, Oxford University Press, London.

Pant, H. C., and Gainer, H., 1980, Properties of a calcium-activated protease in squid axoplasm which selectively degrades neurofilament proteins, *J. Neurobiol.* **11**:1–12.

Pestronk, A., Drachman, D. B., and Griffin, J. W., 1980, Effects of aging on nerve sprouting and regeneration, *Exp. Neurol.* **70**:108–119.

Pfenniger, K. H., and Maylie-Pfenniger, M. F., 1981, Lectin labeling of sprouting neurons. 2. Relative movement and appearance of glycoconjugates during plasmalemmal expansion, *J. Cell Biol.* **89**:547–559.

Pilar, G., and Landmesser, L., 1972, Axotomy mimicked by localized colchicine application, *Science* **177**:1116–1118.

Politis, M. J., Ederle, K., and Spencer, P. S., 1982, Tropism in nerve regeneration *in vivo.* Attraction of regenerating axons by diffusible factors derived from cells in distal nerve stumps of transected peripheral nerves, *Brain Res.* **253**:1–12.

Purves, D., 1975, Functional and structural changes in mammalian sympathetic neurones following interruption of their axons, *J. Physiol. (Lond.)* **252**:429–463.

Rambourg, A., and Droz, B., 1980, Smooth endoplasmic reticulum and axonal transport *J. Neurochem.* **35**:16–25.

Reis, D. J., and Ross, R. A., 1973, Dynamic changes in brain dopamine-β-hydroxylase activity during anterograde and retrograde reactions to injury of central noradrenergic neurons, *Brain Res.* **57**:307–326.

Ross, R. A., Joh, T. H., and Reis, D. J., 1975, Reversible changes in the accumulation and activities of tyrosine hydroxylase and dopamine-β-hydroxylase in neurons of locus coeruleus during the retrograde reaction, *Brain Res.* **92**:57–72.

Sahenk, Z., and Mendell, J. R., 1981, Acrylamide and 2, 5-hexanedione neuropathies: Abnormal bidirectional transport rate in distal axons, *Brain Res.* **219**:397–405.

Schlaepfer, W. W., and Hasler, M. B., 1979, Characterization of the calcium-induced disruption of neurofilaments in rat peripheral nerve, *Brain Res.* **168**:299–309.

Schmidt, R. E., and McDougal, D. B., Jr., 1978, Axonal transport of selected particle-specific enzymes in rat sciatic nerve *in vivo* and its response to injury, *J. Neurochem.* **30**:527–535.

Schmidt, R. E., Yu, M. J. C., and McDougal, D. B., 1980, Turnaround of axoplasmic transport of selected particle-specific enzymes at an injury in control and diisopropylphosphorofluoridate-treated rats, *J. Neurochem.* **35**:641–652.

Schwab, M. E., Heumann, R., and Thoenen, H., 1981, Communication between target organs and nerve cells: Retrograde axonal transport and site of action of nerve growth factor, *Cold Spring Harbor Symp. Quant. Biol.* **46**:125–134.

Schwartz, M., Mizrachi, Y., and Eshhar, N., 1982, Factors for goldfish brain induce neuritic outgrowth from explanted regenerating retinas, *Dev. Brain Res.* **3**:29–35.

Scott, T. M., and Foote, J., 1982, Factors involved in the control of RNA synthesis during regeneration of the optic nerve in the frog. *Neurosci. Lett.* **29**:189–194.

Shecket, G., and Lasek, R. J., 1982, Mg^{2+}- or Ca^{2+}-activated ATPase in squid giant fiber axoplasm, *J. Neurochem.* **38**:827–832.

Singer, P. A., Mehler, S., and Fernandez, H. L., 1982, Blockade of retrograde axonal transport delays the onset of metabolic and morphologic changes induced by axotomy, *J. Neurosci.* **2**:1299–1306.

Sinicropi, D. V., and McIlwain, D. L., 1983, Changes in amount of cytoskeletal proteins within the perikarya and axons of regenerating frog motoneurons, *J. Cell Biol.* **96**:240–248.

Sinicropi, D. V., Michels, K., and McIlwain, D. L., 1982, Acetylcholinesterase distribution in axotomized frog motoneurons, *J. Neurochem.* **38**:1099–1105.

Smith, R. G., and Appel, S. H., 1983, Extracts of skeletal muscle increase neurite outgrowth and cholinergic activity of fetal rat spinal motor neurons, *Science* **219**:1079–1081.

Smith, R. S., 1980, The short term accumulation of axonally transported organelles in the region of localized lesions of single myelinated axons, *J. Neurocytol.* **9**:39–65.

Smith, R. S., 1982, Axonal transport of optically detectable particulate organelles, in: *Axoplasmic Transport* (D. G. Weiss, ed.), pp. 181–192, Springer-Verlag, Berlin, Heidelberg, New York.

Souyri, F., Chretien, M., and Droz, B., 1981, Acrylamide-induced neuropathy and impairment of axonal transport of proteins. I. Multifocal retention of fat-transported proteins at the periphery of axons as revealed by light microscope autoradiography, *Brain Res.* **205**:1–13.

Stearns, M. E., 1982, High voltage electron microscopy studies of axoplasmic transport in neurons—a possible regulatory role for divalent cations, *J. Cell Biol.* **92**:765–776.

Strand, F. G., and Kung, T. T., 1980, ACTH accelerates recovery of neuromuscular function following crush of peripheral nerve, *Peptides* **1**:135–138.

Streit, P., 1980, Selective retrograde labeling indicating the transmitter of neuronal pathways, *J. Comp. Neurol.* **191**:429–463.

Sunderland, S, 1978, *Nerves and Nerve Injuries,* 2nd ed., Churchill Livingstone, London.

Sumner, B. E. H., 1976, Quantitative ultrastructural observations on the inhibited recovery of the hypoglossal nucleus from axotomy response when regeneration of the hypoglossal nerve is prevented, *Exp. Brain Res.* **26**:141–150.

Sumner, B. E. H., 1977, Responses in hypoglossal nucleus to delayed regeneration of transected hypoglossal nerve, a quantitative ultrastructural study, *Exp. Brain Res.,* **29:**219–231.

Sumner, B. E. H., 1979, Ultrastructural data, with special reference to bouton/glial relationships, from the hypoglossal nucleus after a second axotomy of the hypoglossal nerve, *Exp. Brain Res.* **36:**107–118.

Tedeschi, B. and Wilson, D. L., 1983, Modification of a rapidly transported protein in regenerating nerve, *J. Neurosci.* **3:**1728–1734.

Tessler, A., Autiliogambetti, L., Gambetti, P., 1980, Axonal growth during regeneration—a quantitative autoradiographic study, *J. Cell Biol.* **87:**197–203.

Tsukita, S., and Ishikawa, H., 1980, The movement of membraneous organelles in axons. Electron microscopic identification of anterogradely and retrogradely transported organelles, *J. Cell Biol.* **84:**513–530.

Turner, J. E., Schwab, M. E., and Thoenen, H., 1982, Nerve growth factor stimulates neurite outgrowth from goldfish retinal explants: The influence of a prior lesion, *Dev. Brain Res.* **4:**59–66.

Verghese, J. P., Bradley, W. G., Mitsumoto, H., and Chad, O., 1982, A blind controlled trial of adrenocorticotropin and cerebral gangliosides in nerve regeneration in the rat, *Exp. Neurol.* **77:**455–458.

Watson, W. E., 1970, Some metabolic responses of axotomized neurons to contact between their axons and denervated muscle, *J. Physiol. (Lond.)* **210:**321–344.

Watson, W. E., 1973, Some responses of neurones of dorsal root ganglia to axotomy, *J. Physiol. (Lond.)* **231:**41–42P.

Wujek, J. R. and Lasek, R. J., 1983, Correlation of axonal regeneration and slow component *B* in two branches of a single axon, *J. Neurosci.* **3:**243–251.

Zarbin, M. A., Wamsley, J. K. and Kuhar, M. J., 1982, Axonal transport of muscarinic cholinergic receptors in rat vagus nerve: High and low affinity agonist receptors move in opposite directions and differ in nucleotide sensitivity, *J. Neurosci.* **23:**934–941.

Zarbin, M. A., Palacios, J. M., Wamsley, J. K. and Kuhar, M. J., 1983, Axonal transport of beta-adrenergic receptors: Antero- and retrogradely transported receptors differ in agonist affinity and nucleotide sensitivity, *Molec. Pharmacol.* **24:**341–348.

CHAPTER 5

BIOCHEMICAL ASPECTS OF THE REGENERATING GOLDFISH VISUAL SYSTEM

BERNARD W. AGRANOFF and THOMAS S. FORD-HOLEVINSKI

1. INTRODUCTION

Why some nerves regenerate and others do not is a question of direct relevance for investigators who wish to establish a proper treatment of traumatic injuries as well as of degenerative and developmental disorders of the nervous system. At present, knowledge is rapidly unfolding regarding the participation of intrinsic as well as extrinsic factors that have been implicated on the basis of a number of experimental models in a variety of species. An example of the dependence of regeneration on extrinsic factors is the finding that neurites from CNS neurons will grow if provided with PNS supporting cells. This can be

BERNARD W. AGRANOFF and THOMAS S. FORD-HOLEVINSKI ● Department of Biological Chemistry and Mental Health Research Institute, University of Michigan, Ann Arbor, Michigan 48109 seen following implantation of an autograft of sciatic nerve in the rat CNS (Benfey and Aguayo, 1982). Although such experiments can be used to support the hypothesis that extrinsic factors regulate regeneration, it can also be argued that neurons that regenerate following axotomy are able to do so because they possess a genetic potential that is not expressed in neurons that cannot. This concept of an intrinsic neuronal regulation of regeneration is supported by the demonstration of growth-associated proteins (GAPs; see Chapters 10 and 11) that appear in the axons of nerves that can regenerate but not in those that do not. It may eventually be proven that both extrinsic and intrinsic mechanisms play a role (Bunge *et al.*, 1978; Bray *et al.*, 1981), and it is likely to be the case that neuronal and nonneuronal cells interact such that each cell type induces altered metabolism in the other.

In addition to having the potential for applications to clinical problems, regeneration paradigms have proven useful for the study of fundamental questions related to growth and differentiation. The regenerating nervous system permits us to study cell recognition and selective synapse formation within the preexisting scaffolding of a fully differentiated tissue. Specificity of connections can thus be investigated in the absence of the replication and migration of cells characteristic of *de novo* development.

A number of technical advantages contribute to the attractiveness of the teleost visual system for the study of nerve regeneration.

1. It represents a documented instance of recovery of function in the damaged CNS.
2. The optic nerves are crossed, so that the contralateral retina and ipsilateral tectum serve as convenient control tissues.
3. The vitreous humor is a convenient repository for the injection of labeled precursors and drugs. Since the ganglion cells and their axons lie exposed at the vitreal surface, these cells, whose axons comprise the optic nerve, are easily exposed.
4. The retina can easily be removed and used directly for *in vitro* incubations. Its blood supply is largely superficial, so that major vessels are easily detached. Furthermore, long-term maintenance of teleost tissues *in vitro* at lower temperatures than those required for avian or mammalian tissues insures adequate availability of oxygen and removal of CO_2 by diffusion.
5. Retinal explants can be induced to extend neuritic outgrowth under conditions that reflect the regenerative response, as described below.

The above properties indicate the suitability of the goldfish visual system in regeneration research. What, in fact, could be more ideal? Well, quite a bit.

In the best of all possible worlds, the goldfish would have the following additional properties:

6. It would have a rapid generation time, so that mutant stocks could be developed.
7. The retina would consist primarily of large ganglion cells, so that whole-retinal incubations would reflect ganglion cell metabolism, and, in addition, the cells could be easily impaled for neurophysiological studies.
8. The ganglion cell neurotransmitter(s) would be identified.
9. The optic nerve would be surgically accessible in the cranial cavity, so that proximal and distal crushes could be performed with equal ease.

Some of these utopian reveries are in fact realizable among the cold-blooded vertebrates. A number of small fish species have rapid cell cycles (Lagler *et al.*, 1977), and clones are also available (Agranoff *et al.*, 1971; Streisinger *et al.*, 1981). The mudpuppy has large impalable retinal cells (Dowling, 1979). In addition, surgical removal of ganglion cells from the goldfish retina has been reported (Giulian, 1980). Also, there is evidence that acetylcholine is a goldfish ganglion cell neurotransmitter and that the receptor in the tectum is nicotinic (Oswald and Freeman, 1979; Schmidt and Freeman, 1980).

It would seem then that a number of avenues remain to be pursued to exploit fully the teleost visual system as a model for the study of regeneration and development. In the meantime, conventional biochemical techniques can be applied directly to the regenerating teleost visual system to identify metabolic "handles" of neuronal metabolism that follow axotomy. Although there have been extensive morphological studies on the response of the neuronal cell body to axotomy (Cragg, 1970; Grafstein and McQuarrie, 1978) as well as on the subsequent degeneration of the distal segment, biochemical concomitants have also been established recently.

Once identified, it is necessary to determine whether a given biochemical alteration is causally related to regeneration or turns out to be part of an inflammatory or degenerative process secondary to injury and not directly related to regrowth. Proven markers of regeneration can then be used to address questions regarding the nature of their role and their regulation. For example, how is the cell body informed that its processes have been injured? There is considerable evidence that this message is delivered by retrograde flow, although it remains unknown whether the signal is mediated by the return to the cell body of a novel substance such as a protein generated at the injury site, or by the failure of retrogradely transported substances normally produced at the synapse to return to the cell body (see K. Kristensson, M. A. Bisby, this volume). Studies on the nature of this message should also provide indications of the signal for completion of the regenerative process, i. e., how the cell body is informed of the recovery of neuronal function as evidenced by a return to preinjury metabolic patterns. Measured rates of retrograde flow, determined by means of exogenous markers, do not necessarily reflect the rate of flow of the putative messengers that mediate the cell reaction to axotomy. Attempts to label axonal constituents of intact nerves have indicated the presence of retrogradely transported endogenous proteins, but present methods are not sufficiently sensitive to yield detailed information (Fink and Gainer, 1980; Williams and Agranoff, 1983; Logan *et al.*, 1983).

Our laboratory has employed both *in vivo* and *in vitro* preparations of the goldfish visual system to identify biochemical markers of regeneration and to define the cell biology of its regeneration. *In vivo* approaches include behavioral evaluation of recovered visual function and studies of axonal transport of labeled proteins in the intact and regenerating visual system. These approaches are complemented by *in vitro* isotopic incorporation studies in isolated control and postcrush retinas. An *in vitro* explant system is well suited to interventive, i.e., pharmacological investigations, since we can study the enhancement or retardation of the rate of neurite extension in explants in which various substances are added to the culture medium. Whether or not agents proven to be active in the explant system actually accelerate recovery of function can then be addressed via the *in vivo* behavioral measures.

2. BEHAVIORAL EVALUATION OF RECOVERED VISUAL FUNCTION

Although regenerating fibers can be demonstrated returning to the optic tectum within days of crush (Springer and Agranoff, 1977), their presence does not tell us whether there is functional recovery. Electrophysiological correlates of visual function generally examine presynaptic impulses and therefore also do not necessarily indicate recovery of synaptic transmission. We have used a number of indicators of functional recovery, including the optomotor response (Springer *et al.*, 1977), the optokinetic response and food localization (Springer and Agranoff, 1977), respiratory suppression following light-shock classical conditioning (Davis and Benloucif, 1981), and acquisition of shuttlebox behavior (Kohsaka *et al.*, 1981a). The dorsal light reflex and the startle response have also been used (Edwards *et al.*, 1981).

Quite different time courses for the recovery of vision are seen by these various methods. Although some techniques are admittedly more crude than others, the observed differences are largely attributable to the fact that the various techniques measure different aspects of visual function mediated by different anatomic pathways. A refinement of an autonomic conditioning paradigm currently in use by Davis and Schlumpf (1983) would seem to have considerable advantages over previous methods. It is highly automated, reproducible, and does not require removal of the opposite eye. Furthermore, it clearly requires intact retinotectal pathways, whereas a number of other measures, including the startle response, light shock, and the optokinetic response are mediated by retinodiencephalic tracts and therefore can be elicited following removal of the tecta. Even when results are compared between laboratories for a given behavioral paradigm, there may be significant differences in observed recovery times. These are attributable to such variables as the size of the fish, the temperature at which they are maintained, and the nature (i.e., crush, cut) and location (intraorbital, tract) of the optic nerve injury.

3. EXPLANT CULTURE

If fish are dark adapted, the retina becomes separable from the pigment layer and can easily be removed from the eye by dissecting it away at the periphery and cutting the emerging optic nerve from the eye cup. As we have described elsewhere (Landreth and Agranoff, 1976), the retina can thus be removed under sterile conditions and cut into 500-μm squares by means of a McIlwain chopper. These explants are placed as 3×3 or 4×4 arrays in 35-mm petri dishes containing polylysine, polyornithine, or collagen substrata. The culture medium used is Leibowitz L-15 to which is typically added 10% fetal bovine serum and 0.1% gentamycin.

Explants taken from retinas in which the optic nerve had not previously been crushed show minimal or even no neurite outgrowth onto the substratum. If, however, the nerve had been crushed *in vivo* a week prior to the explantation, extensive neurite outgrowth will be seen (Landreth and Agranoff, 1979). This *in vivo* conditioning effect on *in vitro* growth is being used in our laboratory, as well as a number of others (Johnson and Turner, 1982; Koenig and Adams, 1982; Schwartz *et al.*, 1982*b;* Yoon and Baker, 1982; Freeman *et al.*, 1981), to investigate various properties of neurites as well as effects of potential blocking agents and trophic factors (Schwartz *et al.*, 1982*a;* Turner *et al.*, 1981). It has been claimed that the intraocular (IO) injection of NGF will shorten the period following crush after which enhanced explant outgrowth will be observed *in vitro* (Turner *et al.*, 1982).

By adding fluorodeoxyuridine to the medium, fibroblastic outgrowth is retarded, and the neuritic membrane may be investigated in relative isolation. By means of this preparation, we have shown, for example, that Con A, wheat germ, and ricin lectin all bind to the membranes and can be competed with appropriate glycosides (Feldman *et al.*, 1982). Using lectin–antilectin cross linking of the membrane ligand, we were able to show that new membrane is added at the growing tip of the neurites (Feldman *et al.*, 1981). We have also shown that diazacholesterol, a blocker of cholesterol synthesis, will block neuritic outgrowth from explants (Heacock *et al.*, 1983). Tunicamycin can also block outgrowth, but at low concentrations at which it does not, there is a decrease in neuritic Con A receptors as determined by fluorescence techniques (Heacock, 1982). When grown on a polylysine substratum, neurites show a distinctive clockwise pattern (Figure 1), which we believe to reflect an intrinsic helicity of the external neurite membrane (Heacock and Agranoff, 1977). This property could well give rise to spiraling of fibers about one another and lead to the fasciculation of fibers characteristic of the optic nerve.

Neurite outgrowth from explants provides a useful assay for the study of agents purported to accelerate or retard neurite outgrowth. We have made considerable progess in developing a more quantitative measure of neurite outgrowth than the nerve growth index currently in use. This involves the use of a video camera and computer (Ford-Holevinski *et al.*, 1982; Figure 2). This *in vitro* assay can then be used together with the behavioral assay of recovery of vision in order to correlate effects of various interventive agents. For example, colchicine blocks neurite outgrowth in explant culture and has also been shown to retard recovery of visual function (Davis and Benloucif, 1981).

4.   RETINAL INCUBATIONS

4.1.   Protein Synthesis

If one optic nerve is crushed in each fish of a group, pairs of retinas can then be removed at various times in order to address the question of whether there is altered metabolism as a result of the crush and, if so, what its temporal relationship is to the time of crush and to the time of recovery of vision. We have shown elsewhere that retinal tubulin labeling is increased within a few days of crush and that retinal mRNA for tubulin is also increased (Burrell *et al.*, 1979; Heacock and Agranoff, 1976). These labeled proteins return to normal values several weeks later.

Another marker is a labeled doublet with molecular weights of 68–70,000 and isoelectric points of 4.8–4.9 that appears in the soluble fraction of the postcrush retina. The labeling begins about 4 days after crush, becomes increasingly prominent for several weeks (Figure 3), and then recedes by day 36 (not shown), a time at which functional recovery is found to be complete. As discussed below, we have also established that this doublet is axonally transported.

Although these two radiolabeled proteins are not seen in the control ret-

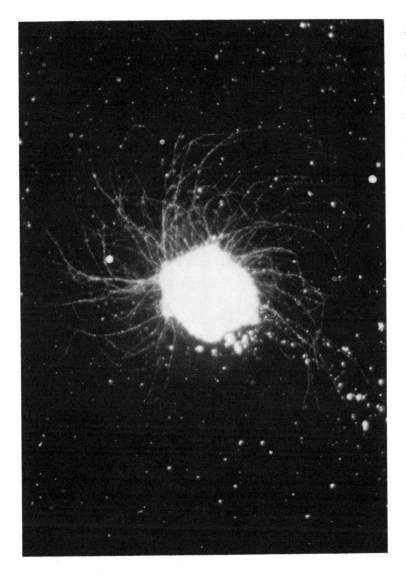

FIGURE 1. Psuedo-dark-field photomicrograph of a growing explant from a postcrush retina after 10 days in culture. The retinal tissue was 500 μm × 500 μm on explantation. Note the marked tendency for neurites to grow in a clockwise direction (see Heacock and Agranoff, 1977).

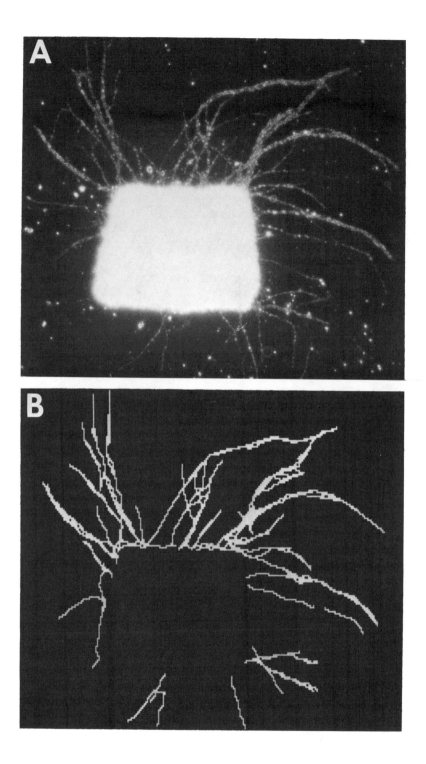

ina, we now have evidence by means of a sensitive silver stain that unlabeled proteins comigrating with the M_r 68–70,000 doublet are present in both postcrush and normal retinas in seemingly equal amounts (Figure 4). It must be noted that at present there is no direct evidence to suggest that this doublet is characteristic of the visual system. When the optic tectum and other regions of the goldfish brain were also examined by two-dimensional PAGE, similar proteins were found in concentrations high enough to allow visualization by Coomassie brilliant blue staining. By mixing small amounts of [^{35}S]methionine-labeled protein from postcrush retina with unlabeled total brain supernatant, we produced a silver-stained gel of brain proteins and a corresponding superimposable autoradiogram of the added labeled retinal protein, indicating that the brain protein and the labeled retinal doublet did in fact comigrate. We are currently examining the possible presence of the doublet in other tissues.

Since the retina appears histologically to be unaffected by optic nerve axotomy except for the chromatolytic changes seen in the ganglion cells, and, further, since the ganglion cells represent only a small fraction of the retinal mass, it is indeed impressive that altered protein synthesis can be detected in incubations of whole retina following optic nerve crush. On the other hand, if one recalls that the ganglion cells must synthesize proteins for the entire neuroplasm of the regenerating optic nerve, a reasonably large structure, it is perhaps not so surprising that prominent increases in labeling of structural proteins such as the α and β subunits of tubulin and actin can be identified in autoradiograms of two-dimensional gels. In the 23-kilodalton region of our gels of retina supernatant, we find additional acidic proteins (isoelectric point 4.8–5.0) that exhibit increases in labeling following axotomy. Unlike the 68,000–70,000 doublet (but like tubulin), the increase in labeling of these proteins persists well beyond 36 days but does eventually decrease (by day 60).

4.2. Altered Enzyme Levels

We have reported increased uridine uptake following crush (Dokas *et al.,* 1981). This can be attributed to an increase in enzymes of uridine metabolism, including uridine kinase, UMP kinase, and UDP kinase (Kohsaka *et al.,* 1981*b*). A 30–40% increase in these enzymes is seen within a few days of crush, and the activities slowly return to normal as vision is regained. Since the

---

FIGURE 2. Photomicrograph of an explant after 5 days in culture (A) and the final computerized image of the same explant (B). The video signal from a camera attached to the microscope was digitized and subjected to image-processing and pattern recognition algorithms to enhance the neurites and eliminate the image of the explant body and floating debris. The remaining white area represents the neuritic outgrowth (Ford-Holevinski *et al.,* 1982).

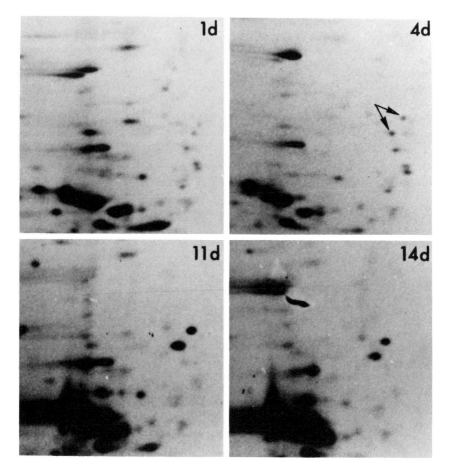

ganglion cells represent only 5% of the total retinal mass, if the changes in the enzymes of uridine metabolism are confined to the ganglion cells, this then represents a seven- to eightfold increase in these enzymes in the ganglion cells.

Increases in retinal ornithine decarboxylase (ODC) are also seen following optic nerve crush (Kohsaka *et al.,* 1981*a*), followed by a return to normal levels within 1 week. Unlike the findings with enzymes of uridine metabolism, in the case of ODC an increase of almost the same magnitude as that in the postcrush retina is seen on the control side. Sham operation did not result in an ODC increase. The axotomy-associated increase was found in brain and kidney in addition to both retinas. When one eye was extirpated, a subsequent ODC

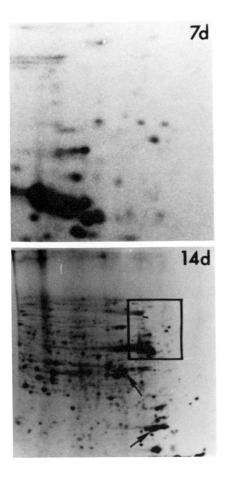

7d

14d

FIGURE 3. Autoradiograms of the soluble proteins obtained from adult goldfish retinas incubated *in vitro* for 1 hr with [³H]leucine at various days post-crush. Note the appearance of the M_r 68–70,000 doublet by day 4, indicated by arrows. A faint triplet observed in this area in the day 1 autoradiogram is actually to the right of the 68–70,000 doublet. The prominent densities in the lower left corner of the enlarged area correspond to tubulin subunits. The lower right 14-day autoradiogram of an entire 140 mm × 160 mm gel indicates the location of the enlarged areas shown in the other panels. The upper arrow indicates actin, and the lower arrow indicates the proteins of the 23K region.

increase was found in the remaining eye. The experiments indicate that the signal that leads to this generalized ODC increase does not originate in the bodies of the retinal ganglion cells but could be related to the degenerating stump of optic nerve distal to the crush. Systemic increases in ODC are well known and in some instances appear to be mediated by growth hormone (Russell, 1973). The question remains whether the increase in ODC triggered by axotomy is causally related to optic nerve regeneration. We approached this question by means of experiments with a blocker of ODC, difluoromethylornithine (DFMO). This substance was administered in the tank water and could be shown to block the increase in ODC seen following crush (Kohsaka *et al.*,

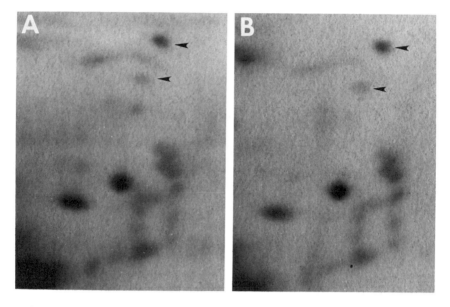

FIGURE 4. Enlargement of the 68,000–70,000 region of silver-stained two-dimensional gels prepared from the soluble fraction of normal (A) and postcrush (B) retinas removed 24 days following axotomy. No significant differences in the 68- to 70-kilodalton doublet (arrows) are apparent despite the differences in labeling seen in this region at this time.

1982). The treatment did not block the behaviorally measured rate of recovery of vision. We concluded that the increase in ODC seen following crush is not likely to play an obligatory role in recovery of function.

Ornithine decarboxylase is a rate-limiting enzyme in the synthesis of polyamines, and it has been shown that axonal transport of polyamines is selectively increased in optic nerve regeneration (Ingoglia *et al.*, 1982). Although the DFMO effectively blocked ODC in our experiments, polyamines were decreased only 50%. It remains possible that a more effective block of polyamine synthesis, such as could be provided by the simultaneous use of an inhibitor of ODC and of methionine decarboxylase, would block recovery of vision effectively.

5. AXONAL TRANSPORT OF PROTEINS ASSOCIATED WITH REGENERATION

Since the ganglion cells represent only a fraction of the retinal mass, we are faced with the dilemma in our retinal studies of sorting out their metabolic alterations from those that may be occurring in other retinal cell types. Fortunately, only ganglion cell components are axonally transported, and by examining the changes in labeled material transported *in vivo* in the optic fibers and their targets, we can verify whether observed retinal alterations are indeed associated with the ganglion cells. Following intraocular injection of labeled amino acid, labeled proteins appear in the contralateral tectum at times characteristic of specific protein classes. In uninjured nerves, rapidly transported proteins arrive 8–24 hr after injection and are found in the particulate (presumably membrane-bound) fraction, whereas slowly transported substances are primarily nonparticulate and may take days or even weeks to make the journey (Willard *et al.*, 1974; Willard and Hulebak, 1977). These latter groups appear to contain mostly the fibrous proteins, including actin, tubulin, and tubulin-associated proteins.

By this technique, alterations in the quantities and rates of transported proteins have been observed following damage to the goldfish retinotectal pathway. For example, Benowitz *et al.* (1981) have reported that there is an increase in a rapidly transported 43-kilodalton membrane-bound protein analogous to a growth-associated protein (GAP) seen in the regenerating toad optic nerve (see Chapters 10 and 11, this volume). We have also observed this GAP in regenerating optic nerve (Heacock and Agranoff, 1982). Among slowly transported, soluble proteins, our laboratory has shown that the labeled 68- to 70-kilodalton doublet is also transported to the tectum under conditions of regeneration (Figure 5). The possible function of this doublet is presently unknown. It does not appear to be associated with the fibrous proteins mentioned above, nor does it appear to be neurofilament related. McQuarrie and Lasek (1981) have reported molecular weights of 60, 80, and 135,000 for the neurofilament protein subunits of this species. In the sense that these labeled proteins are not detected in autoradiograms of gels of the normal retina and are labeled both in the retina and tectum following nerve crush, they may be considered to be growth-associated, or regeneration-associated, proteins. Since the previously described GAPs are rapidly transported, it is speculated that they play a regulatory role in growth and reconnection. It is somewhat more difficult to imagine how such slowly transported substances can regulate events at the growth cone or synapse, since they arrive rather late on the scene. It is possible that the 68- to 70-kilodalton doublet is related primarily to maintenance rather than initiation of growth.

Experiments in progress seem to indicate that the 68- to 70-kilodalton doublet arrives at the tectum sometime after tubulin, believed to be in the most slowly transported group of proteins in intact nerves (Willard *et al.*, 1974; Hoffman and Lasek, 1975, Willard and Hulebak, 1977). This could mean that there is an even slower rate of transport than has previously been established, or at least that tubulin is not in the most slowly transported component in the

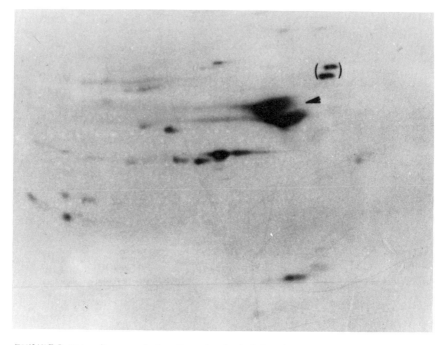

FIGURE 5. Autoradiogram of a two-dimensional gel of the soluble proteins obtained from gold-fish tecta 44 days after optic nerve crush and 30 days after IO injection of [³H]proline (from Heacock and Agranoff, 1982). Arrow marks the position of tubulin subunits; brackets indicate the 68- to 70-kilodalton proteins.

regenerating nerve. When 14-day postcrush fish are injected IO with [³⁵S]methionine and are killed 11 days later, autoradiograms of two-dimensional gels of optic nerve supernatant fractions (Figure 6A) and their corresponding silver- or Coomassie brilliant blue-stained gels show the 68- to 70-kilodalton doublet to be present as well-defined round spots in quantities indicative of major protein components. Tubulin is present in the newly regenerated nerve but is much more prominent in the particulate fraction. At this time, the doublet is not yet autoradiographically detectable in the soluble fraction of the tectum, which does, however, contain labeled tubulin, actin, and the 23-kilodalton soluble GAP proteins (Figure 6B). If 14-day postcrush fish are given a 30-day IO incorporation pulse of [³H]proline, the 68- to 70-kilodalton doublet is prominent in the two-dimensional gel of the tectal supernatant fraction (Figure 5).

Since a systematic study of both soluble and particulate fractions of retina, nerve, and tectum with the same precursor and gel analytical system has not yet been conducted, caution must be exercised in attempts to reconstruct the sequence by which these proteins are transported during regeneration from the existing data. The most parsimonious interpretation of the data at hand is that both slowly and rapidly transported proteins characteristic of the regeneration process can be detected as labeled proteins in the retina within 4 days of intraorbital optic nerve crush. Labeling of tubulin is enhanced severalfold in retina and appears in the soluble fraction of tectal homogenates about 25 days after the nerve has been axotomized, providing the precursor has been injected at least 10 days previously. Labeled tubulin is not prominent in the soluble fraction of the nerve at this time, a result that suggests that it might be transported in a particulate form and then become soluble in the presynaptic region. The 68- or 70-kilodalton doublet appears to be transported in the nerve primarily in the soluble fraction and to arrive in the tectum at some time later than tubulin.

The radiolabeled 68- to 70-kilodalton doublet observed in the tectum appears to have undergone broadening in the IEF direction (Figure 5). This may suggest some posttranslational modification that occurs in the presynaptic region (see Chapter 9). If so, the doublet may play a role in functional reconnection or, by the retrograde transport of its modified form, act as the putative signal to the cell body that regeneration is complete.

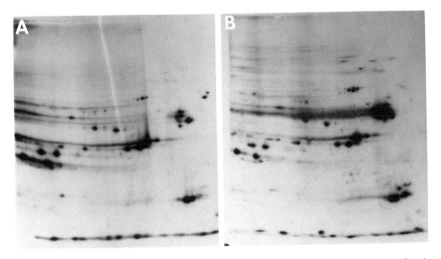

FIGURE 6. Autoradiograms produced from two-dimensional gels of the soluble fractions of optic nerves (A) and tecta (B) removed 25 days post crush and 11 days following IO injection of [^{35}S]methionine.

6. REFERENCES

Agranoff, B. W., Davis, R. E., and Gossington, R. E., 1971, Esoteric fish, *Science* **171**:230.

Benfey, M., and Aguayo, A. J., 1982, Extensive elongation of axons from rat brain into peripheral nerve grafts, *Nature* **296**:150–152.

Benowitz, L. I., Shashoua, V. E., and Yoon, M. G., 1981, Specific changes in rapidly transported proteins during regeneration of the goldfish optic nerve, *J. Neurosci.* **1**:300–307.

Bray, G. M., Rasminsky, M., and Aguayo, A. J., 1981, Interactions between axons and their sheath cells, *Annu. Rev. Neurosci.* **4**:127–162.

Bunge, R., Johnson, M., and Ross, C. D., 1978, Nature and nurture in development of the autonomic neuron, *Science* **199**:1409–1416.

Burrell, H. R., Heacock, A. M., Water, R. D., and Agranoff, B. W., 1979, Increased tubulin messenger RNA in the goldfish retina during optic nerve regeneration, *Brain Res.* **168**:628–632.

Cragg, B. G., 1970, What is the signal for chromatolysis? *Brain Res.* **23**:1–21.

Davis, R. E., and Benloucif, S., 1981, Behavioral investigation of neurotoxicity: The effects of colchicine, lumicolchicine and vincristine sulfate on goldfish optic nerve regeneration, *Neurotoxicology* **2**:419–430.

Davis, R. E., and Schlumpf, B. E., 1983, Circumvention of extraretinal photoresponses in assessing recovery of vision following optic nerve crush in goldfish, *Behav. Brain Res.* **7**:65–79.

Dokas, L. A., Kohsaka, S., Burrell, H. R., and Agranoff, B. W., 1981, Uridine metabolism in the goldfish retina during optic nerve regeneration: Whole retina studies, *J. Neurochem.* **36**:1160–1165.

Dowling, J. E., 1979, Information processing by local circuits: The vertebrate retina as a model system in: *The Neurosciences Fourth Study Program* (F. O. Schmitt and F. G. Worden, eds.), pp. 163–181, MIT Press, Cambridge.

Edwards, D. L., Alpert, R. M., and Grafstein, B., 1981, Recovery of vision in regeneration of goldfish optic axons: Enhancement of axonal outgrowth by a conditioning lesion, *Exp. Neurol.* **72**:672–686.

Feldman, E. L., Axelrod, D., Schwartz, M., Heacock, A. M., and Agranoff, B. W., 1981, Studies on the localization of newly added membrane in growing neurites, *J. Neurobiol.* **12**:591–598.

Feldman, E. L., Heacock, A. M., and Agranoff, B. W., 1982, Lectin binding to neurites of goldfish retinal explants, *Brain Res.* **248**:347–354.

Fink, D. J., and Gainer, H., 1980, Retrograde axonal transport of endogenous proteins in sciatic nerve by covalent labeling *in vivo, Science* **208**:303–305.

Ford-Holevinski, T., Radin, N. S., and Agranoff, B. W., 1982, Applications of a microcomputer-based video analyzer: Neurite outgrowth rates and densitometry, *Soc. Neurosci. Abstr.* **8**:302.

Freeman, J. A., Weiss, J. M., Snipes, G. J., Mayes, B., and Norden, J. J., 1981, Growth cones of goldfish retinal neurites generate DC currents and orient in an electric field, *Soc. Neurosci. Abstr.* **7**:550.

Giulian, D., 1980, Isolation of ganglion cells from the retina, *Brain Res.* **189**:135–155.

Grafstein, B., and McQuarrie, I. G., 1978, The role of the nerve cell body in axonal regeneration, in *Neuronal Plasticity* (C. Cotman, ed.), pp. 155–195, Raven Press, New York.

Heacock, A. M., 1982, Glycoprotein requirement for neurite outgrowth in goldfish retina explants: Effects of tunicamycin, *Brain Res.* **241**:307–315.

Heacock, A. M., and Agranoff, B. W., 1976, Enhanced labeling of a retinal protein during regeneration of the optic nerve in goldfish, *Proc. Natl. Acad. Sci. U.S.A.* **73**:828–832.

Heacock, A. M., and Agranoff, B. W., 1977, Clockwise growth of neurites from retinal explants, *Science* **198**:64–66.

Heacock, A. M., and Agranoff, B. W., 1982, Protein synthesis and transport in the regenerating goldfish visual system, *Neurochem. Res.* **7**:771–788.

Heacock, A. M., Klinger, P. D., Seguin, E. B., and Agranoff, B. W., 1984, Cholesterol synthesis and nerve regeneration *J. Neurochem.* **42**:987–993.

Hoffman, P. N., and Lasek, R. J., 1975, The slow component of axonal transport. Identification of major structural polypeptides of the axon and their generality among mammalian neurons, *J. Cell Biol.* **66**:351–366.

Ingoglia, N. A., Sharma, S. C., Pilchman, J., Baranowski, K., and Sturman, J. A., 1982, Axonal transport and transcellular transfer of nucleosides and polyamines in intact and regenerating optic nerves of goldfish: Speculation on the axonal regulation of periaxonal cell metabolism, *J. Neurosci.* **2**:1412–1423.

Johnson, J. E., and Turner, J. E., 1982, Growth from regenerating goldfish retinal cultures in the absence of serum on hormonal supplements: Tissue extract effects, *J. Neurosci. Res.* **8**:315–329.

Koenig, E., and Adams, P., 1982, Local protein synthesizing activity in axonal fields regenerating *in vitro, J. Neurochem.* **39**:386–400.

Kohsaka, S., Masyuk, A., and Agranoff, B. W., 1981*a*, Nucleoside metabolism in the goldfish retina following optic nerve crush, in: *Abstracts, Eighth Meeting of the International Society for Neurochemistry, Nottingham, England*, p. 396.

Kohsaka, S., Schwartz, M., and Agranoff, B. W., 1981*b*, Increased activity of ornithine decarboxylase in goldfish following optic nerve crush, *Dev. Brain Res.* **1**:391–401.

Kohsaka, S., Heacock, A. M., Klinger, P. D., Porta, R., and Agranoff, B. W., 1982, Dissociation of enhanced ornithine decarboxylase activity and optic nerve regeneration in goldfish, *Dev. Brain Res.* **4**:149–156.

Lagler, K. F., Bardach, J. E., Miller, R. R., and Passino, D. R. M., 1977, *Ichthyology*, John Wiley & Sons, New York.

Landreth, G. E., and Agranoff, B. W., 1976, Explant culture of adult goldfish retina: Effect of prior optic nerve crush, *Brain Res.* **118**:299–303.

Landreth, G. E., and Agranoff, B. W., 1979, Explant culture of adult goldfish retina: A model for the study of CNS regeneration, *Brain Res.* **161**:39–53.

Logan, M. J., McLean, W. G., and Mein, K. F., 1983, Limitations of the usefulness on N-succinimidyl propionate for the study of retrograde axonal flow, *Neurosci. Lett.* **36**:203–210.

McQuarrie, I. G., and Lasek, R. J., 1981, Axonal transport of labeled neurofilament proteins in goldfish optic axons, *J. Cell Biol.* **91**:234a.

Oswald, R. E., and Freeman, J. A., 1979, Characterization of the nicotinic acetylcholine receptor isolated from goldfish brain, *J. Biol. Chem.* **254**:3419–3426.

Russell, H., 1973, Polyamines in growth—normal and neoplastic, in: *Polyamines in Normal and Neoplastic Growth* (D. H. Russell, ed.), pp. 1–13, Raven Press, New York.

Schmidt, J. T., and Freeman, J. A., 1980, Electrophysiologic evidence that retinotectal synaptic transmission in the goldfish is nicotinic cholinergic, *Brain Res.* **187**:129–142.

Schwartz, M., Mizrachi, Y., and Eshhar, N., 1982*a*, Factor(s) from goldfish brain induce neuritic outgrowth from explanted regenerating retinas, *Dev. Brain Res.* **3**:29–35.

Schwartz, M., Mizrachi, Y., and Kimhi, Y., 1982*b*, Regenerating goldfish retinal explants: Induction and maintenance of neurites by conditioned medium from cells originated in the nervous system, *Dev. Brain Res.* **3**:21–28.

Skene, J. H. P., and Willard, M., 1981, Changes in axonally transported proteins during axon regeneration in toad retinal ganglion cells, *J. Cell Biol.* **89**:86–95.

Springer, A. D., and Agranoff, B. W., 1977, Effect of temperature on rate of goldfish optic nerve regeneration: A radioautographic and behavioral study, *Brain Res.* **128**:405–416.

Springer, A. D., Easter, S. S., Jr., and Agranoff, B. W., 1977, The role of the optic tectum in various visually-mediated behaviors of goldfish, *Brain Res.* **128**:393–404.

Streisinger, G., Walker, C., Dower, N., Knauber, D., and Singer, F., 1981, Product of clones of homozygous diploid zebra fish *(Brachydanino rerio)*, *Nature* **291**:293–296.

Turner, J. E., Delaney, R. K., and Johnson, J. E., 1981, Retinal ganglion cell response to axotomy and nerve growth factor antiserum treatment in the regenerating visual system of the gold-fish *(Carassius auratus)*: An *in vivo* and *in vitro* analysis, *Brain Res.* **204**:283–294.

Turner, J. E., Schwab, M. E., and Thoenen, H., 1982, Nerve growth factor stimulates neurite outgrowth from goldfish retinal explants: The influence of a prior lesion, *Dev. Brain Res.* **4**:59–66.

Willard, M. B., and Hulebak, K. L., 1977, The intra-axonal transport of polypeptide H: Evidence for a fifth (very slow) group of transported proteins in the retinal ganglion cells of the rabbit, *Brain Res.* **136**:289–306.

Willard, M., Cowan, W. M., and Vagelos, P. R., 1974, The polypeptide composition of intra-axonally transported proteins: Evidence for four transport velocities, *Proc. Natl. Acad. Sci. U.S.A.* **71**:2183–2187.

Williams, L. R., and Agranoff, B. W., 1983, Retrograde transport of goldfish optic nerve proteins labeled by N-succinimidyl [^{3}H]propionate, *Brain Res.* **259**:207–216.

Yoon, M. G., and Baker, F. A., 1982, Neurites outgrowing from the retinal explant prefer co-cultured tectal tissue to cerebellar tissue *in vitro*, *Soc. Neurosci. Abstr.* **8**:301.

CHAPTER 6

AXONAL TRANSPORT OF GLYCOPROTEINS IN REGENERATING NERVE

JOHN S. ELAM

1. FUNCTIONS AND GROWTH-RELATED CHANGES IN GLYCOPROTEINS OF NONNEURONAL CELLS

Glycoproteins have become increasingly implicated in a variety of cell-to-cell (Rosen *et al.*, 1974; Vacquier and Moy, 1977; Glick, 1979) and cell-to-substrate (Ocklind *et al.*, 1980; Damsky *et al.*, 1982) adhesions. Many of the interactions appear to be at least partially dependent on the carbohydrate portion of the molecules (Kinsey and Lennarz, 1981; Vicker, 1976; Pippia *et al.*, 1980). In addition to mediating interactions at the cell surface, glycosylation has been linked to a number of intracellular processes. Most prominent among these are subcellular routing (Fitting and Kabat, 1982; Rome *et al.*, 1979), secretion (Sidman, 1981), transmembrane transport (Olden *et al.*, 1979), and control of susceptability to proteolysis (Kalish *et al.*, 1979; Milenkovic and Johnson, 1980) [for review see Olden *et al.* (1982)].

A substantial body of evidence has specifically implicated glycoproteins in cellular interactions associated with development and growth. Development-

JOHN S. ELAM ● *Department of Biological Science, Florida State University, Tallahassee, Florida 32306* related characteristics of glycoprotein carbohydrate chains are varied and have been found to include alterations in sulfation (Heiftez *et al.,* 1980*a*; Wenzl and Sumper, 1982), increased fucosylation (Zieske and Bernstein, 1982), presence of high-molecular-weight chains containing repeating N-acetylglucosamine–galactose disaccharide units (Muramatsu *et al.,* 1978; Heifetz *et al.,* 1980*b*), and high concentrations of low-molecular-weight polymannosyl chains (Muramatsu *et al.,* 1976; Hakimi and Atkinson, 1980). Several studies showing extensive binding of concanavalin A (Con A) have independently confirmed high levels of polymannosyl chains in developing systems (Skutelsky and Farquhar, 1976; Maylie-Pfenninger and Jamieson, 1980; Walsh and Phillips, 1981). Endogenous lectins binding to carbohydrate chains have also been isolated from a variety of developing systems (Barondes and Haywood, 1979; Grabel *et al.,* 1979; Roberson and Armstrong, 1980).

Specificity in the type of glycoprotein participating in particular adhesions is inferred from growing hepatocytes, where different cell surface glycoconjugates are involved in cell–cell and cell–substrate adhesion (Ocklind *et al.,* 1980). This is also the case in cultured fibroblasts, where Con-A-binding glycoproteins have been localized in focal adhesion sites, whereas fibronectin (a major adhesive glycorprotein) is concentrated in extracellular matrix contacts (Chen and Singer, 1982). An obligatory role for glycoproteins in cellular development is suggested by several studies in which the glycosylation-blocking antibiotic tunicamycin has blocked differentiation (reviewed by Olden *et al.,* 1982).

2. GLYCOPROTEINS AND NEURONAL GROWTH

Several lines of evidence suggest that changes in glycoprotein composition may also be important to neuronal growth. At the whole-brain level, large increases in glycoprotein content are observed during the period of active neurite outgrowth and synaptogenesis (Kursius *et al.,* 1974; Margolis *et al.,* 1976; Federico and DiBenedetta, 1978). Carbohydrate chains preferentially accumulating during brain development appear to be of the "core segment" type, enriched in glucosamine, mannose, and galactose (Krusius *et al,* 1974; Reeber *et al.,* 1980). More recently, unusual polysialosyl carbohydrate chains have also been found to be characteristic of developing mammalian brain (Finne, 1982).

An alternative to direct compositional analysis of developmental changes in nervous system glycoproteins has been the use of lectins having affinity for particular carbohydrate groups. Developmental stage differences in lectin affinity have been observed on the surfaces of cells from embryonic mouse cerebellum (Huck and Hatten, 1981) and chick retina (Mintz *et al.,* 1981). More specific localization of developmental changes to neurites has been achieved through cytochemical evaluation of lectin binding. Transient appearance of cell surface receptors binding concanavalin A has been reported in several systems including developing photoreceptor cells (McLaughlin and Wood, 1977), parallel fibers of developing cerebellum (Zanetta et al., 1978), and dorsal root ganglion cell axons (Denis-Donini et al., 1978). Interestingly, Con A has been shown to stimulate neurite outgrowth from spinal ganglion cells in vitro (Gombos et al., 1972).

Receptors for wheat germ agglutinin (WGA) and RCA, in addition to Con A, have been found on growing axons of explanted goldfish retina (Feldman et al., 1982), and binding of WGA and RCA has been noted in growing axons of anterior horn cells and superior cervical ganglion (Pfenninger and Maylie-Pfenninger, 1981a,b). These studies confirm the insertion of newly synthesized glycoproteins at the axon tip and, in the case of anterior horn cells, show a differential distribution of lectin receptors between growth cones and maturing axons. It should be noted that the lectin binding studies infer differential exposure of mannose (binding Con A), N-acetylglucosamine or N-acetylneuraminic acid (binding WGA), and galactose or N-acetylgalactosamine (binding RCA) during neurite growth. However, the results do not in themselves permit a precise determination of the chemical differences in cell surface glycans.

A number of additional studies have focused on changes in lectin binding and composition of glycoproteins in developing synaptic membranes. A pattern observed in several studies is a relative increase in sialic acid and corresponding WGA binding as synaptic maturation progresses (DeSilva et al., 1979; McLaughlin et al., 1980; Fu et al., 1981). A failure of cerebellar cells of staggerer mutants to develop WGA binding sites has been hypothesized to be related to defective synaptogenesis in the same animals (Hatten and Messer, 1978). A large number of complex additional changes in binding of lectins and rates of synthesis of synaptic membrane glycoproteins separated on SDS gels have been observed during synaptic maturation (DeSilva et al., 1979; Kelly and Cotman, 1981; Fu et al., 1981).

Of possible relevence to observed developmental changes in lectin binding is the appearance in neonatal rat brain and developing chick optic tectum of endogenous lectins possesing hemagglutinin activity (Simpson et al., 1977; Gremo et al., 1978). Appearance of the lectins is transitory, and, in the case of rat brain, activity is blocked by glycopeptides derived from neonatal brain membranes. Additional evidence for a role of neurite glycoproteins in adhesion derives from the observation of Culp et al. (1980) of a high-molecular-weight polysaccharide in substrate adhesion sites that is specific to neuroblastoma cells that are extending neurites. A major body of evidence produced by Edelman and his colleagues has characterized an adhesion-promoting glycoprotein from developing chick and mammalian brain (Thiery *et al.*, 1977; Hoffman *et al.*, 1982). The glycoprotein is found on the outer surface of growing neurites, and antibodies to the molecule are found to disrupt side-to-side adhesion of growing spinal ganglion fibers (Rutishauser *et al.*, 1978). A failure of the normal embryonic-to-adult modification of the molecules (involving decreased sialic acid content) has been noted in the staggerer mutant (Edelman and Chuong, 1982).

3. AXONAL TRANSPORT OF GLYCOPROTEINS IN MATURE AND GROWING NEURONS

3.1. Mature Nerve

An alternative approach to the evaluation of glycoproteins involved in neurite outgrowth has been to study the molecules exported to the axon by the process of axonal transport. By use of radioactive glycoprotein precursors, most commonly [^{3}H]fucose and [^{3}H]glucosamine, a large number of studies have documented axonal transport of glycoproteins in a variety of experimental systems (for review, see Elam, 1979). Transport rates, after correction for delays in cell body release (Specht and Grafstein, 1977; Goodrum *et al.*, 1979), have been found to be similar to the most rapid movement of amino-acid-labeled proteins. Multiple rapidly migrating peaks of glycoprotein have been observed in a few preparations (Levin, 1977; Goldberg and Ambron, 1981). Retrograde axonal transport of glycoprotein has also been detected in both mammalian peripheral nerve and goldfish optic nerve (Frizell *et al.*, 1976; Whitnall *et al.*, 1982).

Subcellular distribution analysis shows the majority of transported glycoproteins to be particulate, with affiliation of transported label with axolemma (Matthieu *et al.*, 1978; Ambron, 1982, Elam, 1982), smooth endoplasmic reticulum (Markov *et al.*, 1976), synaptic plasma membrane (Marko and Cuenod, 1973; Bennett *et al.*, 1973), and synaptic vesicles (Bennett *et al.*, 1973; Thompson *et al.*, 1976). A soluble fraction with unique molecular properties is also transported, possibly within the membranous organelles (Goodrum *et al.*, 1979; Elam, 1982).

One- and two-dimensional gel electrophoresis has shown that transport in a given nerve includes a large number of individual glycoproteins (Elam, 1979; Wenthold and McGarvey, 1982; Stone and Hammerschlag, 1983). The transported molecules are generally greater than 30,000 daltons and extend to greater than 200,000 daltons. Diversity in the carbohydrate chains attached to the glycoproteins is indicated by binding of transported molecules to a variety of lectins (Karlsson, 1979; Gustavsson *et al.*, 1982; Wenthold and McGarvey,

1982) and the diversity of size and charge of pronase-derived glycopeptides (Ambron, 1982; Elam, 1982). Tract-specific differences in composition of transported glycoproteins have been noted in the rat brain (Padilla and Morell, 1980; Goodrum and Morell, 1982), and, interestingly, most of the identifiable differences in rapidly transported molecules of the guinea pig optic and auditory nerves were in glycoproteins (Wenthold and McGarvey, 1982).

3.2. Growing Nerve

Despite the probable relevance of axonally transported glycoproteins to processes of axonal growth, there have been a very limited number of studies on glycoprotein transport in developing systems and even fewer on regenerating systems. Those investigations that have been conducted allow some preliminary generalizations to be made.

3.2.1. Rates and Amount of Transport

Rapid transport rates, including those for glycoproteins, appear to be unchanged in regenerating peripheral nerve (Frizell and Sjostrand, 1974a; Griffin et al., 1976; Bisby, 1978). This may reflect the fact that normal rapid transport rates already greatly exceed the most rapid rates of neurite elongation. In contrast, the rate of rapid transport of glycoproteins in developing optic nerve has been found to increase with length of growth, possibly in order to provide a relatively constant transit time from cell body to nerve terminals (Marchisio et al., 1973).

Amounts of transported radioactivity in glycoprotein are generally found to increase in growing axons. During regeneration, this represents increases of transported [3H]fucose radioactivity of two- to fourfold in regenerating hypoglossal (Frizell and Sjostrand, 1974a,b; Tessler et al., 1980), sciatic (Griffin et al., 1981), and optic (Giulian et al., 1980; Grafstein and Forman, 1980) nerves. If hypoglossal regeneration is artificially prevented, the expected increase in glycoprotein transport is reduced (Frizell, 1982). An obligatory role of the glycoprotein transport in goldfish optic system is inferred from an observed block of regeneration by tunicamycin (Heacock, 1982). Of probable relevance to the generally increased transport labeling of glycoprotein are recent reports of comparable increases in transport labeling of membrane lipids in regenerating peripheral nerve (Alberghina et al., 1983a,b). This suggests enhanced cotransport of lipids and glycoconjugates as constituents of expanding neurite membranes. Autoradiographic studies indicate a major deposition of transport glycoproteins in axolemma of growing fibers (Tessler et al., 1980; Griffin et al., 1981).

Regeneration is also characterized by a marked increase in the amount of retrograde transport of labeled glycoproteins (Frizell *et al.*, 1976; Whitnall *et al.*, 1982). The magnitude of this increase most likely reflects the combined contribution of increased anterograde transport labeling and premature turnaround of the transported molecules (for a discussion of the possible functional role of altered retrograde transport of endogenous molecules, see M. A. Bisby, this volume).

3.2.2. Composition of Transported Glycoproteins

Two studies that have utilized SDS gel electrophorosis to evaluate changes in the composition of glycoproteins transported in regenerating nerve have detected changes in only a small fraction of isotopically labeled molecules. Guilian *et al.* (1980) noted increased transport of three high-molecular-weight glycoproteins in regenerating goldfish optic axons that were below detectable levels following transport labeling of intact tissue. Skene and Willard (1981*a,b*) reported that one of a few growth-associated proteins (GAPs) of regenerating toad optic nerve is a 50-kilodalton glycoprotein (GAP_{50}). The transported molecule appears to be an integral membrane glycoprotein and is delivered preferentially to the axon terminal (see M. B. Willard, this volume).

3.2.3. Changes Associated with Synaptogenesis

The optic pathway of the embryonic chick has been particularly useful in assessing changes in axonal transport of glycoproteins that appear to be correlated with the synaptogenic phase of growth. Similar studies conducted by Bondy and Madsen (1971) and Marchesio *et al.* (1973) both concluded that relative amounts of glycoprotein transport (based on contralateral/ipsilatral labeling ratios) increase markedly between 13 embryonic days and hatching. This same period marks the transition from fiber outgrowth to active synaptic connection. Another measure of increased transport, the percent of retinal label entering the axon, also increases during synaptogenesis (Sjostrand *et al.*, 1973; Marchisio *et al.*, 1973; Gremo and Marchesio, 1975). These studies reported that the percent of retinal [³H]fucose undergoing transport increases between 13 and 15 embryonic days, subsequently drops, then increases again between day 15 and hatching. The authors speculate that the two periods of increased transport may reflect the needs of both synaptogenesis and electrophysiological maturation. Differences in SDS gel patterns at the various developmental ages were not apparent (Marchesio *et al.*, 1973). A more recent study of developmental changes in hamster optic nerve synaptosomal membrane has shown that [³H]fucose labeling of a 50-kilodalton glycoprotein is delayed until after eye opening (Specht, 1982). A possible additional role of transported glycoproteins in transsynaptic trophic processes in development is suggested by enhanced transsynaptic movement of fucose during the period of optic fiber outgrowth and connection (Specht, 1982; Matthews *et al.,* 1982).

4. AXONAL TRANSPORT OF GLYCOPROTEINS IN REGENERATING OLFACTORY NERVE

4.1. The Olfactory Nerve Preparation

Prior studies have shown that the olfactory nerve has a unique capacity to regenerate *de novo* from neurons produced in the olfactory epithelium (Graziadei and Monti-Graziadei, 1978). An independent body of studies has further demonstrated the particular suitability of the olfactory nerve of the long-nosed garfish for study of axonally transported molecules (Gross and Beidler, 1975; Cancalon and Beidler, 1975; Cancalon *et al.,* 1976). This nerve provides the advantages of considerable length (up to 30 cm), lack of branching, and the absence of myelin. The latter characteristic, combined with the very high proportion of axons in the tissue (Easton, 1971), is of special advantage in performing compositional and subcellular analyses (Cancalon and Beidler, 1975; Elam, 1982). Among the molecules of olfactory nerve that are rapidly transported are glycoproteins that can be labeled with [^{3}H]fucose (Gross and Beidler, 1975; Elam and Peterson, 1979), [^{3}H]glucosamine (Elam, 1982), or $^{35}SO_4$ (Elam and Peterson, 1976).

The combined high regenerative capacity and suitability for transport studies led Paul Cancalon and me to collaboratively investigate the characteristics of fiber regrowth and axonal transport in the gar olfactory nerve (Cancalon and Elam, 1980a,b) (for further details, see P. Cancalon, Chapter 13, this volume). It was found that following a period of pioneer fiber outgrowth, the majority of the newly formed neurons extend axons at a rate of 0.8 mm/day at 21°C. The relatively synchronous outgrowth of this large population of fibers (designated phase III) offered the opportunity to evaluate axonally transported molecules in an unequivocally growing, relatively homogeneous preparation.

4.2. Regeneration-Related Changes in Axonally Transported Glycoproteins

In view of the very limited number of studies on changes in axonal transport of glycoprotein in growing axons, Greg Cole and I undertook an examination of [^{3}H]glucosamine-labeled molecules that are rapidly transported into regenerating garfish olfactory nerve (Cole and Elam, 1981, 1983). We particularly hoped to obtain information on any changes in the carbohydrate chains attached to the transported molecules as well as to assess their subcellular distribution and alteration with stages of axonal growth. Accordingly, groups of fish were subjected to nerve crush 1 cm behind the olfactory mucosa, allowed to regenerate phase III fibers, and labeled with [³H]glucosamine to monitor the axonal transport of glycoproteins.

4.2.1. Extent of Labeling

[³H]Glucosamine-labeled glycoproteins rapidly transported into phase III regenerating fibers contain approximately 30% more transported label per gram of nerve than comparable intact nerves (Cole and Elam, 1983). The magnitude of this increase, although significant, appears to be considerably less than that reported previously for other systems (Frizell and Sjostrand, 1974a; Griffin et al., 1981; Giulian et al., 1980).

4.2.2. Glycoprotein Size Distribution

To assess possible changes in glycoprotein size distribution, labeled nerves were subjected to SDS acrylamide gel electrophoresis (Figure 1). Results

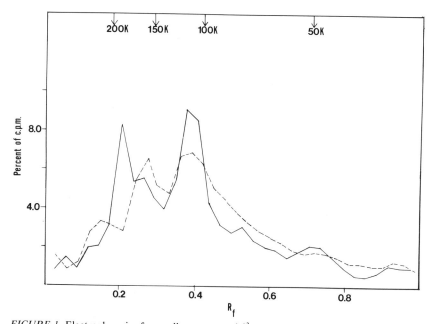

FIGURE 1. Electrophoresis of axonally transported [³H]-glucosamine-labeled glycoproteins of intact and regenerating nerve on 5% SDS polyacrylamide gels. Gels were cut into 2-mm slices, dissolved in 30% hydrogen peroxide, and counted in Aquasol®. Known mol. wt. standards, run in parallel, are indicated on top of graph. Data are expressed as percent of recovered gel radioactivity; and represent an average of three representative gel profiles.

showed general similarity in labeling pattern in intact and regenerating nerve, with a broad distribution of transported molecules above 30 kilodaltons. The exceptions to this similarity were the relatively enhanced labeling in regenerating nerve of molecules in the 100- to 120-kilodalton and 180- to 200-kilodalton ranges.

The observation that major changes in relative transport labeling are confined to a few size groups is in line with the previous results from regenerating optic nerve (Giulian *et al.*, 1980; Skene and Willard, 1981*a,b*). However, there is no detectable enhancement in olfactory nerve labeling of molecules the size of GAP_{50} of the toad optic nerve (Skene and Willard, 1981*a,b*). It also can not be said with certainty if any of the more heavily labeled molecules in olfactory nerve correspond to enhanced high-molecular-weight glycoproteins of regenerating goldfish optic nerve (Giulian *et al.*, 1980). It remains possible that requirements for specific glycoproteins in regeneration show considerable species and/or individual nerve specificity.

4.2.3. Regeneration-Related Changes in Concanavalin A Binding Affinity

Since a number of previous studies had noted enhanced Con A binding during growth of neurites (McLaughlin and Wood, 1977; Zanetta *et al.*, 1978; Denis-Donini *et al.*, 1978), we also wanted to investigate the affinity of regenerating olfactory nerve glycoproteins for this lectin (Cole and Elam, 1983). Results showed a substantial increase (from 21% to 34%) in the percentage of transported [^{3}H]glucosamine-labeled glycoprotein binding to Con A affinity columns in regenerating nerve relative to controls. An even greater proportional increase (from 4.5% to 11%) was observed in the percentage of chemically assayed nerve protein binding the lectin, suggesting major quantitative changes in the types of carbohydrate chains present during regeneration. Studies on SDS gels of transport-labeled Con-A-binding molecules showed that a large variety of different-sized glycoproteins display enhanced Con A binding in regenerating nerve. This observation indicates that the increases in Con A binding are not restricted to the particular subpopulations of glycoprotein showing major increases in transport label on gels of total nerve glycoprotein (Figure 1). Rather, a much broader population of glycoproteins incurs changes in carbohydrate chain structure that promote Con A binding. It should be emphasized that changes in carbohydrate chain structure may have minimal effects on individual glycoprotein molecular weight and might escape detection on gels of the resolution shown in Figure 1.

More direct evidence that enhanced binding of glycoproteins to Con A is related to higher levels of Con-A-binding oligosaccharide was obtained by subjecting transport-labeled nerves to proteolysis and isolating the remaining carbohydrate-enriched glycopeptide chains (Cole and Elam, 1981). An overall twofold increase was observed in glycopeptide radioactivity having some degree of affinity for Con A (from 13.6% to 27.9%) and a five- to sixfold increase in glycopeptides that have low molecular weight (are dialyzable) and bind with high affinity (from 1.8% to 10.2% of label). Compositional analysis shows the latter group to have the *n*-mannose/N-acetylglucosamine composition expected of unsubstituted polymannosyl chains (Cole and Elam, 1983). Furthermore, measurements of absolute levels of glucosamine in low-molecular-weight carbohydrate chains of regenerating nerve showed increases that were proportional to the increased level of transport labeling of these glycopeptides.

The conclusion derived from these observations is that increased Con A binding of intact glycoproteins does reflect the increased presence of Con-A-binding carbohydrate groups (including low-molecular-weight polymannosyl chains) both as constitutents of rapid axonal transport and as residual constituents of the regenerating nerve. Since there is also an overall increase in glycoprotein glucosamine per gram of regenerating nerve, it can be concluded that either growing nerve contains a greater proportion of glycosylated molecules or that there is a greater extent of glycosylation of individual glycoproteins.

4.2.4. Changes in Subcellular Distribution

It was of interest to establish whether the observed increases in Con-A-binding glycopeptides were concentrated in a particular subcellular compartment of the nerve. This question was approached by subjecting the nerve to homogenization and subcellular fractionation into fractions enriched in soluble, plasma membrane (axolemmal), and higher-density membrane fragments (Cole and Elam, 1983). Increases in low-molecular-weight Con-A-binding glycopeptides were found in all subfractions. However, by far the greatest proportional increase in this type of carbohydrate chain (15-fold) was found in a very-high-density subfraction that migrates through 1.4 *M* sucrose. The cellular origin of this fraction remains unknown; however, its appearance in electron micrographs is very similar to a putative "cell coat" or glycocalyx fraction isolated from cultured fibroblasts by similar procedures (Graham *et al.*, 1978). This observation permits the tentative conclusion that one function of the increased polymannosyl chains relates to interactions occurring at the outer surface of the growing axons.

4.2.5. Changes with Stage of Growth

The increased axonal transport of glycoproteins having low-molecular-weight Con-A-binding oligosaccharides occurred in nerves in which all phase III regenerating fibers were still in a state of active growth. This observation is in apparent conflict with the suggestion of McLaughlin and Wood (1977) and

Zanetta *et al.* (1978) that increases in Con-A-binding glycoproteins on grow-ing neurites may be correlated with early stages of target cell recognition and synaptogenesis. When, in fact, olfactory nerve glycopeptides were examined at times when growing axons were closer to but still had not reached the olfactory bulb, there was a significant decrease in the proportion of transported radio-activity in low-molecular-weight Con-A-binding glycopeptides (Figure 2). The reasons for such a shift in glycoprotein transport in axons that are still in an active state of growth are not apparent but may relate to the need for an increased proportion of transported molecules to expand the maturing nerve segment closer to the cell bodies. Since our studies evaluated glycoproteins transported to the entire nerve, our results could not distinguish possible dif-ferences in molecules delivered differentially to growing tips and maturing axons. It also remains possible that alterations in transport are preparatory to synaptogeneses and in this system involve decreases in polymannosyl chains.

4.3. Regeneration-Related Changes in Nonneuronal Glycoproteins

The previously cited observation that proportional increases in regener-ating nerve Con-A-binding glycoprotein somewhat exceeded increases in Con-

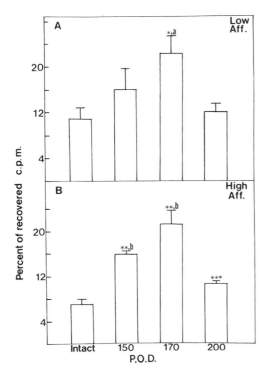

FIGURE 2. Proportion of dialyzable glycopeptide radioactivity binding Con A as a function of postoperative time. Low-affinity binding (disso-ciated with 20 mM methylglucoside) is shown in A. High-affinity binding (dissociated with 200 mM methyl glucoside) is shown in B. Data are graphed as percent of recovered col-umn radioactivity. *Significantly dif-ferent from intact nerve at $P < 0.05$; **Significantly different from intact nerve at $P < 0.001$; ***Significantly different from intact nerve at $P < 0.025$; a, significantly different from 200-P.O.D. nerve at $P < 0.05$; b, sig-nificantly different from 200-P.O.D. nerve at $P < 0.001$.

A-binding transport label suggests a possible extraneuronal contribution to the compositional change. Evaluation of glycoproteins labeled by systemic presentation of [^{3}H]glucosamine to regenerating nerve showed an approximate twofold increase in total glycopeptide label binding to Con A (from 14% to 30.6%) and a corresponding twofold increase in low-molecular-weight glycopeptide (polymannosyl) binding with high affinity (from 2.2 to 4.3%). Although the results bear a similarity to those for transported molecules, it appears that systematically labeled polymannosyl chains undergo a less extensive regeneration-related increase in labeling than those in neurons. Both labeling analysis and morphological observations indicate that nonneuronal elements remain a quantitatively minor constituent of nerve containing phase III regenerating fibers (Cancalon and Elam, 1980a). However, the observed changes in glycoprotein composition may still be of primary importance in extrinsic control of axon outgrowth.

5. CONCLUSIONS

The results of the garfish olfactory nerve study taken in conjunction with the limited number of other studies on glycoprotein transport in growing or regenerating nerve allow a reexamination of the preliminary generalizations previously discussed.

In agreement with the previously cited studies, the amount of glycoprotein transported per unit of nerve increases during regeneration. Much of this increase can be construed as necessary for both elongation and lateral expansion of the axolemma of the growing neurite. Since molecules transported to regenerating olfactory nerve are both deposited along the nerve and transported into the growth cone region (data not shown), it is reasonable to conclude that both elongation and expansion are being supplied simultaneously (see also Tessler et al., 1980; Griffin et al., 1981). The observed increase in amounts of carbohydrate per unit of nerve protein suggests that there are glycoprotein requirements over and above simple replacement of axolemma that may reflect the need for additional protein-bound oligosaccharides to regulate growth.

Also in agreement with previous studies, there are relatively few major changes in amounts of particular sized transported glycoproteins in regenerating olfactory nerve. These findings could again reflect the primary requirement for replacement of axonal constituents, with a relatively limited number of molecules specifically needed for the outgrowth mechanism. Limited numbers of adhesion-mediating glycoproteins have been detected in other systems (Gottlieb and Glaser, 1980); however, the ultimate limit in the number of such molecules required for prolonged in vivo growth in a particular system is not yet known.

The relatively large changes in the amounts of axonally transported Con-A-binding carbohydrate chains have not been elucidated previously in regenerating nerve; however, increases in Con A binding have been seen during neurite development (McLaughlin and Wood, 1977; Zanetta *et al.,* 1978; Denis-Donini *et al.,* 1978). These changes seem to occur in a large number of individual glycoproteins and may reflect roles in any of several processes in which glycoproteins have been implicated. These could include cellular adhesion, routing to particular cellular or subcellular regions, or altering susceptability to proteolysis. The present results do not allow a determination of which of these processes may involve the observed changes in glycoproteins. The large number of glycoproteins showing changes in Con A binding might argue for a more general role, such as in slowing of the proteolytic turnover rate or in routing greater numbers of molecules into the axon (Stone and Hammerschlag, 1983). On the other hand, specific increases in the high-density membrane fraction may point to a role in cell–cell interactions.

The previously discussed correlation of changes in axonal transport with time of synapse formation in the visual system has been somewhat approximate, since the exact time of initial cell–cell contact was not determined. Despite this limitation, a rough correlation of changes in transported protein synthesis and synaptogenesis has been drawn in goldfish optic axons (see L. I. Benowitz, Chapter 10, this volume). Importantly, some of these changes are permanently blocked if synaptogenesis is experimentally prevented. Our studies indicate that decreases in transport of Con-A-binding glycoprotein temporally precedes synaptogenesis and is clearly not induced by contact with postsynaptic cells. It remains possible that such changes "prepare" the growing neurite for impending contact.

Finally, the observed changes in nonneuronal glycoproteins serve as a reminder that outgrowth of regenerating neurons is unlikely to occur in the absence of facilitatory changes in the environment through which growth is occuring (Varon and Adler, 1981). An understanding of the molecular changes outside the axon may ultimately prove of equal or greater importance to those occurring in axonal transport.

6. REFERENCES

Alberghina, M., Viola, M., and Giuffrida, A. M., 1983*a,* Rapid axonal transport of glycero-phospholiphids in regenerating hypoglossal nerve of the rabbit, *J. Neurochem.* **40**:25–31.

Alberghina, M., Moschella, F., Viola, M., Brancati, V., Micali, G., and Giuffrida, A. M., 1983*b,* Changes in rapid transport of phospholipid in the rat sciatic nerve during axonal regeneration, *J. Neurochem.* **40**:32–38.

Ambron, R., 1982, Differences in the distribution of specific glycoproteins among the regions of a single identified neuron, *Brain Res.* **239**:489–505.

Barondes, S. H., Haywood, P. C., 1979, Comparisons of developmentally regulated lectins from three species of cellular slime mold, *Biochim. Biophys. Acta* **550**:297–308.

Bennett, G., DiGiamberardino, L., Koenig, H. C., and Droz, B., 1973, Axonal migration of protein and glycoprotein to nerve endings. II. Radioautographic analysis of the renewal of glycoproteins in nerve endings of chicken ciliary ganglion after intracerebral injection of [^{3}H]fucose and [^{3}H]glucosamine, *Brain Res.* **60**:129–146.

Bisby, M. A., 1978, Fast axonal transport of labeled protein in sensory axons during regeneration, *Exp. Neurol.* **61**:281–300.

Bondy, S. C., and Madsen, C., 1971, Development of rapid axonal flow in the chick embryo, *J. Neurobiol.* **2**:279–286.

Cancalon, P., and Beidler, L. M., 1975, Distribution along the axon and into various subcellular fractions of molecules labeled with [^{3}H]leucine and rapidly transported in the garfish olfactory nerve *Brain Res.* **89**:225–244.

Cancalon, P., and Elam, J., 1980*a*, Study of regeneration in garfish olfactory nerve, *J. Cell Biol.* **84**:779–784.

Cancalon, P., and Elam, J., 1980*b*, Rate and composition of rapidly transported proteins in regenerating olfactory nerve, *J. Neurochem.* **35**:889–897.

Cancalon, P., Elam, J., and Beidler, L. M., 1976, SDS gel electrophoresis of rapidly transported proteins in garfish olfactory nerve, *J. Neurochem.* **27**:687–693.

Chen, W.-T., and Singer, S. J., 1982, Immunoelectron microscopic studies of the sites of cell–substratum and cell–cell contacts in cultured fibroblasts, *J. Cell Biol.* **95**:205–222.

Cole, G., and Elam, J., 1981, Axonal transport of glycoproteins in regenerating olfactory nerve: Enhanced glycopeptide concanavlin A binding, *Brain Res.* **222**:437–441.

Cole, G., and Elam, J., 1983, Characterization of axonally transported glycoproteins in regenerating garfish olfactory nerve, *J. Neurochem.* **41**:691–702.

Culp, L., Ansbacher, R., and Domen, C., 1980, Adhesion sites of neural tumor cells: Biochemical composition, *Biochemistry* **19**:5899–5907.

Damsky, C. H., Knudsen, K. A., and Buck, C. A., 1982, Integral membrane glycoproteins related to cell-substratum adhesion in mammalian cells, *J. Cell Biochem.* **18**:1–13.

Denis-Donini, S., Estenoz, M., and Augusti-Tocco, G., 1978, Cell surface modifications in neuronal maturation, *Cell Diff.* **1**:193–201.

DeSilva, N. S., Gurd, J. W., and Schwartz, C., 1979, Developmental alteration of rat brain synaptic membranes. Reaction of glycoproteins with plant lectins, *Brain Res.* **165**:283–293.

Easton, D. M., 1971, Garfish olfactory nerve: Easily accesible source of numerous long, homogeneous, nonmyelinated axons, *Science* **172**:952–955.

Edelman, G. M., and Chuong, C.-M., 1982, Embryonic to adult conversion of neural cell adhesion molecules in normal and staggerer mice, *Proc. Natl. Acad. Sci. U.S.A.* **79**:7036–7040.

Elam, J., 1979, Axonal transport of complex carbohydrates in: *Complex Carbohydrates of Nervous Tissue* (R. K. Margolis and R. U. Margolis, eds.), pp. 235–267, Plenum Press, New York.

Elam, J., 1982, Composition and subcellular distribution of glycoproteins and glycosaminoglycans undergoing axonal transport in garfish olfactory nerves, *J. Neurochem.* **39**:1220–1229.

Elam, J., and Peterson, N., 1976, Axonal transport of sulfated glycoproteins and mucopolysaccharides in the garfish olfactory nerve, *J. Neurochem.* **26**:845–850.

Elam, J. S. and Peterson, N. W., 1979, Axonal transport of glycoproteins in the garfish olfactory nerve: isolation of high molecular weight glycopeptides labeled with [^{3}H] fucose and [^{3}H] glucosamine, *J. Neurochem.* **33**:571–573.

Federico, A., and DeBenedetta, C., 1978, Glycoprotein changes during the development of human brain, *J. Neurochem.* **31**:797–800.

Feldman, E., Heacock, A., and Agranoff, B., 1982, Lectin binding to neurites of goldfish retinal explants, *Brain Res.* **268**:347–354.

Finne, J., 1982, Occurence of unique polysialosyl carbohydrate units in glycoproteins of developing brain, *J. Biol. Chem.* **257**:11966–11970.

Fitting, R., and Kabat, D., 1982, Evidence for a glycoprotein "signal" involved in transport between subcellular organelles, *J. Biol. Chem.* **257**:14011–14017.

Frizell, M., 1982, The effect of ligation combined with section on anterograde axonal transport in rabbit hypoglossal nerve, *Brain Res.* **250**:65–69.

Frizell, M., and Sjostrand, J., 1974*a*, Transport of proteins, glycoproteins and cholinergic enzymes in regenerating hypoglossal neurons, *J. Neurochem.* **22**:845–850.

Frizell, M., and Sjostrand, J., 1974*b*, The axonal transport of (^{3}H)fucose labeled glycoproteins in normal and regenerating peripheral nerves., *Brain Res.* **78**:109–123.

Frizell, M., McLean, W. G., and Sjostrand, J., 1976, Retrograde axonal transport of rapidly migrating labeled proteins and glycoproteins in regenerating peripheral nerves, *J. Neurochem.* **27**:191–196.

Fu, S. C., Cruz, T. F., and Gurd, J. W., 1981, Development of synaptic glycoproteins: Effect of postnatal age on the synthesis and concentration of synaptic membrane and synaptic junctional fucosyl and sialyl glycoproteins, *J. Neurochem.* **36**:1338–1351.

Giulian, D., Des Ruisseaux, H., and Cowburn, D., 1980, A study of proteins from ganglion cells of the goldfish retina, *J. Biol. Chem.* **255**:6486–6493.

Glick, M. C., 1979, Membrane glycopeptides from virus-transformed hamster fibroblasts and the normal counterpart, *J. Biol.. Chem.* **18**:(12):2523–2532.

Goldberg, D. J., and Ambron, R. T., 1981, Two rates of fast axonal transport of [^{3}H]glycoprotein in an identified invertebrate neuron, *Brain Res.* **229**:445–455.

Gombos, S., Hermetet, J. C., Reeber, A., Zanetta, J.-P., and Treska-Ciesielski, J., 1972, The composition of glycopeptides, derived from neural membranes, which affect neurite growth *in vitro*, *FEBS Lett.* **24**:247–250.

Goodrum, J. F., and Morell, P., 1982, Axonal transport, deposition, and metabolic turnover of glycoproteins in the rat optic pathway, *J. Neurochem.* **38**:696–704.

Goodrum, J. F., Toews, A. D., and Morell, P., 1979, Axonal transport and metabolism of [^{3}H]fucose- and [^{35}S]-sulfate-labeled macromolecules in the rat visual system, *Brain Res.* **176**:255–272.

Gottlieb, D., and Glaser, L., 1980, Cellular recognition during neural development, *Annu. Rev. Neurosci.* **3**:303–318.

Grabel, L. B., Rosen, S. D., and Martin, G. R., 1979, Teratocarcinoma stem cells have a cell surface carbohydrate-binding component implicated in cell–cell adhesion, *Cell* **17**:477–484.

Grafstein, B., and Forman, D. S., 1980, Intracellular transport in neurons, *Physiol. Rev.* **60**:1167–1283.

Graham J. M., Hynes, R. O., Rowlatt, C., and Sandall, J. K., 1978, Cell surface coat of hamster fibroblasts, *Ann. N.Y. Acad. Sci.* **312**:221–239.

Graziadei, P. P. C., and Monti-Graziadei, G. A., 1978, The olfactory system: A model for the study of neurogenesis and axon regeneration in mammals, in *Neuronal Plasticity*, (C. W. Cotman ed.), pp. 131–152, Raven Press, New York.

Gremo, R., and Marchisio, P. C., 1975, Dynamic properties of axonal transport of proteins and glycoproteins: A study based on the effects of metaphase blocking drugs in the developing optic pathway of chick embryos, *Cell Tissue Res.* **161**:303–316.

Gremo, R., Kobiler, D., and Barondes, S. H., 1978, Distribution of an endogenous lectin in the developing chick optic tectum, *J. Cell Biol.* **79**:491–499.

Griffin, J. W., Drachman, D. B., and Price, B. L., 1976, Fast axonal transport in motor nerve regeneration, *J. Neurobiol.* **7**:355–370.

Griffin, J. W., Price, D. L., Drachman, D. B., and Morris, J., 1981, Incorporation of axonally transported glycoproteins into axolemma during nerve regeneration, *J. Cell Biol.* **88**:205–214.

Gross, G. W., and Beidler, L. M., 1975, A quantitative analysis of isotope concentration profiles and rapid transport velocities in the C-fibers of the garfish olfactory nerve, *J. Neurobiol.* **6**(2):213–232.

Gustavsson, S., Ohlson, C., and Karlsson, J. O., 1982, Glycoproteins of axonal transport: Affinity chromatography on fucose-specific lectins, *J. Neurochem.* **38**:852–855.

Hakimi, J., and Atkinson, P. H., 1980, Growth-dependent alterations in oligomannosyl glyco-peptides expressed in Sindbis virus glycoproteins, *Biochemistry* **19**:5619–5624.

Hatten, M. and Messer, A., 1978, Postnatal cerebellar cells from staggerer mutant mice express embryonic cell surface characteristics, Nature **276**:504–506.

Heacock, A. M., 1982, Glycoprotein requirements for neurite outgrowth in goldfish retina explants: Effects of tunicamycin, *Brain Res.* **241**:307–315.

Heifetz, A., Kinsey, W., and Lennarz, W., 1980*a*, Synthesis of a novel class of sulfated glyco-proteins in embryonic liver and lung, *J. Biol. Chem.* **255**:4528–4534.

Heifetz, A., Lennarz, W. J., Libbus, B., and Hsu, Y.-C., 1980*b*, Synthesis of glycoconjugates during the development of mouse embryos *in vitro, Dev. Biol.* **80**:398–408.

Hoffman, S., Sorkin, B. C., White, P. C., Brackenbury, R., Mailhammer, R., Rutishauser, U., Cunningham, B. A., and Edelman, G. M., 1982, Chemical characterization of a neural cell adhesion molecule purified from embryonic brain membranes, *J. Biol. Chem.* **257**:7720–7729.

Huck, S., and Hatten, M. E., 1981, Developmental stage-specific changes in lectin binding to mouse cerebellar cells *in vitro, J. Neurosci.* **1**:1075–1084.

Kalish, F., Chovick, N., and Dice, J. F., 1979, Rapid *in vivo* degradation of glycoproteins isolated from cytosol, *J. Biol. Chem.* **254**:(11):4475–4481.

Karlsson, J. O., 1979, Proteins of axonal transport: Interaction of rapidly transported proteins with lectins, *J. Neurochem.* **32**:491–494.

Kelly, P. T., and Cotman, C. W., 1981, Developmental changes in morphology and molecular composition of isolated synaptic junctional structures, *Brain Res.* **206**:251–271.

Kinsey, W. H., and Lennarz, W. J., 1981, Isolation of a glycopeptide fraction from the surface of the sea urchin egg that inhibits sperm–egg binding and fertilization, *J. Cell Biol.* **91**:325–331.

Krusius, R., Finne, J., Karkkainen, J., and Jarnefelt, J., 1974, Neutral and acidic glycopeptides in adult and developing rat brain, *Biochim. Biophys. Acta* **365**:80–92.

Levin, B. E., 1977, Axonal transport of [^{3}H]fucosyl glycoproteins in noradrenergic neurons in the rat brain, *Brain Res.* **120**:421–432.

Marchisio, P. C., Sjostrand, J., Aglietta, M., and Karlsson, J.-O., 1973, The development of axonal transport of proteins and glycoproteins in the optic pathway of chick embryos, *Brain Res.* **63**:273–284.

Margolis, R. K., Preti, C., Lai, D., and Margolis, R. U., 1976, Developmental changes in brain glycoproteins, *Brain Res.* **112**:363–369.

Marko, P., and Cuenod, M., 1973, Contributions of the nerve cell body to renewal of axonal and synaptic glycoproteins in the pigeon visual system, *Brain Res.* **62**:419–423.

Markov, D., Rambourg, A., and Droz, B., 1976, Smooth endoplasmic reticulum and fast axonal transport of glycoproteins, an electron microscope radioautographic study of thic sections after heavy metals impregnation, *J. Microsc. Biol.* **25**:57–60.

Matthews, M. A., West, L. C., and Clarkson, D. B., 1982, Inhibition of axoplasmic transport in the developing visual system of the rat. II. Quantitative analysis of alterations in transport of tritiated proline or fucose, *Neuroscience* **7**:385–404.

Matthieu, J.-M., Webster, H. D., DeVries, G. H., Corthay, S., and Koellreutter, B., 1978, Glial versus neuronal origin of myelin proteins and glycoproteins studied by combined iontraocu-lar and intracranial labelling, *J. Neurochem.* **31**:93–102.

Maylie-Pfenninger, M.-F., and Jamieson, J. D., 1980, Development of cell surface saccharides on embryonic pancreatic cells, *J. Cell Biol.* **86**:96–103.

McLaughlin, B. J., and Wood, J. G., 1977, The localization of concanavalin A binding sites during photoreceptor synaptogenesis in the chick retina, *Brain Res.* **119**:57–71.

McLaughlin, B. J., Wood, J. G., and Gurd, J. W., 1980, The localization of lectin binding sites during photoreceptor synaptogenesis in the chick retina, *Brain Res.* **191**:345–357.

Milenkovic, A. G., and Johnson, T. C., 1980, The relationship between glycosylation and gly-coprotein metabolism of mouse neuroblastoma N18 cells, *Biochem. J.* **191**:21–28.

Mintz, G., Gottlieb, D. I., Reitman, M. L., Derby, M., and Glaser, L., 1981, Developmental changes in glycoproteins of the chick nervous system, *Brain Res.* **206**:51–70.

Muramatsu, T., Koide, N., Ceccarini, C., and Atkinson, P. M., 1976, Characterization of man-nose-labeled glycopeptides from human diploid cells and their growth-dependent alterations, *J. Biol. Chem.* **251**:(15):4673–4679.

Muramatsu, T., Gachelin, G., Nicholas, J. F., Condamine, H., Jakob, H., and Jakob, F., 1978, Carbohydrate structure and cell differentiation: Unique properties of fusocyl-glyco-peptides isolated from embryonal carcinoma cells, *Proc. Natl. Acad. Sci. U.S.A.* **75**:2315–2319.

Ocklind, C., Rubin, K., and Obrink, B., 1980, Different cell surface glycoproteins are involved in cell–cell and cell–collagen adhesion of rat hepatocytes, *FEBS Lett.* **121**:47–50.

Olden, K., Pratt, R., Jaworski, C., and Yamada, K., 1979, Evidence for role of glycoprotein carbohydrates in the membrane transport: Specific inhibition by tunicamycin, *Proc. Natl. Acad. Sci. U.S.A.* **76**:791–795.

Olden, K., Parent, J. B., and White, S. L., 1982, Carbohydrate moieties of glycoproteins. A reevaluation of their function, *Biochim. Biophys. Acta* **650**:209–232.

Padilla, S. S., and Morell, P., 1980, Axonal transport of [³H]fucose-labeled glycoproteins in two intra-brain tracts of the rat, *J. Neurochem.* **35**:444–450.

Pfenninger, K. H., and Maylie-Pfenninger, M.-F., 1981*a*, Lectin labeling of sprouting neurons. I. Regional distribution of surface glycoconjugates, *J. Cell Biol.* **89**:536–546.

Pfenninger, K. H., and Maylie-Pfenninger, M.-F., 1981*b*, Lectin labeling of sprouting neurons. II. Relative movement and appearance of glycoconjugates during plasmalemmal expansion, *J. Cell Biol.* **89**:547–559.

Pippia, P., Ivaldi, G., and Cogoli, A., 1980, Identification of carbohydrates and functional groups involved in the adhesion of neoplastic cells, *FEBS Lett.* **116**:281–284.

Reeber, A., Vincendon, G., and Zanetta, J.-P., 1980, Transient concanavalin A-binding glycopro-teins of the parallel fibres of the developing rat cerebellum: Evidence for the destruction of their glycans, *J. Neurochem.* **35**:1273–1277.

Roberson, M. M., and Armstrong, P. B., 1980, Carbohydrate-binding component of amphibian embryo cell surfaces: Restriction to surface regions capable of cell adhesion, *Proc. Natl. Acad. Sci. U.S.A.* **77**:3460–3463.

Rome, L., Weissman, B., and Neufeld, E., 1979, Direct demonstration of binding of a lysosomal enzyme, α-L-iduronidase, to receptors on cultured fibroblasts, *Proc. Natl. Acad. Sci. U.S.A.* **76**:2331–2334.

Rosen, S. D., Simpson, D. L., Rose, J. E., and Barondes, S. H., 1974, Carbohydrate-binding protein from *Polyspondylium pallidum* implicated in intercellular adhesion, *Nature* **252**:(128):149–150.

Rutishauser, U., Gall, W. E., and Edelman, G. M., 1978, Adhesion among neural cells of the chick embryo. IV. Role of the cell surface molecule cam in the formation of neurite bundles in cultures of spinal ganglia, *J. Cell Biol.* **79**:382–393.

Sjostrand, J., Karlsson, J. O., and Marchisio, P. C., 1973, Axonal transport in growing and mature retinal ganglion cells, *Brain Res.* **62**:395–397.

Skene, J. H. P., and Willard, M., 1981*a*, Characteristics of growth-associated polypeptides in regenerating toad retinal ganglion cell axons, *J. Neurosci.* **1**:419–426.

Skene, J. H. P., and Willard, M., 1981*b*, Electrophoretic analysis of axonally transported proteins in toad retinal ganglion cells, *J. Neurochem.* **37**:79–87.

Skutelsky, E., and Farquhar, M. G., 1976, Variations in distribution of Con A receptor sites and anionic groups during red blood cell differentiation in the rat, *J. Cell Biol.* **71**:218–231.

Sidman, C., 1981, Different requirements for glycosylation is determined neither by the producing cell nor by the relative number of oligosaccharide units, *J. Biol. Chem.* **256**:9374–9376.

Simpson, D. L., Thorne, D. R., and Loh, H. H., 1977, Developmentally regulated lectin in neonatal rat brain, *Nature* **266**:367–369.

Specht, S. C., 1982, Postnatal changes in [^{3}H]fucosyl glycopeptides of hamster optic nerve synaptosomal membrane, *Dev. Brain Res.* **4**:109–114.

Specht, S. C., and Grafstein, B., 1977, Axonal transport and transneuronal transfer in mouse visual system following injection of [^{3}H]fucose into the eye, *Exp. Neurol.* **54**:352–368.

Stone, G., and Hammerschlag, R., 1983, Glycosylation as a criterion for defining subpopulations of fast-transported proteins, *J. Neurochem.* **40**:1124–1133.

Tessler, A., Autilio-Gambetti, L., and Gambetti, P., 1980, Axonal growth during regeneration: A quantitative autoradiographic study, *J. Cell Biol.* **27**:197–203.

Thiery, J.-P., Brackenbury, R., Rutishauer, U., and Edelman G. M., 1977, Adhesion among neural cells of the chick embryo. II. Purification and characterization of a cell adhesion molecule from neural retina, *J. Biol. Chem.* **252**:(19):6841–6845.

Thompson, E. B., Schwartz, J. H., and Kandel, E. R., 1976, A radioautographic analysis in the light and electron microscope of identified *Aplysia* neurons and their processes after intrasomatic injection of L-[^{3}H]fucose, *Brain Res.* **112**:251–281.

Vacquier, V. D., and Moy, G. W., 1977, Isolation of Bindin: The protein responsible for adhesion of sperm to sea urchin eggs, *Proc. Natl. Acad. Sci. U.S.A.* **74**:2456–2460.

Varon, S., and Adler, R., 1981, Trophic and specifying factors directed to neuronal cells, *Adv. Cell Neurobiol.* **2**:115–163.

Vicker, M. G., 1976, BHK21 Fibroblast aggregation inhibited by glycopeptides from the cell surface, *J. Cell Sci.* **21**:161–173.

Walsh, F., and Phillips, E., 1981, Specific changes in cellular glycoproteins and surface proteins during myogenesis in clonal muscle cells, *Dev. Biol.* **81**:229–237.

Wenthold, R. J., and McGarvey, M. L., 1982, Different polypeptides are rapidly transported in auditory and optic neurons, *J. Neurochem.* **39**:27–35.

Wenzl, S., and Sumper, M., 1982, The occurrence of different sulphated cell surface glycoproteins correlates with defined developmental events in *Volvox, FEBS Lett.* **143**:311–315.

Whitnall, M. H., Currie, J. R., and Grafstein, B., 1982, Bidirectional axonal transport of glycoproteins in goldfish optic nerve, *Exp. Neurol.* **75**:191–207.

Zanetta, J.-P., Roussel, G., Ghandour, M. S., Vincendon, G., and Gombos, G., 1978, Postnatal development of rat cerebellum: Massive and transient accumulation of concanavalin A binding glycoproteins in parallel fiber axolemma, *Brain Res.* **142**:301–319.

Zieske, J., and Bernstein, I., 1982, Modification of cell surface glycoprotein: Addition of fucosyl residues during epidermal differentiation, *J. Cell Biol.* **95**:626–631.

CHAPTER 7

TRANSPORT OF TRANSMITTER-RELATED ENZYMES
Changes after Injury

DAVID B. MCDOUGAL, JR.

1. INTRODUCTION

Dramatic changes in the axonal transport of several enzymes involved in transmitter metabolism occur following axotomy (for an extensive review see Grafstein and Forman, 1980). Axonal transport of transmitter-related enzymes has generally been found to be reduced, as is nerve content of these enzymes. Similarly, the amount of enzyme activity present in the perikarya of the cells of origin of the damaged axons is decreased. As we shall see, there are exceptions to each of these statements. These changes are thought to reflect a change in emphasis in the neuronal economy from that of a functioning cell carrying out its essential role in the life of the organism to that of a convalescent invalid. Because the neuron has lost its efferent connections, the enzymes involved in transmitter metabolism are presumed to be, at least temporarily, useless, and

DAVID B. MCDOUGAL, JR. ● Department of Pharmacology, Washington University School of Medicine, St. Louis, Missouri 63110 the production of some of them in the perikaryon and their export from it are curtailed.

Information available on the extent of the changes and their timing leads to several questions that cannot be answered on the basis of the available data:

1. Is the decrease in nerve content merely a reflection of the decrease in axonal transport, or are content and transport regulated independently?
2. Is the decrease in axonal transport merely a reflection of decreases in perikaryal enzyme content, or are perikaryal enzyme levels and axonal transport regulated independently?
3. Is a decrease in axonal transport after injury unique to proteins involved primarily in synaptic function and therefore a characteristic by which such proteins may be recognized?

One aim of the present chapter is to describe, briefly, what is known of the responses of the axonal transport, nerve content, and perikaryal or nuclear content of transmitter-related enzymes to axonal injury and the methods used to achieve this knowledge. A second aim is to point out at least some of the reasons why a more comprehensive description of the relationships between axonal and perikaryal enzyme content and axonal enzyme transport implied in the questions listed above cannot yet be given. It is hoped that if these aims have been achieved in what follows, the way to experimental solutions of the problems will become clearer.

2. METHODS

Enzyme transport has been studied by measuring the accumulation of enzyme activity at a site of interruption of transport in a nerve or tract. The interruption is usually mechanical, a ligature, crush, or transection, but is occasionally thermal or chemical. The methods of determining transport rate have recently been reviewed (Brimijoin, 1982).

2.1. Single Ligation

The rate of accumulation of enzyme activity at a tie gives an estimate of the rate at which enzyme activity is leaving the cells of origin of the nerve or tract under study and of the rate at which the activity is being delivered to the axonal terminals. Various factors affect the accuracy of the estimate. Both the rate of delivery to the terminals and the rate at which the enzyme is leaving the perikaryon will be underestimated if turnaround at the site of injury is appreciable. Turnaround is defined as the reversal of direction of materials in transit at a site of axonal interruption. It has been observed to occur with enzymes (Partlow *et al.*, 1972; Schmidt *et al.*, 1980) and with radiolabeled proteins (Bray *et al.*, 1971; Bisby and Bulger, 1977). Because some enzymes, notably acetylcholinesterase (AChE), are also an integral part of the axolemma with a characteristic half-life (Brimijoin *et al.*, 1978; Schmidt *et al.*, 1980), resupply of axolemmal enzyme may result in overestimation of the amount of enzyme being delivered to the axonal terminals and underestimation of the amount leaving the perikaryon. This effect would be particularly large in long axons and would be expected to be greater the farther the site of enzyme accumulation was from the location of interest—cell body or axonal terminal.

If the amount of enzyme remaining in the nerve distal to and at some distance (3 mm or more) from the site of injury is measured, one obtains, by difference from control nerve, the amount of enzyme in orthograde motion. This difference is a true measure only if the activity is moving sufficiently rapidly to clear the segment before the sample is taken and before motion of the activity ceases for lack of energy or some other essential component.

From these data the transport rate can be calculated:

$$(\text{accumulation/unit time})/(\text{activity/mm nerve}) \times 1/\text{fraction in motion} = \text{mm/unit time}$$

The orthograde transport rate calculated in this manner may still be too slow because of turnaround.

Similar measurements of accumulation of activity distal to the site of injury enable calculation of the rate of retrograde transport. Turnaround of retrogradely transported material does not seem to occur (Schmidt *et al.*, 1980). The estimate can be improved, and the rate increased, if the fraction in retrograde motion can be determined.

2.2. Double Ligation

2.2.1. In Vivo

Two ties are applied to a nerve simultaneously, and accumulation of enzyme proximal to each tie is measured as a function of time. The proximal tie has a large supply of enzyme activity from the perikaryon; the distal tie has only the enzyme trapped between the ties. When accumulation proximal to the distal tie lags behind that proximal to the proximal tie and stops, the interligature supply of enzyme is presumed to be exhausted. The transport rate = length of nerve between ties (minus length of collection segment)/time to stop (clearance time). It is not clear why turnaround proximal to the distal tie has not been shown in such experiments. Were turnaround active, the apparent clearance time would be too short, and the calculated transport rate too fast. The method depends upon maintenance of viability of the transport system beyond the time needed to clear the axons of the enzymes in question. This is not a problem with substances in rapid transit but has been an insurmountable obstacle for materials moving by slow flow.

2.2.2. In Vitro

Double-tied nerve segments incubated *in vitro* have been used to obtain transport rates for enzymes located in several different classes of organelles and to establish the fact of turnaround (Partlow *et al.*, 1972; Schmidt *et al.*, 1980). The method has the same dependence on viability as the method of Section 2.2.1.

2.3 Stop-Flow

Blockade of axonal transport by local cooling (not freezing) has also been used to produce an accumulation of enzyme activity in nerve (Brimijoin, 1975). After rewarming, the orthograde or retrograde progress of the peak of activity along the nerve can be followed to give a direct measure of transport rates that appears to be unambiguous. This is particularly useful where determination of the fraction of enzyme activity in motion is difficult. Unfortunately, if cooling is continued for more than a few hours, damage to the nerve ensues. Therefore, if the amount of enzyme in motion is too small, or the rate at which it is moving is too slow, the accumulation of enzyme at the site of cooling in the allowable time will be too small to follow.

2.4. Effect of Injury

In the work reviewed below, the effect of prior, distal injury on the accumulation of enzyme activity per unit time at a (proximal) test site of axonal interruption is reported, often without calculating a transport rate in millimeters per hour or day. No apology need be made for such reporting, since the amount of enzyme activity arriving at a test site of interruption in a fixed time period and the way in which this amount changes as a function of time after injury are useful measures of the neuronal enzyme economy whatever the transit rate.

The injury used was most often a crush or ligation, but other injuries were studied. The changes seem to vary predictably with regard to severity of injury. Greater changes are seen after transection than after crush, for example. Problems in reaching firm conclusions are caused by discrepancies among the results obtained in the various studies, which are not easily explained.

3. "CHOLINERGIC" ENZYMES

3.1. Choline Acetyltransferase

3.1.1. Nerve Content

Nerve content is the same as "intrinsic activity," defined as all the activity in nerve, whether in axon or Schwann cell and whether stationary or in motion, at sufficient distance from any lesion to be unaffected by local changes (Schmidt and McDougal, 1978). It is usually expressed in units of enzyme activity per unit length of nerve, often in millimeters, occasionally kilometers. After injury to the nerve, the changes that may be seen are characteristic of the enzyme activity measured and perhaps the species of animal and the nerve in which the observations are made. In the case of choline acetyltransferase (ChAT), nerve content falls 35 to 50% within 1 or 2 weeks in mouse sciatic, rat sciatic, rabbit peroneal, and rabbit hypoglossal nerves (Jablecki and Brimijoin, 1975; Ranish *et al.,* 1979; Heiwall *et al.,*1979; O'Brien, 1978; Frizell and Sjöstrand, 1974). If no change in axoplasmic enzyme concentration occurs, a relatively small reduction in axon diameter (30% or so) proximal to the injury would result in a reduction in enzyme content of the magnitude observed. The decrease in axonal diameter reported by Aitken and Thomas (1962) was only 17%, but the first observation was made 100 days after injury. A more extensive report of the postinjury changes in axonal diameters is given in Chapter 14 of this book.

Confusingly, Heiwall *et al.* (1979) found a significant increase in the nerve content of enzyme activity during the first 3–5 days after injury, but Ranish *et al.*(1979) did not. The other investigators studying this enzyme did not look before 6 days. It is not clear how much ChAT activity is stationary, if any. Partlow *et al.* (1972) in frog and Jablecki and Brimijoin (1975) in mouse assume that all ChAT activity is in motion. Fonnum *et al.* (1973) conclude on the basis of their experiments that only 8 to 10% of the activity is in motion, but their experiments and conclusion appear to be based on the assumption that ChAT moves by rapid transport, which may not be so. At a time when axonal transport of the enzyme had essentially stopped in rabbit peroneal (13 days), nerve content was still nearly 40% of control (O'Brien, 1978). Perhaps this 40% represents stationary enzyme in this nerve, since the transport process itself was in good order as evidenced by the accumulation of

AChE. It is unfortunate that efforts to measure the rate of transport of this enzyme by stop-flow have been unsuccessful (Brimijoin, 1982). An independent measure of transport rate would enable calculation of the fraction of motion.

3.1.2. Axonal Transport

Investigators disagree regarding the response of ChAT transport to injury. In mouse, the amount of ChAT activity accumulating at a test tie on the sciatic nerve from 10 to 80 days after transection was equal to that in control nerves (Jablecki and Brimijoin, 1975). Because there was a fall in nerve enzyme content, and because it was assumed that all of the ChAT activity was in motion, the rate of transport was calculated to have doubled 10 and 20 days into the recovery period. In rabbit peroneal nerve, however, the amount of enzyme accumulating at a test tie was reduced to undetectable levels 13 days after crush, recovering to more than 50% of control after 51 days (O'Brien, 1978). Functional recovery, based on a nonquantitative test, was estimated to have occurred at 39 days. In rat sciatic nerve, there was a depression of transport of ChAT activity (similarly measured) at 11 days that was greater in cut or ligated nerves (75–80%) than in crushed or frozen nerves (35–50%) (Heiwall et al., 1979). The transport in these nerves had recovered to 75 or 80% of control at 21–29 days. Similarly, transport of ChAT activity was depressed 50% 1 week after crush of the rabbit hypoglossal nerve (Frizell and Sjöstrand, 1974). Recovery was complete at 4 weeks, but intermediate times were not tested.

Since there are gaps in some of the data, these reports may not be as discrepant as they seem. For example, it may be that at 2 weeks or so transport of ChAT fails in rabbit hypoglossal nerve, as it appears to do in rabbit peroneal nerve. If events proceed more rapidly in mouse than in rat or rabbit, it may be that an early fall in ChAT transport was missed by choosing 10 days as the first time after injury at which to make an assessment in mouse. However, in rabbit peroneal nerve, the time courses of the changes in nerve content and axonal transport were very similar (O'Brien, 1978), although the magnitudes of the changes were quite different. Since the time course of the changes in nerve enzyme content in mouse sciatic nerve parallels that in rabbit peroneal, it is perhaps more likely that there is indeed a fundamental difference between the axonal transport of ChAT in mouse and that in rabbit and rat. Therefore, the response of ChAT transport to injury in peripheral nerve may in fact vary from species to species and even from nerve to nerve. It appears that further experiments would be justified.

3.1.3. Cells of Origin

In order to understand the changes following axotomy, it is useful to review what is known of the economy of enzyme production and distribution in the normal neuron. These have been studied in only a few instances where anatomic arrangements are particularly favorable.

Choline acetyltransferase has been studied most comprehensively, for present purposes, in the tongue, hypoglossal nucleus, and nerve of the rabbit. Fonnum *et al.* (1973) estimated that of the total enzyme activity in the system (5.5 μmol/hr), only 2% was in the 2 hypoglossal nuclei, 42% was in the nerves, and the remainder (56%) was in the fine intramuscular nerve branches and axon terminals in the tongue. From measurements of the accumulation of ChAT activity at a tie on the hypoglossal nerve, it was estimated that 49 nmol/ hr of enzyme activity were exported from one nucleus each day, a little more than the nuclear content. From this it was calculated that the half-life of the enzyme in the tongue was 16–21 days.

Fonnum *et al.* (1973) showed that ChAT activity in the hypoglossal nucleus fell 60% in the 2 weeks after transection of the hypoglossal nerve. On the basis of experimental evidence and assumptions that appear reasonable, they suggest that perhaps all of the enzyme in the hypoglossal neurons had disappeared at 2 weeks. It is unfortunate that the experiments of Frizell and Sjöstrand (1974) on axonal transport of ChAT were not better correlated with their earlier experiments with Fonnum (Fonnum *et al.*, 1973). In the 1973 study, the nerve was injured by transection, and the first postinjury time studied was 2 weeks. In the 1974 study, the nerve was crushed, and the first postinjury time was 1 week. The nerve was not studied 2 weeks after injury. Therefore, even the simplest sort of correlation between nuclear enzyme content and axonal enzyme transport cannot be attempted.

3.2. Acetylcholinesterase

3.2.1. Nerve Content

The intrinsic AChE activity decreases after injury in frog, rat, and rabbit nerves (Carlsen *et al.*, 1982; Sinicropi *et al.*, 1982; Ranish *et al.*, 1979; Heiwall *et al.*, 1979; Frizell and Sjöstrand, 1974; O'Brien, 1978). In rabbit peroneal nerve, 75% of the enzyme content remains at 2 weeks, and 50% at 50 days (O'Brien, 1978). In rat sciatic nerve, Ranish *et al.* (1979) observed an increase (40%) during the first 2 or 3 days after injury, with a subsequent decrease. Heiwall *et al.* (1979), working on the same preparation, did not observe the early increase. The reason for the discrepancy is not clear. In frog, activity in ventral roots dropped to 80% of control at 20 days and to 65% of control at 35 days. The decrease in nerve content must have been substantial. However, because the sample included the site of injury, the time of onset of the decrease and its magnitude cannot be determined from the data (Sinicropi *et al.,* 1982). Since it appears that 25% or less of the AChE activity is in rapid motion in the nerves of frog, rabbit, rat, and chicken (Partlow *et al.,* 1972; Fonnum *et al.,* 1973; Schmidt *et al.,* 1980; Couraud and diGiambardino, 1980), the changes observed in nerve enzyme content are not fully accounted for by changes in the amount of activity in motion (see below). A reduction in axonal diameter (Aitken and Thomas, 1962; Chapter 14, this volume) might help in the accounting if the concentration of AChE activity in axolemma remained unchanged or was decreased.

3.2.2. Axonal Transport

The effect of injury on the amount of AChE activity in motion is profound. Schmidt and McDougal (1978) reported that after nerve crush, transport of AChE activity in rat sciatic nerve was maintained at control levels for 24 hr and then fell to 40% of control at 48 hr. Heiwall *et al.* (1979) reported a 30– 50% decrease in transported activity 1 day after various sorts of injury in rat sciatic. It is not clear why the results obtained by these two groups in the same animal are not in better agreement. At 6–8 days, accumulation at a test tie was only 20–25% of control in rat sciatic nerve (Schmidt and McDougal, 1978; Heiwell *et al.,* 1979) and rabbit peroneal nerve (O'Brien, 1978) and 50% in rabbit hypoglossal nerve (Frizell and Sjöstrand, 1974). There appears to be a significant difference in the magnitude of the decrease in axonal transport of AChE in the two rabbit nerves, hypoglossal and peroneal. O'Brien (1978) found recovery to 44% of control by 13 days and to 60–70% at 51 days in rabbit peroneal nerve.

3.2.3. Cells of Origin

A detailed examination of AChE activity in cell bodies of rat hypoglossal neurons after axonal injury (nerve crush) was undertaken by Watson (1966). He found a decrease in activity starting 4 days after injury. By 8 to 11 days, neuronal AChE activity had fallen to 40% of control. Recovery to control levels appeared to be complete in about 3 weeks. As in frog spinal motor neurons (Sinicropi *et al.,* 1982; see below), there was no evidence for an increase in neuronal AChE levels at any time after axotomy. When the whole hypoglossal nucleus was examined in rabbit, AChE activity fell to 60% of control at 2 weeks and was equally depressed at 4 weeks after nerve section (Fonnum *et al.,* 1973). The discrepancy between these results and those of Watson (1966) may depend on the difference in method of nerve injury or in species of animal or on the inclusion of sources of enzyme activity in whole nucleus that are not present in single cells.

Sinicropi *et al.* (1982) showed that in frog, the amount of AChE activity that was delivered to ventral roots 9 and 10 each day was 0.7 to 2 times the amount contained in the appropriate number of motor neuronal perikarya isolated from spinal cord. The sciatic nerve and roots together were shown to contain about 14 times as much AChE activity as contained in the perikarya of the neurons of origin. No estimate of the intramuscular content of AChE activity of neural origin was attempted, doubtless because neuronal and muscular AChEs cannot yet be assayed separately in whole tissue containing both enzymes. After injury to their axons, AChE activity in the perikarya was maintained at control levels for 2 or 3 days. At 20 days, a 27% decrease in activity was observed (Sinicropi *et al.*, 1982). Again, because of problems with sampling times and, in addition, differences in species used for observations in nerve and neurons of origin, the contribution of changes in perikaryal enzyme activity to enzyme content or transport in nerve cannot be assessed.

The experiments of Sinicropi *et al.* (1982) were undertaken in part to discover whether an increase in neuronal AChE activity would occur as a result of premature return of the enzyme to the perikaryon from the site of injury. The expectation appears to be based on a misunderstanding of the results of experiments using radiolabeled amino acids and is worthy of comment.

When proteins or other substances are pulse-labeled in the cells of origin and transported "down" the nerve, proteins traveling at the same rate in different axons will pass any point on the nerve in approximate synchrony. However, when the proteins return from the periphery, unless all the axons in the nerve are the same length, the distances that the proteins have traveled, and hence the times taken for them to return to a test tie, will be longer for long axons than for short ones. Consequently, the returning labeled proteins will be distributed in a low peak, broadly distributed in time or distance, and the fraction of the total returning protein collected by a tie briefly applied will be relatively small. However, when a nerve is crushed, the experimenter has assumed the role of Procrustes: he has shortened the extremities of all the neurons in the nerve to fit the same bed. Therefore, the return of labeled materials after turnaround in the periphery (now the crush site) has been synchronized, the peak of returning protein has been sharpened, and larger amounts of label appear at the test tie in a short time (Bisby and Bulger, 1977). This is a problem only for pulse-labeled materials and hence does not occur in measurements of enzyme activity, which depend on a marker that is in a steady state of transport. It should be noted that this argument does not eliminate the possibility that injured axons return more transported materials by turnaround than do normal ones. But it does demonstrate that the question cannot be asked by monitoring pulse-labeled material in a nerve whose axons in the uninjured state are not all of approximately the same length. For AChE transport, insofar as the experiments of Watson (1966) and Sinicropi *et al.* (1982) are a test of this question, the results suggest that injured axons do not return more transported enzyme than do uninjured axons.

4. ADRENERGIC ENZYMES

Studies of the responses of these enzymes to axonal injury have taken quite a different form from the studies of the cholinergic enzymes. There are no published studies of nerve enzyme content and only a few of axonal transport, but there are many of nuclear and ganglionic enzyme content.

4.1. Cells of Origin

The levels of both tyrosine hydroxylase (TOH) and dopamine-β-hydroxylase (DβH) rose 50% in locus coeruleus 2 days after an electrolytic lesion in the posterolateral hypothalamus interrupting the dorsal ascending adrenergic bundle (Ross *et al.*, 1975). At the end of a week, both enzymes had fallen below 75% of control, and at the end of 2 weeks, they were near 50% of control. Recovery was relatively prompt. Levin (1981) also found an early rise in both enzymes after a selective lesion to the bundle by 6-hydroxydopamine.

The response of peripheral autonomic ganglia to nerve injury is quite different. There was no increase in either enzyme in stellate ganglion after systemic injection of 6-hydroxydopamine (Brimijoin and Molinoff, 1971) but instead a prompt decrease in DβH, which lasted at least 7 days. The decrease in TOH activity was much smaller. Activities of both enzymes were elevated after treatment with reserpine, but these elevations were blocked by pretreatment with 6-hydroxydopamine. Cheah and Geffen (1973) found a more substantial fall in the TOH levels in lumbar sympathetic ganglia after sciatic ligation. It seems likely that the difference reflects a difference in the severity of the two types of injury.

4.2. Axonal Transport

Wooten and Coyle (1973) calculated orthograde rates of 138–185 mm/day for DβH and 106–167 mm/day for TOH in uninjured rat sciatic nerve, corrected for fraction in motion, 26% for TOH and 33% for DβH. Using cold block followed by rewarming (stop flow), Brimijoin and Wiermaa (1977) found a rate of 336 mm/day for DβH in rabbit sciatic nerve, suggesting that the fraction in motion for DβH found by Wooten and Coyle (1973) may have been too large. A small amount of TOH was found to progress at the same rate, but the bulk of the enzyme traveled more slowly (120 mm/day). Wooten and Coyle (1973) found a decrease in the calculated rate of axoplasmic transport of 52% for TOH and 65% for DβH in sciatic nerve 2 days after ligation injury. The data presented make it unclear whether the decreases in calculated rate were produced by decreases in the amount of enzyme traveling at normal rates or by normal amounts of enzyme activity traveling at reduced rates.

Similarly, 3 days after rat sciatic nerves were injured by ligation, accumulation of DβH activity proximal to a test tie was decreased 70% (R. E. Schmidt, personal communication). At the same time, nerve content of the enzyme activity was reduced 30%. Seventeen hours after parenteral 6-hydroxy-dopamine R. E. Schmidt (personal communication) found no change in the amount of activity accumulating at a test tie on rat sciatic nerve, but after 3 days, the 12-hr accumulation proximal to the test tie was only 50% of control.

It is apparent that these studies represent only a beginning and that an examination of the full time course of changes both of axonal enzyme content and transport and of ganglionic enzyme content is required before the relationships between them can be ascertained.

5. OTHER ENZYMES

Cheah and Geffen (1973) found a 30% decrease in monoamine oxidase activity in rat lumbar sympathetic ganglia at 3 and 7 days after injury and 40% at 2 weeks. But no change was found in the proximal or distal accumulation of this enzyme at a test tie on rat sciatic nerve as a function of time after injury (Schmidt and McDougal, 1978), nor was there a change in the accumulation of another mitochondrial enzyme, glutamic acid dehydrogenase. At least two-thirds of the monoamine oxidase activity in motion in rat sciatic nerve is in sympathetic axons (Schmidt *et al.*, 1978), but only one-third of the glutamic acid dehydrogenase in transit is in these axons (McDougal *et al.*, 1983).

There was a decrease in the accumulation of acid phosphatase activity at a test tie after injury to rat sciatic nerve, however (Schmidt and McDougal, 1978). This was somewhat puzzling, since histochemical studies had suggested an increase in the activity of lysosomal acid phosphatase in the perikarya of axotomized neurons (Bodian and Mellors, 1945; Cerf and Chacko, 1958; Barron and Tuncbay, 1964; Holtzman *et al.*, 1967). More recently, we have devised analytical methods that enable quantitation of several different acid phosphatase activities in homogenates of whole tissue (Schmidt *et al.*, 1980; McDougal *et al.*, 1981). The presumptive lysosomal enzyme activity, isolated analytically by tartrate inhibition, accounts for 25 to 30% of the fluoride-inhibitable acid phosphatase activity in motion (McDougal *et al.*, 1983).

At least 70% of the remaining fluoride-inhibitable acid phosphatase activity in motion in rat sciatic nerve (resistant to inhibition by tartrate) travels in the axons of capsaicin-sensitive neurons (McDougal *et al.*, 1983). These are small dorsal root ganglion cells that appear to be chemogenic nociceptors (Jancsó *et al.*, 1977). Their central processes contain the so-called fluoride-resistant acid phosphatase activity (FRAP) that has been demonstrated histochemically in the substantia gelatinosa Rolandi (Coimbra *et al.*, 1970; Knyihár and Gerebtzoff, 1973; Jancsó and Knyihár, 1975). The activity of the histochemically demonstrated fluoride-resistant acid phosphatase is probably measured in our assay as tartrate-resistant acid phosphatase (McDougal *et al.*, 1983; D. B. McDougal, Jr. and E. M. Johnson, unpublished data). Preliminary experiments suggest that it is reduction in the activity of the tartrate-resistant acid phosphatase that is responsible for the decrease seen earlier with the non-discriminative assay (Schmidt and McDougal, 1978). Three days after an injury, accumulation of tartrate-resistant acid phosphatase activity proximal to a 12-hr test tie was reduced 68%. Accumulation of the tartrate-sensitive activity was only slightly reduced if at all (D. B. McDougal, Jr. and R. E. Schmidt, unpublished data).

6. CONCLUSIONS

It is clear that in order to answer the first two of the questions with which this chapter began much work is still necessary. The relationships for a given enzyme of the three variables, nerve content, perikaryal content, and axonal transport, must be examined as a function of time after injury in the same system. It may be that comparing two or more neuronal systems with respect to the same enzyme (for example, mouse sciatic *vs.* rat sciatic nerves; hypoglossal *vs.* peroneal nerve, both in rabbit) may give insights that examination of a single system would not. It seems likely that techniques other than simple enzyme activity assays will be required. For example, only by a combination of radioactive labeling in the cells of origin with immunoprecipitation in the nerve does it seem likely that an unequivocal answer to the question of the rate of transport of ChAT will be obtained. Similar methods will be needed to discover how an enzyme in transit is used to replenish stationary activity as, for example, in the case of AChE.

Finally, the behavior of the tartrate-resistant acid phosphatase after injury raises the third question that was presented at the beginning. From its histochemically defined location, the tartrate-resistant acid phosphatase may well have a synaptic function (Knyihár and Gerebtzoff, 1973). Its axoplasmic transport appears to be greatly depressed after injury. If, as has been suggested several times, transport of transmitter-related enzymes is depressed after injury because they have no function until recovery is completed, it could be that the synthesis and transport of other proteins involved primarily in synaptic function will also be depressed while the synapse is disabled. It might, then, be possible that a depression of transport of a protein after injury could serve to identify that protein as being primarily involved in synaptic function.

ACKNOWLEDGMENTS

I thank Dr. E. M. Johnson for stimulating discussions and helpful criticisms.

7. REFERENCES

Aitken, J. T., and Thomas, P. K., 1962, Retrograde changes in fibre size following nerve section, *J. Anat. (Lond.)* **96**:121–129.
Barron, K. D., and Tuncbay, T. O., 1964, Phosphatase histochemistry of feline cervical spinal cord after brachial plexectomy, *J. Neuropathol. Exp. Neurol.* **23**:368–386.
Bisby, M. A., and Bulger, V. T., 1977, Reversal of axonal transport at a nerve crush, *J. Neurochem.* **29**:313–320.
Bodian, D., and Mellors, R. C., 1945, The regenerative cycle of motoneurons, with special reference to phosphatase activity, *J. Exp. Med.* **81**:469–488.
Bray, J. J., Kon, C. M., and Breckenridge, B. McL., 1971, Reversed polarity of rapid axonal transport in chicken motoneurons, *Brain Res.* **33**:560–564.
Brimijoin, S., 1975, Stop-flow: A new technique for measuring axonal transport, and its application to the transport of dopamine-β-hydroxylase, *J. Neurobiol.* **6**:379–394.
Brimijoin, S., 1982, Axonal transport in autonomic nerves: Views on its kinetics, in: *Trends in Autonomic Pharmacology*, Volume 2 (S. Kalsner, ed.), pp. 17–42, Urban & Schwarzenberg, Munich, Baltimore.
Brimijoin, S., and Molinoff, P. B., 1971, Effects of 6-hydroxydopamine on the activity of tyrosine hydroxylase and dopamine-β-hydroxlase in sympathetic ganglia of the rat, *J. Phamacol. Exp. Ther.* **178**:417–424.
Brimijoin, S., and Wiermaa, M. J., 1977, Rapid axonal transport of tyrosine hydroxylase in rabbit sciatic nerves, *Brain Res.* **120**:77–96.
Brimijoin, S., Skau, K., and Wiermaa, M. J., 1978, On the origin and fate of external acetylcholine esterase in peripheral nerve, *J. Physiol. (Lond.)* **285**:143–158.
Carlsen, R. C., Kiff, J., and Ryugo, K., 1982, Suppression of the cell body response in axotomized frog spinal neurons does not prevent initiation of nerve regeneration, *Brain Res.* **234**:11–25.
Cerf, J. A., and Chacko, L. W., 1958, Retrograde reaction in motoneuron dendrites following ventral root section in the frog, *J. Comp. Neurol.* **109**:205–216.
Cheah, T. B., and Geffen, L. B., 1973, Effects of axonal injury on norepinephrine, tyrosine hydroxylase and monoamine oxidase levels in sympathetic ganglia, *J. Neurobiol.* **4**:443–452.
Coimbra, A., Magalhães, M. M., and Sodré-Borges, B. P., 1970, Ultrastructural localization of acid phosphatase in synapatic terminals of the rat substantia gelatinosa Rolandi, *Brain Res.* **22**:142–146.
Couraud, J. Y., and DiGiamberardino, L., 1980, Axonal transport of molecular forms of acetylcholinesterase in chick sciatic nerve, *J. Neurochem.* **35**:1055–1066.

Fonnum, F., Frizell, M., and Sjöstrand, J., 1973, Transport, turnover and distribution of choline acetyltransferase and acetylcholinesterase in the vagus and hypoglossal nerves of the rabbit, *J. Neurochem.* **21**:1109–1120.

Frizell, M., and Sjöstrand, J., 1974, Transport of proteins, glycoproteins and cholinergic enzymes in regenerating hypoglossal neurons, *J. Neurochem.* **22**:845–850.

Grafstein, B., and Forman, D. S., 1980, Intracellular transport in neurons, *Physiol. Rev.* **60**:1167–1283.

Heiwall, P.-O., Dahlström, A., Larsson, P.-A., and Bööj, S., 1979, The intra-axonal transport of acetylcholine and cholinergic enzymes in rat sciatic nerve during regeneration after various types of axonal trauma, *J. Neurobiol.* **10**:119–136.

Holtzman, E., Novikoff, A. B., and Villaverde, H., 1967, Lysosomes and GERL in normal and chromatolytic neurons of the rat ganglion nodosum, *J. Cell Biol.* **33**: 419–435.

Jablecki, C., and Brimijoin, S., 1975, Axoplasmic transport of choline acetyltransferase activity in mice: Effect of age and neurotomy, *J. Neurochem.* **25**:583–593.

Jancsó, G., and Knyihár, E., 1975, Functional linkage between nociception and fluoride-resistant acid phosphatase activity in the Rolando substance, *Neurobiology* **5**:42–43.

Jancsó, G., Kiraly, E., and Jancsó-Gábor, A., 1977, Pharmacologically induced selective degeneration of chemosensitive primary sensory neurons, *Nature* **270**:741–743.

Knyihár, E., and Gerebtzoff, M. A., 1973, Extra-lysosomal localization of acid phosphatase in the spinal cord of the rat, *Exp. Brain Res.* **18**:383–395.

Levin, B. E., 1981, Reserpine effect on the axonal transport of dopamine-β-hydroxylase and tryosine hydroxylase in rat brain, *Exp. Neurol.* **72**:99–112.

McDougal, D. B., Jr., Yuan, M. J. C., Dargar, R. V., and Johnson, E. M., Jr., 1983, Neonatal capsaicin and guanethidine and axonally transported organelle-specific enzymes in sciatic nerves and in sympathetic and dorsal root ganglia, *J. Neurosci.* **3**:124–132.

O'Brien, R. A. D., 1978, Axonal transport of acetylcholine, choline acetyltransferase and cholinesterase in regenerating peripheral nerve, *J. Physiol. (Lond.)* **282**:91–103.

Partlow, L. M., Ross, C. D., Motwani, R., and McDougal, D. B., Jr., 1972, Transport of axonal enzymes in surviving segments of frog sciatic nerve, *J. Gen. Physiol.* **60**:388–405.

Ranish, N. A., Kiauta, T., and Dettbarn, W.-D., 1979, Axotomy induced changes in cholinergic enzymes in rat nerve and muscles, *J. Neurochem.* **32**:1157–1164.

Ross, R.A., Joh, T. H., and Reis, D. J., 1975, Reversible changes in the accumulation and activities of tyrosine hydroxylase and dopamine-β-hydroxylase in neurons of nucleus locus coeruleus during the retrograde reaction, *Brain Res.* **92**:57–72.

Schmidt, R. E., and McDougal, D. B., Jr., 1978, Axonal transport of selected particle-specific enzymes in rat sciatic nerve *in vivo* and its response to injury, *J. Neurochem.* **30**:527–535.

Schmidt, R. E., Ross, C. D., and McDougal, D. B., Jr., 1978, Effects of sympathectomy on axoplasmic transport of selected enzymes including MAO and other mitochondrial enzymes, *J. Neurochem.* **30**:537–541.

Schmidt, R. E., Yu, M. J. C., and McDougal, D. B., Jr., 1980, Turnaround of axoplasmic transport of selected particle-specific enzymes at an injury in control and diisopropylphosphorofluoridate-treated rats, *J. Neurochem.* **35**:641–652.

Sinicropi, D. V., Michels, K., and McIlwain, D. L., 1982, Acetylcholinesterase distribution in axotomized frog motoneurons, *J. Neurochem.* **38**:1099–1105.

Watson, W. E., 1966, Quantitative observations upon acetylcholine hydrolase activity of nerve cells after axotomy, *J. Neurochem.* **13**:1549–1550.

Wooten, G. F., and Coyle, J. T., 1973, Axonal transport of catecholamine synthesizing and metabolizing enzymes, *J. Neurochem.* **20**:1361–1371.

CHAPTER 8

TRANSFER-RNA-MEDIATED POSTTRANSLATIONAL AMINOACYLATION OF PROTEINS IN AXONS

N. A. INGOGLIA, M. F. ZANAKIS, and
G. CHAKRABORTY

1. INTRODUCTION

Successful regeneration requires a neuron to accomplish a complex series of biochemical steps, few of which are well understood. One metabolic event that has been studied in some depth and is the subject of a good portion of this text is the change in the types of molecules the soma exports into the growing axon during regeneration. In general, attention has been directed towards the proteins that are transported axonally in regenerating axons, but several years ago

N. A. INGOGLIA, M. F. ZANAKIS, and G. CHAKRABORTY ● *Department of Physiology, University of Medicine and Dentistry of New Jersey, New Jersey Medical School, Newark, New Jersey 07103*

we found that 4 S (later shown to be transfer) RNA was transported axonally in large amounts during regeneration of the optic nerve of goldfish (reviewed by Ingoglia and Zanakis, 1982). The function of this lone species of RNA found in growing axons as well as in axonal growth cones (Gambetti *et al.,* 1978) has been difficult to understand, especially since axons are likely to be incapable of protein synthesis. However, as early as 1971, it was suggested that although protein synthesis probably does not occur in axons, it might be that protein modification by amino acid addition was occurring (Droz and Koenig, 1971). It was proposed that this might be responsible for the observation of a low level of incorporation of [^{3}H]amino acids into proteins in synaptosomes.

We have been investigating this possibility over the past several years and, using axoplasm isolated form the giant axon of the squid, have found evidence that the axoplasm does contain the elements necessary for the addition of a variety of amino acids to endogenous axonal proteins. This reaction appears to be dependent on the presence of transfer RNA and is not confined to squid axons but occurs in axons of higher vertebrates as well. Thus, the evidence leads us to conclude that a function of transfer RNA in axons in general, and particularly during nerve regeneration, is to serve as an amino acid donor in a reaction involving the posttranslational addition of amino acids to endogenous proteins. The evidence supporting the presence of tRNA in regenerating axons and its role in posttranslational protein modification is the subject of this chapter.

2. RNA IS PRESENT IN AXONS

It is clear that a large portion of the proteins required by the axon are synthesized in the neuron soma and delivered to the axon by axonal transport (reviewed by Grafstein and Forman, 1980). An alternate view of axonal metabolism is that although much of the protein requirement of axons is met by axonal transport, a significant portion of the proteins can be synthesized within the axon itself (see for example, Koenig, 1979). For the latter view to be tenable, it is necessary to demonstrate the presence of RNA in axoplasm. The concept of local protein synthesis in axons is not easily reconcilable with the morphological observations of a lack of ribosomes beyond the initial segment of the axon (Peters *et al.,* 1976). However, a variety of studies have reported the presence of RNA in axons of invertebrate (Anderson *et al.,* 1970; Lasek, 1970) and vertebrate (Koenig, 1965; Hartmann *et al.,* 1968) neurons.

The most unequivocal evidence for an axonal locus of RNA can be obtained using invertebrate giant axons. These axons, the giant axon of the squid stellate nerve and the median giant axon of the sea worm, *Myxicola,* are large enough so that axoplasm can be obtained from them without contamination from surrounding cells. When this axoplasm was analyzed for nucleic acids, it was found that it contained a significant amount of extramitochondrial RNA (Lasek, 1970; Lasek *et al.,* 1973). What was even more important was the finding that this RNA was at least 85%, and perhaps exclusively, 4 S RNA, (Figure 1). More recently this study has been repeated, and although evidence is presented for trace amounts of high-molecular-weight RNA in squid axoplasm, the vast majority of the RNA was verified as 4 S (Giuditta *et al.,* 1980). Thus, it seems clear that RNA is present in axoplasm of squid and *Myxicola* nerves and that the predominant if not the only species present is 4 S RNA.

The principal difficulty in establishing the presence of 4 S RNA in ver-

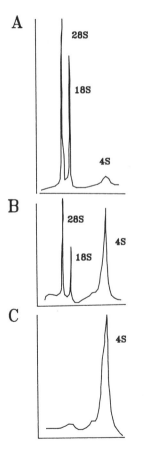

FIGURE 1. Optical density tracings of electrophoretic profile of RNA extracted from (A) squid ganglia, (B) squid giant axons (containing axoplasm and adaxonal glia), and (C) axoplasm obtained from the giant axon. Analyses were performed on SDS polyacrylamide (2% acrylamide, 1% agarose) gels for 150 min at 50 V. Note the typical profile for RNA in cells in A (10–15% of the total RNA is 4 S), the disproportionate amount of 4 S RNA in B (the sample contains large amounts of axoplasm and small amounts of cellular material), and the presence of only 4 S RNA and no high-molecular-weight RNA in C (containing only axoplasm). Electrophoresis is from left to right, and the ordinate represents optical density at 260 nm. (Modified from Lasek *et al.,* 1973.)

tebrate nerves has been that direct analysis of the content of axons has been technically impossible because of their small size and close physical association with supporting cells. One way to circumvent these problems is to use isotopic tracer techniques to label intraaxonal molecules but not those in surrounding cells. This technique is routinely used to differentiate axonally transported proteins from those synthesized in cells surrounding the axon, since the introduction of labeled amino acids to neuronal cell bodies labels proteins in axons but not in surrounding cells (reviewed by Grafstein and Forman, 1980). The difficulty in applying this technique to the study of intraaxonal RNA is that when [³H]RNA precursors are administered to a neuronal cell body, the precursor rapidly migrates down the axon and is transferred out of the axon to surrounding cells (reviewed by Ingoglia *et al.*, 1982a). These cells then utilize labeled precursors in the synthesis of nucleic acids (Figure 2). Thus, any attempt to identify labeled RNA in the axon necessarily identifies to a large extent [³H]RNA synthesized in cells surrounding the axon and not only axonal RNA. This problem has led to misinterpretation of data in some of the earlier experiments and resulted in the erroneous conclusion that all molecular species of RNA are transported axonally in vertebrate axons (reviewed by Ingoglia and Zanakis, 1982).

    We began to study the phenomenon of RNA transport in the visual system of goldfish utilizing [³H]uridine and [³H]adenosine, but in our first series of experiments, we were also not able to distinguish convincingly between the synthesis of [³H]RNA by glial cells surrounding the axons and [³H]RNA that might be intraaxonal and axonally transported. In subsequent experiments, we decided to examine the phenomenon during regeneration of the optic nerve of goldfish to see if this change in the functional state of the axon resulted in any changes in the characteristics of putative RNA transport.

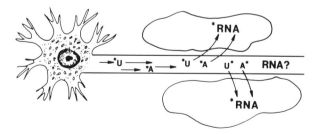

FIGURE 2. Schematic representation of the axonal transport and transcellular transfer of RNA precursors in vertebrate neurons. These labeled precursors are used for RNA synthesis by cells surrounding the axon.

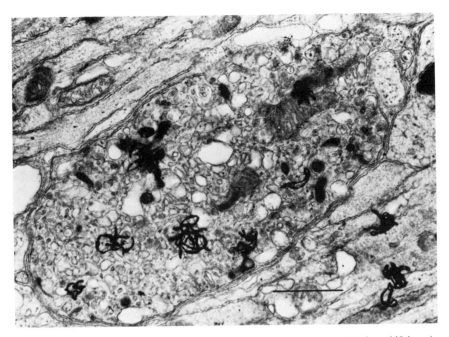

FIGURE 3. Electron microscopic autoradiogram of an axonal growth cone in the goldfish optic tectum 24 days after crushing of the optic nerve and 6 days following the intraocular injection of [³H]uridine. Note the presence of several reduced silver grains (RNA) in the growth cone. Bar, 1 μm. (Reproduced from Gambetti *et al.,* 1978.)

The changes we observed were so startling and so consistent that they led us to a series of experiments spanning the subsequent 8–10 years. The finding was that the amount of ³H radioactivity transported as [³H]nucleotides and presumptive [³H]RNA was increased 10–15 times as the nerve was regenerating when compared with intact controls (Ingoglia *et al.,* 1975). Also, light autoradiographic examination of the optic tectum showed the presence of reduced silver grains in areas of the tectum containing regenerating optic axons. The linear distribution of the grains in this region strongly suggested an intraaxonal locus for some of the radioactivity. This suggestion was borne out several years later in a collaborative electron microscopic autoradiographic study (EMAR) with the laboratory of Pierluigi Gambetti. These experiments unequivocally demonstrated the presence of silver grains within regenerating axons including axonal growth cones (Gambetti *et al.,* 1978) (Figure 3). Free nucleotides were removed from the tissue prior to microscopy, and SDS-PAGE showed the remaining activity to be in [³H]RNA. Several other experiments ruled out a mitochondrial or glial site of synthesis of axonal RNA. We concluded that the radioactivity localized in axons was in RNA whose origin must have been the cell body of the retinal ganglion cell.

Thus, we arrived at a model for the axonal transport of RNA in regenerating optic nerves of goldfish (Figure 4).

3.   RNA IN AXONS IS 4 S RNA

While the experiments cited above provided evidence that RNA was contained within regenerating optic axons of goldfish, they shed no light on the possible species of RNA present. However, these experiments did confirm observations made previously (Ingoglia *et al.,* 1975) that whereas intraocular injections of [³H]uridine resulted in [³H]RNA in both glia and axons, intracranial injections of [³H]uridine led to [³H]RNA localized only over glia (Gambetti *et al.,* 1978). Using this information, we designed experiments in which [³H]uridine was injected either intraocularly or intracranially and [³H]RNA in the tectum was analyzed using SDS-PAGE.

Results showed a striking difference in radioactivity profiles when only glia were labeled compared with those obtained when both regenerating axons and glia were labeled (Figure 5). The profile for glial cell labeling (5B) was similar to the labeling pattern of retinal RNA (5A). However, in experiments in which both axons and glia were labeled, we found inordinately large 4 S RNA peaks (5C, D). We reasoned that the excess [³H]4 S RNA (shaded areas, Figure 5C, D) was likely to have originated from the regenerating axons, whereas the other molecular RNA species represented all species of [³H]RNA synthesized by cells surrounding the axon (Ingoglia and Tuliszewski, 1976; Ingoglia, 1979). Thus, we concluded that although all molecular species of RNA could be synthesized by glia using [³H]nucleotides derived by axonal transport, only 4 S RNA was undergoing axonal transport. This conclusion has withstood several experimental tests (Ingoglia, 1979, 1982) and appears to be as unequivocal as one can be using indirect measurement techniques. It is fur-

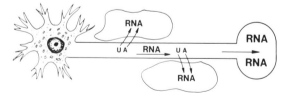

FIGURE 4. Schematic representation of the axonal transport of RNA and RNA precursors in regenerating optic axons of goldfish. As in intact axons (see Figure 2), RNA precursors are transported and transferred to periaxonal cells, where they are used for RNA synthesis. However, these regenerating axons also transport large amounts of RNA that remains intraaxonal.

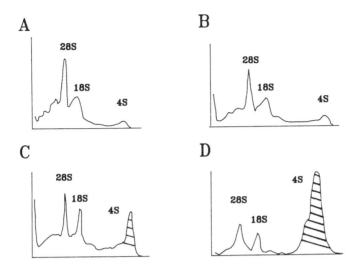

FIGURE 5. Analysis by SDS-PAGE on 2.0% gels of radioactive RNA in (A) goldfish retinas 1 day after the intraocular injection of [³H]uridine, (B) goldfish optic tecta 1 day after intracranial injection of [³H]uridine, (C) goldfish optic tecta 6 days after intraocular injection of [³H]uridine and 24 days after crushing of the optic nerves, and (D) goldfish optic tecta 12 days after intraocular injection of [³H]uridine and 30 days after crushing of the optic nerves. Electrophoresis is from left to right, and the ordinate represents percent of total radioactivity present in each gel slice. (Figure shows data presentation modified from Ingoglia and Tuliszewski, 1976; Ingoglia, 1978; and Ingoglia, 1979.)

ther supported by the finding that axoplasm taken from invertebrate axons contains mostly, if not exclusively, 4 S RNA (see Figure 1; Lasek *et al.*, 1973; Giuditta *et al*, 1980).

This finding has been extended by us and others (Por *et al.*, 1978; Gunning *et al.*, 1979) to include a variety of vertebrate nerves, both regenerating and mature, peripheral and central (Ingoglia and Zanakis, 1982). To summarize these studies, it appears that *all axons from invertebrates to the higher vertebrates contain 4 S RNA* and that *the amount of 4 S RNA transported axonally is greatly increased during nerve regeneration.*

4. THE 4 S RNA IN AXONS IS TRANSFER RNA

In squid axoplasm, 4 S RNA has the properties of transfer RNA (Black and Lasek, 1977; Giuditta *et al.*, 1977; Ingoglia and Giuditta, 1982). These experiments showed that axoplasmic 4 S RNA could be charged with radioactive amino acids, that charging was dependent on ATP, and that the aminoacylated product could be deacylated by incubation at alkaline pH. This was true for several amino acids tested, and the results indicate that squid axoplasm contains a variety (and perhaps a full complement) of aminoacylated transfer RNAs as well as their cognate synthetase enzymes.

Since the 4 S RNA in squid axons includes tRNA, it is quite likely that the 4 S RNA in vertebrate axons also includes transfer RNA. We have, in fact, come to this conclusion, again using indirect techniques similar in principle to those described above. In these experiments, we injected [^{3}H]uridine intraocularly and [^{14}C]uridine intracranially in fish with regenerating optic nerves. Then we removed all the high-molecular-weight RNA by DEAE cellulose chromatography, leaving only 4 S RNA (^{3}H and ^{14}C). The [^{14}C]-labeled 4 S RNA is derived from tectal cells, whereas the [^{3}H]-labeled 4 S RNA is primarily from optic axons. The latter conclusion is based on EMAR data (Gambetti *et al.,* 1978) and PAGE results (Ingoglia, 1982) indicating that 50% of the [^{3}H]RNA is within axons and 50% is extraaxonal. In addition, all of the intraaxonal RNA is 4 S RNA, but only 10–15% of the extraaxonal RNA is 4 S. Thus, when high-molecular-weight RNA is removed from the preparation, greater than 90% of the [^{3}H]4 S RNA is intraaxonal.

The double-labeled RNA mixture was then passed over methylated albumin kieselguhr (MAK) or BD cellulose columns to separate species of tRNA. The chromatographic profiles typical of tRNA of each were identical, indicating that intraaxonal 4 S RNA is similar to tRNA derived from glia (see Zanakis *et al.,* 1984*a*) and is likely to be composed of a variety of species of transfer RNA. These data are consistent with the view that, as in invertebrates, the 4 S RNA present in vertebrate axons is composed of a variety of species of transfer RNA.

Similar experiments have recently been performed in the chick optic system. Axonal 4 S RNA was labeled by intraocular injection and was compared with cellular 4 S RNA labeled by intracranial injection of [^{3}H]uridine. A comparison of the radioactivity profiles on gradient SDS slab gels showed similar distributions for each, indicating the presence within optic axons of the chick of a variety of species of 4 S RNA. Aminoacylation experiments show that this RNA is capable of accepting a range of amino acids, indicating that it contains transfer RNA. Thus, these investigators have reached the same conclusion that we reached for regenerating optic axons of goldfish, i.e, that the 4 S RNA transported axonally in chick optic axons is composed of a variety of species of transfer RNA (Scheffer *et al.,* 1984).

As mentioned earlier, one of the most compelling reasons for pursuing this line of research is the finding that large amounts of RNA are transported axonally when nerves are regenerating. Thus, the question that arises now is: What is the function of the relatively large amounts of transfer RNA found in axons of regenerating nerves?

5. TRANSFER RNA IN AXONS SERVES AS AN AMINO ACID DONOR IN POSTTRANSLATIONAL PROTEIN MODIFICATION

5.1. Squid Axoplasm

We have attempted to address the function of tRNA in axons by turning from our work on vertebrate axons to the squid giant axon. This sytsem was chosen so that we could be sure that what we were measuring was axonal transfer RNA and not a nonaxonal tRNA contaminant. Our working hypothesis was that the function of transfer RNA in axons was to serve as an amino acid donor in the posttranslational addition of amino acids to axonal proteins. The possibility that this reaction might occur in axons was first raised by Droz and Koenig (1971), on the basis of their observations that a low level of incorporation of amino acids into proteins occurred following incubation of synaptosomes with labeled amino acids. The addition of certain amino acids to proteins in a ribosomal RNA-free 105,000 g supernatant fraction of rat liver homogenates had been described by Kaji *et al.* (1963). Barra *et al* (1973) described a similar reaction in rat brain homogenates and reported that the addition of tyrosine to proteins could occur in the absence of transfer RNA but that argininylation of proteins was tRNA dependent. The tyrosylation reaction was later shown to be the addition of tyrosine to the α subunit of tubulin (Barra *et al.,* 1980), but the acceptor proteins for arginine have not been described. Transfer-RNA-dependent posttranslational arginylation of proteins appears to be ubiquitous in eukaryotic cells, and the acceptor proteins appear to be heterogeneous (Soffer, 1980).

Whereas Leu, Met, and Phe are able to be added posttranslationally to proteins in prokaryotes, only arginine has been reported to be added to the amino terminus of an acceptor protein in a reaction that is dependent on the presence of transfer RNA. Recently, it has been shown that leucine can be added to brain proteins posttranslationally in a reaction that is tRNA dependent and ribosomal RNA independent; this addition is not a terminal addition, however, but appears to be the result of an ester bond between Leu and Ser, Thr, or Tyr residues in the acceptor protein (Laughrea, 1982).

Our finding that axoplasm contains a variety of tRNA species as well as their cognate aminoacyl-tRNA synthetases (Ingoglia and Giuditta, 1982) would seem to argue against a function for axonal tRNA as a donor of a single amino acid to protein. However, as we were beginning these studies, Dr. G. Chakraborty working in our laboratory in Newark began finding that under the appropriate experimental conditions a variety of amino acids (and not just arginine) could be added to protein in a purified fraction of a 150,000 g supernatant of a rat brain homogenate (G. Chakraborty, unpublished data). Thus, we continued our efforts to attempt to demonstrate the posttranslational addition of amino acids to proteins in axoplasm.

A series of experiments were designed in which we prepared [³H]aminoacylated tRNA from squid optic lobe tRNA and then either incubated it with fresh axoplasm or injected it directly into the giant axon of the squid. In the incubation studies, [³H]Arg, [³H]Lys, and [³H]Asp tRNAs were incubated with 5 μl of fresh axoplasm (extruded from the giant axon) and a reaction mixture containing an energy source (ATP and CTP), MgCl₂, and dithiothreitol. Following 2 hr of incubation, the distribution of radioactivity in the reaction product was determined by precipitation with cold and hot 5% trichloroacetic acid (TCA). Results showed that no radioactivity was transferred to the protein fraction in any of the reactions (Figure 6), indicating that under the *in vitro* conditions used in these experiments, protein modification by amino acid addition was not occurring (Ingoglia *et al.*, 1983).

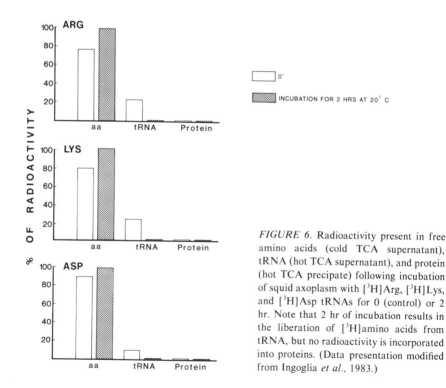

FIGURE 6. Radioactivity present in free amino acids (cold TCA supernatant), tRNA (hot TCA supernatant), and protein (hot TCA precipate) following incubation of squid axoplasm with [³H]Arg, [³H]Lys, and [³H]Asp tRNAs for 0 (control) or 2 hr. Note that 2 hr of incubation results in the liberation of [³H]amino acids from tRNA, but no radioactivity is incorporated into proteins. (Data presentation modified from Ingoglia *et al.*, 1983.)

This conclusion was also reached by us following injection of the same [^{3}H]aminoacylated tRNAs directly into the axon. In these experiments, [^{3}H]aminoacylated tRNA was injected into isolated giant axons by Dr. I. Tasaki at the Marine Biological Laboratories, Woods Hole, Mass. and incubated for 1 hr at 30°C in Millipore®-filtered sea water, and then the axoplasm was extruded and analyzed for radioactivity as in the previous experiment. Following incubation, the radioactivity was distributed in the free amino acid and tRNA fractions, but no radioactivity was associated with proteins of axoplasm (Figure 7) (Ingoglia *et al.*, 1983), confirming the findings of Lasek *et al.* (1977). Low levels of incorporation into glia of the sheath indicates that the preparation was metabolically active. Thus, both *in vitro* and *in situ* experiments failed to reveal the transfer of amino acids either from a free amino acid pool or from aminoacylated tRNA to proteins.

We next examined the transfer of amino acids to proteins in a 150,000 *g* supernatant of squid axoplasm. Axoplasm was pooled and stored in 50% glycerol until a volume of 50 to 100 μl was reached. These samples were then centrifuged at 150,000 *g* for 1 hr at 4°C, and the supernatant was either analyzed directly for the ability to incorporate [^{3}H]amino acids into proteins or passed through a Sephacryl S200 column prior to the same analysis.

Incubation of aliquots of the supernatant containing endogenous tRNAs with a variety of [^{3}H]amino acids resulted in no incorporation of radioactivity into proteins when compared with heat-inactivated controls. However, in the eluent of the S200 Sephacryl column, large amounts of radioactivity were incorporated into proteins following incubation with each of the amino acids tested (Figure 8), (Ingoglia *et al.*, 1983). The Sephacryl column removes all molecules of less than 25,000 mol. wt. from the supernatant, so it appears that the partial purification of the supernatant removes a substance of less than 25,000 daltons that is capable of inhibiting this reaction. We do not yet know what this inhibitor is, but preliminary evidence indicates that it is neither a protein nor calcium (G. Chakraborty, unpublished findings).

5.2. Rat Sciatic Nerve

We have repeated these experiments in homogenates of rat sciatic nerves and have obtained similar results (Zanakis *et al.*, 1984b). In these experiments, we analyzed portions of a nerve proximal (with respect to the soma) to a constriction applied 7 days earlier and another portion distal to that ligature. The logic for this approach was that if the reaction we are measuring occurs only in Schwann cells, then the two segments of nerve should have similar levels of activity. However, if the reaction is taking place in axons (as well as in

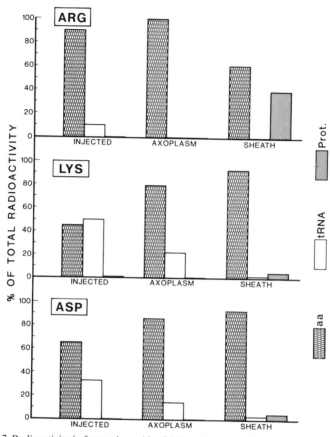

FIGURE 7. Radioactivity in free amino acids, tRNA, and proteins in the injection solution (left), axoplasm extruded 1 hr after incubation (middle), and the sheath (tissue remaining after extrusion, right). As in the *in vitro* experiment (Figure 6), incubation resulted in the release of [³H]amino acids from tRNA but not in the transfer of that radioactivity to proteins. Note that some radioactivity is incorporated into proteins in the sheaths. This is likely to be the result of the transfer of [³H]amino acids to sheath cells, where they are utilized for protein synthesis. (Values are the means of two or three points. Data presentation modified from Ingoglia *et al.*, 1983.)

Schwann cells), then there should be greater activity in the proximal segment of the nerve (containing axons and dammed up axonally transported material) than in the distal segment (in which most of the axons have disappeared through Wallerian degeneration). Results of these experiments were identical to those in squid in that no radioactivity was incorporated into proteins in the 150,000 *g* supernatant containing endogenous tRNAs, but all amino acids tested (Arg, Lys, Leu, Try, and Asp) were incorporated into proteins in the S200 eluent (lacking molecules of less than 25,000 daltons). Also, activity was always greater in the proximal nerve segment (between two and ten times greater) than in the distal segment, suggesting that the elements necessary for the posttranslational addition of amino acids to proteins are found in axons of the sciatic nerve of rats (Zanakis *et al.*, 1984*b*).

It appears, then, that this reaction is a tRNA-dependent, ribosomal RNA-independent posttranslational addition of amino acids to proteins. To conclude this with more certainty, several additional experiments were performed. First, we attempted to show that the reaction cannot occur in the absence of tRNA and, second, that the radioactivity that is present in the hot TCA precipitate is still present as the parent amino acid and that it is, in fact, incorporated into protein.

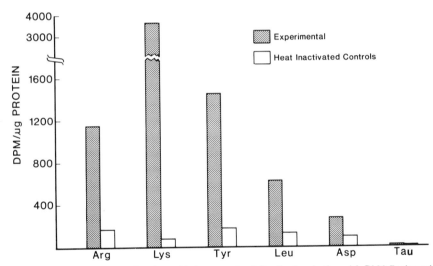

FIGURE 8. Incorporation of amino acids into proteins following incubation with S200 Sephacryl fractions of squid axon supernatant. Squid axoplasm was centrifuged at 150,000 *g* and then passed through a sephacryl S200 column. The graph shows the radioactivity associated with the protein fraction (hot TCA insoluble) following incubation of a high-molecular-weight (>120,000) fraction of the S200 column with [³H]amino acids and an appropriate reaction mixture. Controls were heated to 100°C for 20 min prior to incubation. Taurine, a sulfonic amino acid that is not incorporated into protein, is used here as a control to rule out the possibility that the incorporation of [³H]amino acids into protein was by means of nonspecific binding. All of the carboxylic amino acids, but not taurine, were incorporated into protein in amounts severalfold greater than in heat-inactivated controls. (Data presentation modified from Ingoglia *et al.*, 1983.)

5.3. Evidence That the Reaction Is Dependent on the Presence of tRNA

In an attempt to determine if this reaction is dependent on the presence of tRNA, we have used rat sciatic nerve homogenates to analyze the fraction of the S200 eluent for the presence of tRNA. The active fraction was subjected to phenol extraction and ethanol precipitation. The precipitate was then dissolved in buffer and subjected to SDS-PAGE on 10% gels. Absorption at 260 nm was measured and compared with the optical density profile of *E. coli* tRNA. The peaks were superimposable, indicating that the S200 fraction contained a species of RNA with the mobility of 4 S RNA. This RNA is very likely to be transfer RNA. Thus, the fraction of the S200 column capable of incorporating [^{3}H]amino acids into proteins contains tRNA.

We next removed tRNA from that fraction by passing it through a DEAE cellulose column under conditions that allow proteins to pass through but retain tRNA on the column. This procedure resulted in the loss of 93% of the capability for the incorporation of [^{3}H]Lys into protein. When the fraction containing tRNA was added back to it, 64% of the original activity could be recovered (Zanakis *et al.,* 1984*b*). These studies indicate that the incorporation of [^{3}H]Lys into proteins is dependent on the presence of tRNA.

5.4. Evidence That the Radioactivity in the Product Is Amino Acid Enzymatically Incorporated into Protein

The reaction product was examined in squid axoplasm and rat sciatic nerve by first allowing for the incoporation of [^{3}H]Lys or Arg into TCA-precipitable material and then hydrolyzing it and analyzing the radioactivity on an amino acid analyzer. Results showed that the majority of the radioactivity was still present as the injected amino acid (Ingoglia *et al.,* 1983). In other experiments, we treated the hot-TCA-precipitable material with proteinase K for 30 min at 37°C. Radioactivity that was not liberated from the precipitate by successive treatments with cold 5% TCA or chloroform–methanol (4:1) was liberated by proteinase K incubation. These experiments indicate that the radioactivity incorporated into a TCA-precipitable product is still the parent amino acid and that the incoproration represents the covalent binding of [^{3}H]amino acids to proteins (Zanakis *et al.,* 1984*b*). When the active fraction is treated with proteinase K, virtually all of the ability of the fraction to incorporate [^{3}H]Lys into protein is lost, suggesting that the incorporation of [^{3}H]Lys into protein is enzymatically driven (G. Chakraborty, unpublished data).

Thus, we conclude *that axoplasm of the squid giant axon and axons of the rat sciatic nerve contain elements capable of the enzymatic incorporation of amino acids into endogenous proteins. This reaction is not protein synthesis since it occurs in a purified fraction of the 150,000 g supernatant that is free of ribosomes and of molecules of less than 25,000 daltons and hence devoid of free amino acids. This reaction does represent (at least in part) the tRNA-dependent posttranslational incorporation of a variety of amino acids into proteins.*

5.5. Regenerating Optic Axons of Goldfish

We have also extended this work to the system in which we made the original observations on the transport of RNA, the goldfish visual system. In these experiments, we have cut the optic nerve and waited 6 days for the nerve to begin growing. Then the stump of the regenerating optic nerve was removed and analyzed for its ability to incorporate [³H]amino acids into proteins in the same way as described for squid axoplasm and the rat sciatic nerve. Preliminary evidence indicates that the regenerating optic nerve of goldfish, like rat sciatic nerves and squid axoplasm, incorporates a variety of [³H]amino acids into proteins in the S200 Sephacryl eluent of the high-speed supernatant but not in the supernatant itself (G. Chakraborty, T. Leach, and N. A. Ingoglia, unpublished data).

Thus, the posttranslational addition of amino acids to proteins is not confined to squid axoplasm but is also a property of axons of the rat sciatic nerve and regenerating optic nerves of goldfish.

Since tRNAs are probably present in most if not all axons (Ingoglia and Zanakis, 1982), it is likely that posttranslational modification occurs in all axons. Also, since the amount of tRNA in axons is increased during nerve regeneration, it can be assumed that this is indicative of an increase in posttranslational protein modification during regeneration. The question that is raised now is: What is the role of tRNA-mediated posttranslational addition of amino acids to protein in regenerating axons?

6. POSTTRANSLATIONAL MODIFICATION OF PROTEINS BY tRNA-DEPENDENT AMINO ACID ADDITION OCCURS IN GROWTH CONES OF REGENERATING OPTIC AXONS OF GOLDFISH

To begin to answer this question, let us first return to the EMAR studies of Gambetti *et al.* (1978). In these experiments, of the total [³H]RNA in the tectum, approximately 50% was found in regenerating axons. As mentioned earlier, many of those silver grains ([³H]RNA) were localized to the tips of the growing axons, the axonal growth cones (Figure 3). In 1978, we could state with certainty that these silver grains represented [³H]RNA. Now, we conclude that this RNA is transfer RNA and that it is involved in posttranslational protein modification. Thus, elements found in the advancing tip of the growing axon are actively transforming axonal proteins. The question posed now is why. At present, we can only speculate on the answer to this question (see Figure 9), and we have no reason to favor one possibility over another.

Perhaps the most intriguing aspect of this finding is that by allowing for local changes in proteins in the axon, the neuron is capable of a certain degree of axonal autonomy not dictated by the soma. Thus, axonally transported proteins can be modified at sites distant from their synthetic origins and likely in response to local environmental cues. Injury to the axon could result in protein modifications (by the removal of the so far unidentified inhibitor) that lead to the formation of the end bulbs characteristic of axonal injury (Ramon y Cajal, 1928) or perhaps in modification of a protein that is then transported retrogradely (D. L. Wilson, Chapter 9, this volume) to signal the soma that injury

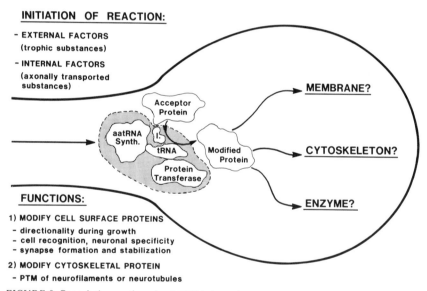

FIGURE 9. Speculation on the role of tRNA-dependent posttranslational protein modification by amino acid addition in growth cones of regenerating axons. Results of experiments currently in progress strongly indicate that there is in regenerating axons transport of tRNA, aminoacyl tRNA synthetases, protein transferases, and an inhibitor (I) as part of a high-molecular-weight complex. The function of these elements is to modify endogenous acceptor proteins. What remains speculative is (1) the nature of the substances that can initiate the reaction (external trophic substances or endogenous axonal elements), (2) the destination of the modified proteins (membranous, cytoskeletal, or perhaps an enzyme that is either activated or inactivated as a result of modification), and (3) the ultimate purpose of the modification (perhaps for roles in determining directionality, cell recognition, or synaptic specificity).

has occurred. In the regenerative phase, the reaction might be triggered by changes in the external milieu, perhaps by neuronal or glial trophic substances (reviewed by Barde *et al.,* 1983) or by chemical gradients produced by target cells. The changes in axonal proteins induced by these substances might play a role in guidance and directionality during growth. Finally, modification of proteins in growth cones may be linked to synaptogenesis, as has been suggested by Skene *et al.* (1982).

There are many other areas where one could speculate on the roles of tRNA-dependent protein modification reactions in axonal metabolism. What seems certain, however, is that whatever the function of these reactions, they will undoubtedly be shown to play key roles in the ability of a nerve to regenerate successfully following injury.

7. REFERENCES

Anderson, E., Edstrom, A., and Jarlstedt, J., 1970, Properties of RNA from giant axons of the crayfish, *Acta Physiol. Scand.* **78**:491–502.

Barde, Y. A., Edgar, D., and Thoenen, H., 1983, New neurotropic factors, *Annu. Rev. Physiol.* **45**:601–612.

Barra, H. S., Rodriquez, J. A., Arce, C. A., and Caputto, R., 1973, A soluble preparation from rat brain that incorporates into its own proteins ^{14}C-arginine by a ribonuclease sensitive system and ^{14}C-tyrosine by a ribonuclease insensitive system, *J. Neurochem.* **20**:97–108.

Barra, H. S., Arce, C. A., and Caputto, R., 1980, Total tubulin and its aminoacylated and non-aminoacylated forms during development of rat brain, *Eur. J. Biochem.* **109**:439–446.

Black, M. M., and Lasek, R. J., 1977, The presence of transfer RNA in the axoplasm of the squid giant axon, *J. Neurobiol.* **8**:229–237.

Droz, B., and Koenig, H. L., 1971, Dynamic condition of protein in axons and axon terminals, *Acta Neuropathol. (Berl.)* **5**:109–118.

Gambetti, P., Ingoglia, N. A., Autilio-Gambetti, L., and Weiss, P., 1978, Distribution of ^{3}H-RNA in goldfish optic tectum following intraocular or intracranial injection of ^{3}H-uridine: Evidence of axonal migration of RNA in regenerating optic fibers, *Brain Res.* **154**:284–300.

Guiditta, A., Metatory, S., Felsami, A., and del Rio, A., 1977, Factors of protein synthesis in the axoplasm of squid giant axons, *J. Neurochem.* **28**:1393–1395.

Giuditta, A., Cupello, A., and Lazzarini, G., 1980, Ribosomal RNA in the axoplasm of the squid giant axon, *J. Neurochem.* **34**:1756–1760.

Grafstein, B., and Forman, D. S., 1980, Intracellular transport in neurons, *Physiol. Rev.* **60**:1167–1283.

Gunning, P. W., Por, S. B., Langford, C. J., Scheffer, J., Austin, L., and Jeffery, P. L., 1979, The direct measurement of the axoplasmic transport of individual RNA species: Transfer but no ribosomal RNA is transported, *J. Neurochem.* **32**:1737–1743.

Hartmann, H. A., Lin, I., and Shively, M. C., 1968, RNA of nerve cell bodies and axons after β,β'-iminodipropionitrile, *Acta Neuropathol. (Berl.)* **11**:275–281.

Ingoglia, N. A., 1979, 4S RNA is present in regenerating optic axons of goldfish, *Science* **206**:73–75.

Ingoglia, N. A., 1982, 4S RNA in regenerating opic axons of goldfish, *J. Neurosci.* **2**:331–338.

Ingoglia, N. A., and Giuditta, A., 1982, Multiple species of transfer RNA are present in squid axoplasm, *Trans. Am. Soc. Neurochem.* **13**(1):235.

Ingoglia, N. A., and Tuliszewski, R., 1976, Transfer RNA may be axonally transported during regeneration of goldfish optic nerves, *Brain Res* 112:371–381.

Ingoglia, N. A., and Zanakis, M. F., 1982, Axonal transport of 4S RNA, in: *Axoplasmic Transport* (D. G. Weiss, ed.), pp. 161–169, Springer-Verlag Berlin, Heidelberg, New York.

Ingoglia, N. A., Weis, P., and Mycek, T., 1975, Axonal transport of RNA during regeneration of the optic nerve of goldfish, *J. Neurochem.* 6:549–563.

Ingoglia, N. A., Sharma, S. C., Pilchman, J., Baranowski, K., and Sturman, J. A., 1982a, Axonal transport and transcellular transfer of nucleosides and polyamines in intact and regenerating optic nerves of goldfish: Speculation on the axonal regulation of periaxonal cell metabolism, *J. Neurosci.* 2(10):1412–1423.

Ingoglia, N. A., Sturman, J. A., Jaggard, P., and Perez, C., 1982b, Association of spermine and 4 S RNA during axonal transport in regenerating optic nerve of goldfish, *Brain Res.* 238:341–351.

Ingoglia, N. A, Giuditta, A., Zanakis, M. F., Babigian, A., Tasaki, I., Chakraborty, G., and Sturman, J., 1983, Incorporation of ^{3}H-amino acids into proteins in a partially purified fraction of axoplasm: Evidence for transfer RNA mediated, post-translational protein modification in squid giant axons, *J. Neurosci.* 3:2463–2473.

Kaji, H., Novelli, G. D., and Kaji, A., 1963, A soluble amino acid-incorporating system from rat liver, *Biochim. Biophys. Acta* 76:477–479.

Koenig, E., 1965, Synthetic mechanisms in the axon. II. RNA in myelin . . . free axons of the cat, *J. Neurochem.* 12:357–361.

Koenig, E., 1979, Ribosomal RNA in Mauthner axon: Implications for a protein synthesizing machinery in the myelinated axon, *Brain Res.* 175:95–107.

Lasek, R. J., 1970, The distribution of nucleic acids in the giant axon of the squid *(Loligo pealei),* *J. Neurochem.* 17:103–109.

Lasek, R. J., Dabrowski, C., and Nordlander, R., 1973, Analysis of axoplasmic RNA from invertebrate giant axons, *Nature* 244:1188–1192.

Lasek, R. J., Gainer, H., and Barker, J. I., 1977, Cell to cell transfer of glial proteins to the squid giant axons, *J. Cell Biol.* 74:501–523.

Laughrea, M., 1982, Transfer ribonucleic acid dependent but ribosome independent leucine incorporation into rat brain protein, *Biochemistry* 21:5694–5700.

Peters, A., Palay, S. L., and Webster, H. de, 1976, *The Fine Structure of the Nervous System,* W. B. Saunders, Philadelphia.

Por, S., Gunning, P. W., Jeffery, P. L., and Austin, L., 1978, The axoplasmic transport of 4S RNA in the chick optic system, *Neurochem. Res.* 3:411–422.

Ramon y Cajal, S., 1928, *Degeneration and Regeneration of the Nervous System,* Volume 1 (translated by R. M. May), Oxford University Press, London.

Scheffer, J. W., Howe, N., Gunning, P. W., and Austin, L., 1983, The axoplasmic transport of transfer RNA in the chick optic system, *J. Neurochem.* 42:698–704.

Skene, P., Willard, M., and Freeman, J. A., 1982, Modification of axonally transported protein in toad retinotectal terminals, *Soc. Neurosci. Abstr.* 8:864.

Soffer, R. L., 1980, Biochemistry and biology of aminoacylated tRNA protein transferase, in: *Transfer RNA: Biological Aspects* (D. Soll, J. N. Abelson, and P. R. Shimmel, eds.), pp. 493–505, Cold Spring Harbor Laboratory, New York.

Zanakis, M. F., Eskin, B., and Ingoglia, N. A., 1984a, Evidence that multiple species of aminoacylated transfer RNA are present in regenerating optic axons of goldfish *Neurochem. Res.* Vol. 9 (No. 2): 249–262.

Zanakis, M. F., Chakraborty, G., Sturman, J. A., and Ingoglia, N. A., 1984b, Posttranslational and regenerating axons of the rat sciatic nerve, *J. Neurochem.,* in press.

MOLECULAR EVENTS ASSOCIATED WITH PERIPHERAL NERVE REGENERATION

DAVID L. WILSON

1. INTRODUCTION

The early events associated with nerve regeneration probably involve strong neuron–environment interactions. Observations on axonally transported proteins can aid in exploring such interactions at a number of levels.

The neuron appears to play a primary role in some of the early events associated with axon regrowth. This can be inferred from observations such as the following: (1) neurons in culture, isolated from other cells, can initiate neurite outgrowth; (2) even in the environment of the central nervous system (CNS) of mammals, where regeneration usually is abortive, some outgrowth of short processes can be observed; (3) in some cases, isolated axon segments can sprout (Carbonetto and Muller, 1982). In sustaining axon outgrowth, the neuron also plays a crucial role as the source of the major materials required

DAVID L. WILSON ● Department of Physiology and Biophysics, University of Miami School of Medicine, Miami, Florida 33101 for regrowth ("building blocks"). The major elements of axoplasm and cytoskeleton are largely supplied by slow transport, whereas axonal membrane appears to be inserted at growing tips (Pfenninger, 1982) after rapid transport from nerve cell bodies.

The environment, including glia, extracellular matrix, target cells, etc., appears to be involved both in providing proper surfaces for axonal attachment and regrowth and in possibly supplying trophic and chemotatic factors that could play a role in sustained, directed regrowth. The general importance of environmental surfaces or trophic factors in nerve regrowth has been demonstrated in many studies. Mammalian sensory and motor neuron axons do not regrow if damaged in the CNS, whereas the same neuron axons do regrow if damaged in the peripheral nervous system (PNS) (Guth, 1956). Indeed, after dorsal root damage, mammalian sensory neurons will regrow axons up to, but not into, the CNS. At the point at which the Schwann cells and fibroblasts of the PNS give way to oligodendrocytes and neuroglia of the CNS, the axons cease growth or actually reverse direction of growth (Hare and Hinsley, 1940). The recent, elegant studies from Aguayo's laboratory (David and Aguayo, 1981) again emphasize the strong role of environment in axon regrowth. Studies on neurons in culture also support the concept of a dual role of environment (surfaces and substances) in neurite outgrowth (Carbonetto and Muller, 1982).

The task of unraveling the complex set of interactions among the cells that participate in nerve regeneration has just begun. Studies on axonally transported proteins in regrowing neurons are contributing to the understanding of these relationships. In this chapter I consider two issues. One is the relationship between the materials synthesized and supplied for maintenance of normal nervous tissue and the materials needed by neurons regrowing after nerve damage. Are massive increases in the amount of materials required during regeneration? Are new kinds of materials required? Can there be axon regrowth without changes in the materials normally being supplied through axonal transport?

The second issue concerns the utilization and fate of the materials that are transported from nerve cell bodies to the damaged and regrowing axon tips. Are any of the materials modified at the tips to meet the special needs of a regrowing axon? Are any of the transported proteins released at the tips, perhaps to play interactive roles with other cells or with the extracellular environment? Are there new "signal" proteins returning to the cell bodies of the neurons by retrograde transport?

2. METHODS

Rat (Sprague–Dawley) or frog *(Rana catesbeiana)* peripheral nerves are damaged by cut or crush *in situ* under anesthesia. Animals are returned to cage or tank for varying lengths of time, as indicated below. Animals are killed by decapitation, and the damaged nerve with attached ganglia is removed for *in vitro* labeling of the ganglia with radioactive amino acids and, when appropriate, axonal transport of the labeled material. The labeled protein and protein-containing materials from ganglia and nerve are examined by autoradiography or fluorography after separation by two-dimensional polyacrylamide gel electrophoresis (2-D PAGE). All of the procedures have been described in detail in published papers (Wilson *et al.*, 1977; Hall *et al.*, 1978; Stone *et al.*, 1978; Perry and Wilson, 1981; Wilson, 1982).

3. PROTEIN SYNTHESIS AFTER NERVE DAMAGE

Michael Hall and I performed a series of studies on superior cervical ganglia (SCG) from rats. Our analysis of changes in protein synthesis in the ganglion at from 1 to over 100 days following postganglionic cut of its principal nerves detected no change in overall incorporation and no new polypeptides, but significant changes in the relative abundance of a number of proteins was detected (Hall *et al.*, 1978). Tubulin, whose synthesis has been shown to increase dramatically following optic nerve crush in goldfish (Heacock and Agranoff, 1976), was not significantly affected in the rat SCG.

A study of the effects of preganglionic damage (deafferentation) on the SCG revealed many changes in the rates of synthesis of specific proteins similar to those seen after postganglionic nerve damage (Hall and Wilson, 1979). Since the principal neurons of the ganglion are not directly damaged by deafferentation, these changes probably are not directly related to nerve regeneration. Interestingly, all of the proteins that changed significantly in synthesis rates after deafferentation when compared with controls were not significantly different in rate of synthesis from postgangionic axotomy values. It thus appears that deafferentation induces a subset of the changes produced by axotomy. The additional changes produced exclusively by axotomy remain candidates for polypeptides playing significant roles in nerve regeneration. The one of these that shows the most profound alteration in synthesis rate (a fourfold increase) we designated as 3C2. Its position on two-dimensional gels suggests that it might correspond to the rapidly transported GAP 23 of Skene and Willard (1981) and to the transported protein C23, which increases in abundance after frog sciatic nerve damage (Perry and Wilson, 1981).

Michael Hall (1982) has completed a similar analysis of rat dorsal root ganglia following sciatic nerve crush. The conclusions were basically similar: no new proteins were detected, but a number of individual polypeptides showed significant changes in rate of synthesis, some increasing while others decreased. Many but not all of the protein species exhibiting change were the same as seen in the SCG.

Gary Perry and I have examined protein synthesis in frog dorsal root gan-
i (DRG) after sciatic nerve damage (Perry and Wilson, 1981). As with rat
SCG and DRG, no significant change in overall rate of incorporation of radioactive precursor ([^{35}S]methionine) into TCA-insoluble material was observed
in the ganglia, and no new species of protein were detected on fluorographs
after protein separation by 2-D PAGE. Eighty polypeptides were analyzed
quantitatively, and only a minority showed significant changes in synthesis
rates. The magnitude of such changes (20 to 40%) were not as great as seen in
the rat (Hall, 1982).

4. PROTEINS TRANSPORTED AFTER NERVE DAMAGE

Rapidly transported proteins are a small subset of the proteins synthesized
by nervous tissue and appear to be present in minor abundance (Stone *et al.*,
1978). These transported proteins could be undergoing more significant
changes, which would not be detected in the studies of proteins synthesized in
ganglia. After sciatic nerve damage, a number of such proteins show significant
changes in abundance in transport when the amount of radioactivity in transport is used as a guide to abundance levels (Perry and Wilson, 1981). The most
profound change in a transported protein observed after sciatic nerve damage
was a threefold increase in label in one spot. Again, new species were not
detected, and there was no significant change in overall levels of transported
radioactivity. Interestingly, after sciatic nerve damage, changes in transport
from DRG seen in the sciatic nerve were also observed in the dorsal root. Thus,
the sensory neurons, in response to sciatic nerve damage, make the same
changes in what is being transported in both branches. Bisby (1981) has made
a similar observation.

The studies described thus far permit us to conclude that, at least in some
nerve cells, axon regrowth can occur without massive increases in the materials
normally being supplied to axons. If new materials are required, these must be
found in quite low abundance in the nerve.

5. AXON REGROWTH WITHOUT CHANGES IN SYNTHESIS OR TRANSPORT

Are the changes in synthesis and transport of proteins that are observed
after nerve damage necessary for axon elongation? We have attempted to
answer this question by studying DRG protein synthesis and fast transport in
sciatic nerve after damage of dorsal roots. We were unable to detect changes
in synthesis or transport of any proteins while demonstrating that regrowth in
the damaged roots did occur (Perry *et al.*, 1983).

At the other extreme, some researchers have described more profound alterations in protein synthesis and transport than we have observed (Skene and Willard, 1981; Benowitz *et al.*, 1981; Giulian *et al.*, 1980; Heacock and Agranoff, 1976). The reason for such different responses in different systems is not at all clear. Also, the role of the proteins that show profound alterations in abundance in synthesis or transport after damage in some neurons is not yet clear.

6. THE FATE OF AXONALLY TRANSPORTED PROTEINS AT REGROWING TIPS

In our studies on transported proteins, Dr. Perry and I were careful not to allow the transported proteins to reach the sites of damage and regrowth. Bruce Tedeschi and I have now carried out some studies on the fate of rapidly transported proteins after their arrival at sites of regeneration. We (Tedeschi and Wilson, 1983a) have detected a set of polypeptide-containing molecules that only appears on the two-dimensional gels if proteins have reached regions of nerve containing regrowing axon tips. The new spots (designated A25) are heavily labeled by [^{35}S]methionine and therefore appear to be the product of posttranslational modification in a rapidly transported protein (Tedeschi and Wilson, 1983a). The A25 set first appears a few days after nerve damage, at a time when large numbers of axons are just starting to regrow. After their arrival at sites of damage or regrowth, a sizable fraction of rapidly transported proteins return, via retrograde transport, towards the cell bodies of the neurons (Bisby, 1982). Interestingly, A25 also appears among the retrogradely transported materials (Tedeschi and Wilson, 1983a). This is the first time that a new species not normally present in retrograde transport has been detected after nerve damage.

The role of A25 in nerve regrowth can only be a subject of speculation today. By being retrogradely transported, it could play a role in signaling the cell body about the state of axon tips. Another possibility is that A25 serves as a surface molecule, giving modified properties to growing tips. There is a correlation between the first appearance of A25 and the time of appearance of significant numbers of outgrowing axons, both in crushed nerve and after conditioning lesions (Krayanek *et al.*, 1984).

Tedeschi and I (Wilson and Tedeschi, 1983) have recently detected a different fate for some of the rapidly transported proteins. There is a subset of the transported proteins that is selectively released from axon tips after nerve crush. Although a release of transported proteins from undamaged segments of nerve has been reported (Hines and Garwood, 1977), it was not confirmed (Tedeschi *et al.*, 1981). Even during the first 24 hr after nerve crush, we have been unable to detect release of fast-transported proteins from frog sciatic nerve. However, we now have good evidence for such release after that time, which continues for a period of weeks. The released label is enriched in a number of proteins that comigrate with a subset of the fast-transported polypeptides on two-dimensional gels.

Why is such release from whole nerve only detected after nerve damage? Perhaps the amount of such release is greatly increased as new membrane is added at growing axon tips. Thus, these proteins could be the more soluble contents of membrane-limited packages and could be released as the membrane is inserted at the tip. Alternatively, such release could always be occurring along axons but go undetected in intact nerve if surrounding tissues effectively scavenge the material before it can exit the whole, intact nerve.

The proteins that are enriched in release include B14, first identified as a transported protein several years ago (Stone and Wilson, 1979). We now have evidence that B14 is also synthesized and released by a number of cell types other than neurons (Wilson and Tedeschi, 1983). B14 has been a relatively conserved protein during evolution, as B14 from rat and frog comigrate on two-dimensional gels (Perry and Wison, 1983). It also appears to be ubiquitous in neurons, as it has been found not only in dorsal root ganglion neurons but also in motoneurons (Stone and Wilson, 1979) and may be the same protein that Wentholt and McGarvey (1982) described as the 36,000-dalton HC protein in auditory nerve. Such a common protein could play a role in the extracellular environment. After nerve damage, more of B14 appears to be released from nerve at and peripheral to the site of the damage (Wilson and Tedeschi, 1983).

7. CONCLUSIONS

At least some neurons can regrow axons without major changes in the materials being supplied by axonal transport. This observation points to the importance of events occuring at the damaged or regrowing axon tips. We have just begun to identify some of the biochemical events occurring at regrowing axon tips. Such events include posttranslational modification of rapidly transported protein (see also N. A. Ingoglia *et al.,* this volume), release of some rapidly transported proteins from nerve, and significant changes in proteins synthesized and released by nonneuronal nervous system cells. A long-term goal of these studies is to have a complete enough description of such events in the regenerating peripheral nerve to approach the problem of identifying the event(s) that cause attempts at regeneration in the central nervous system to fail.

ACKNOWLEDGMENTS

The support of NIH grant NS 18263 and NSF grant BNS 81-17817 is gratefully acknowledged.

8. REFERENCES

Benowitz, L. I., Shashousa, V. E., and Yoon, M. G., 1981, Specific changes in rapidly transported proteins during regeneration of the goldfish optic nerve, *J. Neurosci.* **1**:300–307.

Bisby, M. A., 1981, Axonal transport in the central axons of sensory neurons during regeneration of their peripheral axon, *Neurosci. Lett.* **21**:7–11.

Bisby, M. A., 1982, Retrograde axonal transport of endogenous proteins, in: *Axoplasmic Transport* (D. G. Weiss, ed.), pp. 193–199, Springer-Verlag, Berlin, Heidelberg, New York.

Carbonetto, S., and Muller, K. J., 1982, Nerve fiber growth and the cellular response to axotomy, *Curr. Top. Dev. Biol.* **17**:33–76.

David, S., and Aguayo, A. J., 1981, Axonal elongation into peripheral nervous-system bridges after central nervous system injury in adult rats, *Science* **214**:931–933.

Giulian, D., Des Ruisseaux, H., and Conburn, D., 1980, Biosynthesis and axonal transport of proteins during neuronal regeneration, *J. Biol. Chem.* **255**:6494–6501.

Guth, J., 1956, Regeneration in the mammalian peripheral nervous system, *Physiol. Rev.* **36**:441–478.

Hall, M. E., 1982, Changes in synthesis of specific proteins in axotomized dorsal root ganglia *Exp. Neurol.* **76**:83–93.

Hall, M. E. and Wilson, D. L., 1979, Modification of protein synthesis by deafferentation of rat sympathetic ganglia, *Brain Res.* **168**:414–418.

Hall, M. E., Wilson, D. L., and Stone, G. C., 1978, Changes in synthesis of specific proteins following axotomy: Detection with two-dimensional gel electrophoresis, *J. Neurobiol.* **9**:353–366.

Hare, K., and Hinsey, J. C., 1940, Reactions of dorsal root ganglion cells to section of peripheral and central processes, *J. Comp. Neurol* **73**:489–502.

Heacock, A., and Agranoff, B., 1976, Enhanced labeling of a retinal protein during regeneration of optic nerve in goldfish, *Proc. Nat., Acad. Sci. U.S.A.* **73**:828–832.

Hines, J. F., and Garwood, M. M., 1977, Release of proteins from axons during axonal transport: An *in vitro* preparation, *Brain Res.* **125**:141–148.

Krayanek, S. R., Tedeschi, B., and Wilson, D. L., 1984, Protein modification in regenerating nerve is correlated with the presence of axon regrowth, in preparation.

Perry, G. W., and Wilson, D. L., 1981, Protein synthesis and axonal transport during nerve regeneration, *J. Neurochem.* **37**:1203–1217.

Perry, G. W., and Wilson, D. L., 1983, Polypeptides in frog and rat: Evolutionary changes in rapidly transported and abundant nerve proteins, *J. Neurochem.* **4**:772–779.

Perry, G. W., Krayanek, S. R., and Wilson, D. L., 1983, Protein synthesis and rapid axonal transport during regeneration of dorsal roots, *J. Neurochem.* **40**:1590–1598.

Pfenninger, K. H., 1982, Axonal transport in the sprouting neuron: Transfer of newly synthesized membrane components to the cell surface, in: *Axoplasmic Transport in Physiology and Pathology* (D. G. Weiss and A. Gorio eds.), pp. 52–61, Springer-Verlag, Berlin, Heidelberg, New York.

Skene, J. H. P., and Willard, M., 1981, Axonally transported proteins associated with growth in rabbit central and peripheral nervous systems, *J. Cell Biol.* **89**:96–103.

Stone, G. C., and Wilson, D. L., 1979, Qualitative analysis of proteins rapidly transported in ventral horn motoneurons and bidirectionally from dorsal root ganglia, *J. Neurobiol.* **10**:1–12.

Stone, G. C., Wilson, D. L., and Hall, M. E., 1978, Two dimensional gel electrophoresis of proteins in rapid axonal transport, *Brain Res.* **144**:287–302.

Tedeschi, B. W., and Wilson, D. L., 1983*a*, Modification of a rapidly transported protein in regenerating nerve, *J. Neurosci.* **3**:1728–1734.

Tedeschi, B. W., and Wilson, D. L., 1983*b*, Release of fast-transported proteins from regenerating nerve, *Soc. Neurosci. Abstr.* **8**:48.

Tedeschi, B., Wilson, D. L., Zimmerman, A., and Perry, G. W., 1981, Are axonally transported proteins released from sciatic nerves? *Brain Res.* **211:**175–178.

Wentholt, R. J., and McGarvey, M. L., 1982, Changes in rapidly transported proteins in the auditory nerve after hair cell loss, *Brain Res.* **253:**263–269.

Wilson, D. L., 1982, Two-dimensional polyacrylamide gel electrophoresis of proteins, in: *Handbook of Neurochemistry,* 2nd edition, Vol. 2 (A. Lajtha, ed.), pp. 133–146, Plenum Press, New York.

Wilson, D. L., and Tedeschi, B., 1983, Release of non-neuronal proteins from regenerating nerve, *Soc. Neurosci. Abstr.* **8:**48.

Wilson, D. L., Hall, M. E., Stone, G. C., and Rubin, R. W., 1977, Some improvements in two-dimensional gel electrophoresis of proteins: Protein mapping of eucaryotic tissue extracts, *Anal. Biochem.* **83:**33–44.

TARGET-DEPENDENT AND TARGET-INDEPENDENT CHANGES IN RAPID AXONAL TRANSPORT DURING REGENERATION OF THE GOLDFISH RETINOTECTAL PATHWAY

LARRY I. BENOWITZ

1. INTRODUCTION

Unlike mammals, in which most pathways of the adult central nervous system fail to regenerate if injured, neurons in fish and amphibia retain the capacity to regenerate their axons even in the mature animal. Of particular interest, both to the clinical and basic neuroscience communities, has been lower ver-

LARRY I. BENOWITZ ● *Department of Psychiatry, Harvard Medical School and Mailman Research Center, McLean Hospital, Belmont, Massachusetts 02178*

tebrates' ability to regenerate the optic nerve, a phenomenon first described by Matthey in 1925. Despite the enormous number of fibers that must reconnect from the eye to the brain and the apparent disarray of these fibers within the optic nerve, visually guided behaviors return to a level indistinguishable from that seen before surgery within 1–2 months (Sperry, 1943). In a classic series of experiments, Sperry (1948, 1963; Attardi and Sperry, 1963) demonstrated that this return of vision is predicated on the reestablishment of a precise, topographically organized mapping of the retinal ganglion cells' nerve terminals onto appropriate brain structures, the optic tectum of the midbrain in particular. Numerous studies have subsequently used the regenerating retinotectal pathway of lower vertebrates as a model system for studying the events that underlie the development and regeneration of complex neural systems (Grafstein, 1975; Jacobson, 1978; also, Murray, 1976, 1982; Springer et al., 1977; Ingoglia and Tuliszewski, 1976; Giulian et al., 1980; Quitschke et al., 1980; McQuarrie and Grafstein, 1982; Heacock and Agranoff, 1976, 1982; Meyer, 1980; Benowitz et al., 1981, 1982, 1983).

Within a few days of axotomy, the nucleoli of the retinal ganglion cells enlarge and a proliferation of ribosomal RNA, associated with free ribosomes, occurs (Murray and Grafstein, 1969; Murray, 1973; Murray and Forman, 1971). Within 2 weeks, the cell body begins to enlarge as the amount of protein synthesis increases; in this period, the ribosomes are now associated primarily with a hypertrophied rough endoplasmic reticulum as the amount of protein transported down the regenerating axon, both in the slow and fast phases of transport, increases (Grafstein and Murray, 1969; Murray and Forman, 1971; McQuarrie and Grafstein, 1982). These changes reach their maxima at 3–4 weeks before declining and eventually returning to normal levels at 2–3 months (Grafstein, 1975). Optic axons first appear in the tectum by 10–14 days but do not descend and begin forming synapses with tectal neurons for another 2–3 weeks, at which time visually guided behaviors mediated by retinotectal connections begin to return (Springer et al., 1977a,b; Murray, 1976; Yoon, 1975).

Throughout this process, the nerve terminal membrane plays a central role as the site of axon elongation and of much of the neuron's interaction with its environment (Bray, 1976; Feldman et al., 1979; Barondes, 1976). At early stages, the membrane must remain in a fluid state, allowing for the continuous movement of the growth cone; later on, the nerve ending becomes the site of adhesion to target cells and of the development of synaptic specializations. Molecular species involved in the recognition of appropriate target cells are generally believed to be localized on these endings (Barondes, 1970). Thus, to understand the regeneration of the retinotectal pathway or, for that matter, the development of any brain connections at a molecular level, it is essential to identify the constituents of the nerve terminal membranes at various stages of development and to characterize the significance of these components for the growth process.

Many of the constituents of the nerve terminals are synthesized in the cell body and then transported down the axon as parts of preassembled membranous organelles (Hammerschlag and Stone, 1982; Schwartz, 1979; Droz et al., 1975; Bennett et al., 1973). These organelles are conveyed down the axon at a much higher velocity than other cellular constituents such as mitochondria or the subunits of neurofilaments, microtubules, or microfilaments (Willard et al., 1974; Lorenz and Willard, 1978; Schwartz, 1979; Grafstein and Forman, 1980). Consequently, although membranous material in transit to the terminals constitutes only a small fraction of the total contents of the nerve (McEwen and Grafstein, 1968), these components can be studied in relative isolation by introducing radiolabeled precursors into the cell bodies and then analyzing the labeled products present in the nerve at short survival times.

Taking advantage of the characteristically high transport rate of membrane-bound components in the nerve, our studies have combined isotopic labeling with one- or two-dimensional gel electrophoretic separation of proteins to study constituents of the nerve terminal membranes associated with the regenerative process. Our initial concern was to determine whether regeneration involves a qualitative shift in the complement of material that is transported to the nerve terminal membranes or whether the same gene products present in the normal, mature nerve are sufficient to allow for regrowth of the axon and reformation of its synaptic relations. After establishing that the program of protein metabolism and/or transport is in fact altered during regeneration, we next attempted to characterize the principal molecular changes that occur in greater detail. Finally, we have begun to study the mechanisms that regulate the changes in protein transport during regeneration, particularly those mediated by interactions between the developing nerve terminals and their appropriate target tissue, the optic tectum.

2. QUALITATIVE STUDIES ON THE CHANGES IN RAPIDLY TRANSPORTED PROTEINS DURING REGENERATION

2.1. Unidimensional Gel Studies

Our initial studies (Benowitz et al., 1981) examined whether regeneration of the goldfish optic nerve involves a change in the molecular composition of the rapid phase of axonal transport and attempted to identify which proteins might be selectively increased or decreased at various stages of the growth process. For these studies, we used double-isotope labeling combined with one-dimensional gel separation methods to contrast the rapidly transported proteins in intact and regenerating optic nerves.

In 4-inch (total length) Comet variety goldfish, one optic nerve was crushed 1–2 mm behind the eye, whereas the other was left intact to serve as a control. At times ranging from 8 to 62 days after surgery, [³H]proline was injected into one eye, and an equimolar amount of [¹⁴C]proline into the other. Five hours later, at which time most labeling in the nerve is associated with rapidly transported components (moving at ~2 mm/hr; Forman *et al.*, 1971), control and regenerating nerves were dissected out, combined, homogenized, and the proteins separated by one-dimensional gel electrophoresis. Gels were cut at 1-mm intervals and counted for ³H and ¹⁴C activity. Radioactivity in each slice was normalized by the overall amount of each isotope on the gel.

Figure 1 illustrates the disparity between the labeling profiles of rapidly transported proteins in an optic nerve regenerating for 8 days and in the contralateral control side. The greatest relative increases on the regenerating side, indicated in the figure by strippling (1A), are seen for components with apparent molecular masses of 210 kilodaltons (K), 44 K, and 27 K. These changes can also be represented in a plot of normalized [¹⁴C]/[³H] ratios (1B). The counting errors in these experiments, reflecting the probabilisitic nature of the radioactive decay process, translate into errors of ± 10–15% for the [¹⁴C]/[³H] ratios (95% confidence limits), and many of the differences between the regenerating and intact sides far exceed this statistical error range. A repetition of this experiment, done in another animal under similar conditions (Fig. 1C), shows the replicability of these results, with the principal labeling increases on day 8 of regeneration again appearing for components with approximate molecular masses of 210 K, 44 K, and 27 K; relative decreases on the regenerating side include proteins in the 35-K range. We have shown that the same relative labeling profiles appear regardless of which isotope is injected into the regenerating or control sides, thus demonstrating the absence of isotope artifacts in this experimental system (Benowitz *et al.*, 1981).

A time course series (Figure 2) shows a qualitative shift in the composition of the rapid phase of transport at about 1 month after surgery. The enhanced labeling of the 210-, 44-, and 27-K proteins that had appeared on day 8 remains prominent up to 3–4 weeks. These peaks then begin to decline, and between 4 and 6 weeks, the greatest increases are associated with proteins between 110 and 140 kilodaltons. Synaptogenesis in the retinotectal pathway is occurring in this period (Yoon, 1975; Murray, 1976, 1982), and in the studies described in Section 3, we have examined the possibility that the transition in labeling pattern seen at about 1 month may actually be initiated by target contact. By day 62, most of the regeneration-related changes have subsided, as shown by the relatively small magnitude of the deviations in the isotope ratios on the bottom of Figure 2.

As anticipated from earlier investigations on the nature of rapid axonal transport (e.g., Lorenz and Willard, 1978; Droz *et al.*, 1973), the proteins visualized in these studies appear to become associated with nerve terminal mem-

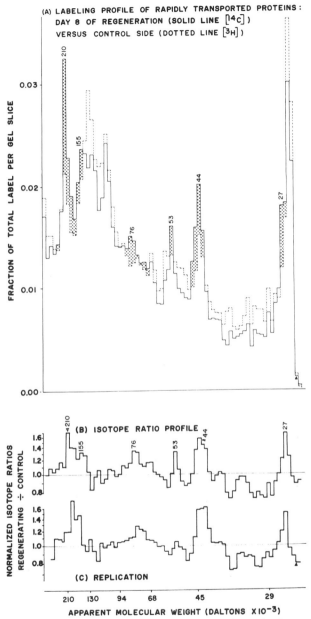

FIGURE 1. Comparison of double-labeled rapidly transported proteins in regenerating and intact optic nerves by unidimensional gel electrophoresis. Proteins synthesized in retinal ganglion cells undergoing axonal regeneration for 8 days were labeled by intraocular injection of [^{14}C]proline, the contralateral control side with [^{3}H]proline. Relative increases in the regenerating nerve are indicated by stippling (A) and correspond (B) to regions of the gel with normalized [^{14}C]/[^{3}H] ratios greater than 1. A similar isotope ratio profile is seen in C, a replication of the experiment in which the principal labeling increases again involve components with approximate molecular masses of 210, 44, and 24–27 kilodaltons.

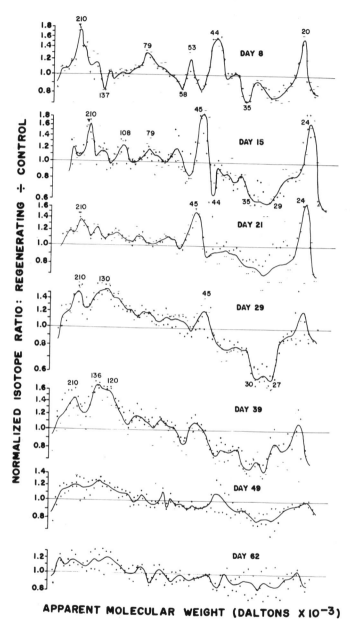

FIGURE 2. Changes in rapidly transported proteins during the course of optic nerve regeneration. At each postoperative time, proteins transported in regenerating and control nerves were compared as in Figure 1, and normalized isotope ratio profiles from two to four cases were averaged together. Values for individual gels are represented by the various symbols.

branes. To demonstrate this, proteins synthesized in regenerating and intact retinal ganglion cells were differentially labeled with [³H]- or [¹⁴C]proline. After allowing 15 hr for rapidly transported proteins to accumulate in the nerve terminals, optic tecta receiving either intact or regenerating optic fibers were dissected out, combined, and subjected to standard subcellular fractionation procedures (Whittaker and Greengard, 1971), in which components of a lysed crude membrane (P_2) fraction (obtained by centrifugation at 17,000 × g for 20 min) were separated by centrifugation on a discontinuous sucrose density gradient (Figure 3). At both 19 and 35 days after surgery, material that is selectively enriched in regenerating nerve sediments at the 0.6/0.8 and 0.8/1.0 M sucrose interfaces, consistent with their association with membranous components (Lorenz and Willard, 1978). When this membranous fraction is separated on one-dimensional gels, a striking peak is seen at ∼44 K and a lesser one at ∼210 K. Thus, at least some of the proteins that increase during regeneration do appear to be associated with nerve terminal membranes.

2.2. Two-Dimensional Gel Analyses

Having established that regeneration does in fact involve a shift in the composition of rapid axonal transport, we next explored some of the protein changes in greater detail, combining high-resolution two-dimensional gel electrophoresis (2DGE) with single- and double-isotope labeling, subcellular fractionation, and silver staining methods (Benowitz and Lewis, 1982, 1983). In particular, we were interested in (1) determining whether the proteins that increase during regeneration coincide with identified molecular species, (2) quantifying the magnitude of the changes, and (3) examining whether these

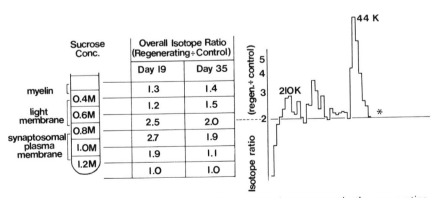

FIGURE 3. Subcellular fractionation of rapidly transported components in the regenerating visual pathway.

changes reflect increased turnover or a net accumulation of the proteins during regeneration.

A 2DGE comparison of the rapidly transported proteins in intact and regenerating retinotectal pathways is shown in Figure 4. In this study, retinal ganglion cells were labeled with [^{35}S]methionine; after allowing 16 hr for rapidly transported components to accumulate in the nerve terminals, we dissected out the optic tecta and subjected them to subcellular fractionation. Material collected in the light membrane fraction (0.6/1.0 sucrose interface) was subjected to two-dimensional gel electrophoresis using a modification of the method of O'Farrell (1975). The fluorograms of this material (Figure 4) show a general increase in protein labeling in regenerating nerves, particularly at the earlier time point, a finding consistent with several other reports (Forman *et al.*, 1971; Heacock and Agranoff, 1982; McQuarrie and Grafstein, 1982). However, over and above this general increase is a qualitative change for the acidic proteins at 48 K and 49 K. These proteins are prominently labeled in the day 19 case, subside on day 40 of regeneration, and are not seen at all in controls. Presumably, this group of proteins corresponds to the labeling peak at around 44 K that had been observed in the earlier one-dimensional gel studies but whose magnitude may have been obscured by comigrating species that are not differentially increased during regeneration.

Other differences between regenerating and intact nerves of a quantitative nature are also suggested in the gels of Figure 4 but are difficult to evaluate because of uncontrolled experimental variables, e.g., overall radioactivity levels on the gels, exposure times, or possible differences in gel runs. Additional studies show that during regeneration, the 44 to 49 K acidic proteins appear in the soluble fraction in the optic tectum as well as in the particulate fraction. This suggests that these proteins may normally be only loosely bound to membranous components and are readily liberated or that they may be sequestered within vesicles that are partially ruptured during subcellular fractionation.

Increases in the total amount of the 48-K acidic protein present in the retinotectal pathway during regeneration can be seen using sensitive protein-staining methods. On the gels shown in Figure 5, membranous proteins from tecta receiving either intact (A) or regenerating (B) optic nerves were separated by two-dimensional gel electrophoresis and then stained by the reduced silver method (Oakley, 1980). Only a small portion of the material on these gels derives from the terminals of the retinotectal pathway, the remainder being associated with other neural systems and with glia of the tectum. Nevertheless, the enhancement of the 48-K acidic protein during regeneration is quite evident. The small amount of this protein also seen in tecta receiving intact nerves may be associated either with low levels that may normally be present in the intact optic nerve or with other cells of the tectum (e.g., interneurons).

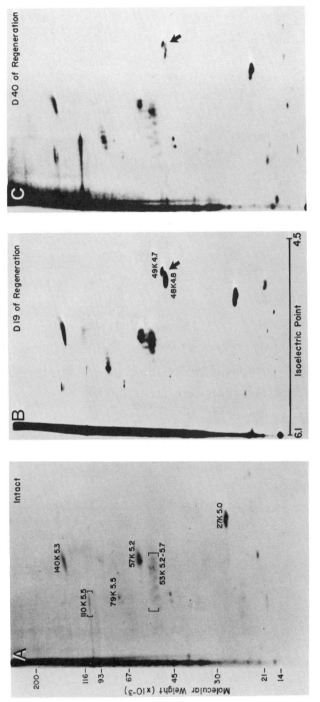

FIGURE 4. Evaluation of rapidly transported proteins in regenerating and intact retinotectal pathways by two-dimensional gel electrophoretic (2DGE) analysis. Arrows indicate the prominent labeling of the acidic 48-K and 49-K proteins during regeneration compared with the absence of their labeling in the controls. Brackets delineate groups of similar-sized proteins that differ in pI. Protein was pooled from seven animals in each group.

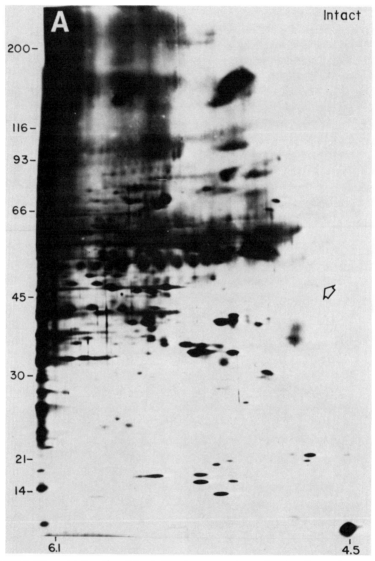

FIGURE 5. Silver staining of proteins in the plasma membrane fraction of tecta innervated by K acidic protein in the reinnervated tectum.

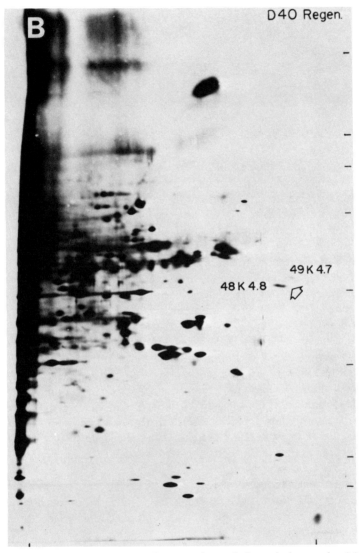

intact (A) and regenerating (B) optic nerves. Arrows indicate the increased staining of the 48-

In order to quantify the labeling changes associated with regeneration, double-isotope methods were combined with 2DGE. As in the one-dimensional gel studies of Section 2.1, regenerating and control retinal ganglion cells were differentially labeled with [^{3}H]- and [^{14}C]proline, and the proteins rapidly transported to the nerve terminals of the optic tecta (P$_2$ fraction) were coseparated on two-dimensional gels. Gels were fluorographed to identify the positions of labeled components, a template of the fluorogram was prepared, and this was then used to cut proteins from the gels. Gel segments were counted for ^{3}H and ^{14}C activities, the ratio of which, when normalized by the overall ratio of the two isotopes in the total sample, reflects the extent to which the metabolism of each molecular species is relatively increased or decreased during regeneration.

Figure 6 shows double-labeling experiments comparing the rapidly transported proteins in regenerating and intact optic nerves at two different times after surgery. One striking feature of the fluorograms is the intensity of labeling of the group of acidic proteins between 44 and 49 K when proline is used as a metabolic precursor rather than methionine (cf. Figure 4). With proline, these proteins become the most heavily labeled components on the two-dimensional gels of acidic, rapidly transported proteins. Even more remarkable, however, is the selective enrichment of these proteins in regenerating nerves. Relative to the amounts of [^{3}H]- and [^{14}C]proline injected into the two eyes of these animals, the 44 to 49 K acidic proteins have a normalized isotope ratio greater than 100-fold on day 19 and ~30-fold on day 40.

As a control to verify that the 44 to 49 K acidic proteins are truly of neuronal origin and not associated with changes that may be occurring in the glial sheath cells, optic nerve segments were dissected from day 30 post-crush material and incubated in the presence of [^{35}S]methionine under conditions favorable to survival of the nonneuronal cells (Nixon, 1980). Gels of the soluble and particulate protein fractions labeled under these conditions show no evidence of the 44 to 49 K acidic proteins. Thus, the 44 to 49 K acidic proteins would appear to be neuron specific and are visualized in the previous experiments by virtue of axonal transport.

In sum then, the results of our 2-D gel studies show that among the rapidly transported proteins, the most prominent change that occurs during regeneration involves a group of acidic proteins with molecular weights between 44 and 49,000. At early stages of regeneration, these proteins increase ~100-fold relative to intact controls; they are present in both membrane and soluble fractions and appear to be relatively abundant in proline while having few methionine residues. In this group of proteins are components that are likely to correspond to the protein GAP-43 described by Skene and Willard (1981*a–c*), a rapidly transported species whose labeling increases greatly during regeneration of the toad optic nerve and which is prominent in early developmental

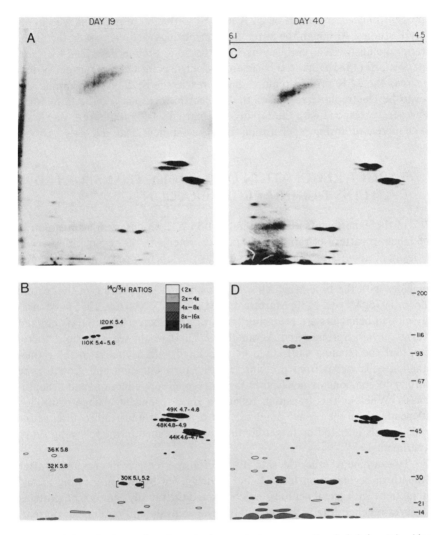

FIGURE 6. Quantitative studies of protein changes during regeneration. Labeled proteins, identified on the gels by fluorography (A and C) were cut out and counted for $[^3H]/[^{14}C]$ ratios (B and D). The acidic proteins between 44 and 49 K have a normalized ratio >100 on day 19 of regeneration and ~30 on day 40. Other, less striking molecular changes are also visualized on these gels as indicated. Note the high labeling of the 44- to 49-K acidic proteins with proline relative to methionine (cf. Figure 4).

stages of the mammalian visual pathway. Skene and Willard have also found specific increases in the regenerating toad visual pathway for proteins with apparent molecular masses of 24 K and 50 K that were not visualized in our 2DGE studies. Although the latter components may well increase in the regenerating goldfish visual pathway as well, the 50-K protein described by Skene and Willard (1981 *a*) has too basic an isoelectric point to enter our gel system, whereas the 24-K protein requires high urea in the SDS-polyacrylamide slab gel to be electrophoresed out of the isoelectric focusing gel; the latter may, however, correspond with the rapidly transported 24-K protein that was found to be increased during regeneration in our one-dimensional gel analyses.

3. TARGET REGULATION OF RAPIDLY TRANSPORTED PROTEINS DURING REGENERATION

In the experiments described in Section 2.1, we observed a transition in the labeling pattern of rapidly transported proteins in the regenerating visual pathway at about 1 month after surgery, as the labeling peaks at 210, 44, and 24 K declined and new ones between 110 and 140 K appeared. This change coincides with the time at which synapses are first reappearing in the tectum (Yoon, 1976; Meyer, 1980; Marotte and Mark, 1975; Murray, 1976) and visually guided behaviors are returning (Attardi and Sperry, 1963; Grafstein and Murray, 1969; Springer and Agranoff, 1977). It would seem possible, therefore, that the labeling shift could be associated with a change in the retinal ganglion cells' needs from proteins required for elongation and growth cone motility to components involved in target recognition, adhesion, and synaptogenesis. Whether this transition reflects a time-dependent change controlled independently in the retinal ganglion cells, or whether it instead requires retrograde signals initiated by target contact, was examined in the following set of experiments.

To examine whether the transition in transported proteins occurring after 1 month of regeneration may in fact be triggered by the outgrowing axons' interactions with tectal neurons, we contrasted the rapidly transported proteins in nerves regenerating with and without the contralateral optic tecta present. In one set of experiments, this comparison was carried out using two different groups of fish; in one of these groups, both optic tecta were removed at the time of optic nerve crush, so that the regenerating fibers would not encounter their normal central target field [regeneration without tecta (R − T)]; in the second group, nerves were crushed at the same time as in the first group, but the optic tecta were left intact [regeneration with tecta (R + T)]. Comparisons between such groups were made at ten time points ranging from 10 days to 5 months after surgery. As before, double-isotope methods were used to contrast the labeling patterns in the two experimental conditions at each time point. Proteins synthesized in the R + T and R − T groups were differentially labeled by intraocular injections of [^{3}H]- and [^{14}C]proline, and components present in the optic nerves after 5 hr were analyzed by one- or two-dimensional gel electrophoresis (Benowitz *et al.*, 1983; Yoon *et al.*, in preparation).

In the experiment shown in Figure 7, [^{3}H]-labeled proteins from R + T nerves (36 days post-surgery) were coseparated on two-dimensional gels with [^{14}C]-labeled proteins from R − T nerves. The staining pattern of these gels, shown in Figure 7A, is dominated by the principal constituents of the glial sheath cells and of the optic fibers, including tubulin, actin, and intermediate filaments. A fluorogram showing the mixed [^{3}H]- and [^{14}C]proline incorporation profiles in the nerves 5 hr after labeling is shown in Figure 7B and demonstrates the distinctiveness of the rapid phase of transport from the major structural components of the nerve. The normalized [^{3}H]/[^{14}C] ratios for the rapidly transported proteins, illustrated in Figure 7C for components separated on a two-dimensional gel of neutral proteins and in Figure 7D for the acidic proteins shown in Figure 7A and 7B, reflect the extent to which individual proteins are selectively increased or decreased when regenerating fibers are allowed to interact with the optic tectum. These ratios can be seen to vary over a fourfold range, a result that demonstrates that interactions between the optic fibers and the tectum do in fact selectively increase or decrease particular rapidly transported components.

The greatest positive change associated with target contact is for the protein that migrates at 140,000 daltons with an isoelectric point between 5.2 and 5.4. Increases of a nearly equal magnitude also appear in several less prominent constituents, several of which migrate in the vicinity of the 140-K 5.2–5.4 protein, possibly having some precursor–product relationship to it. The most prominent decreases associated with tectal interactions involve a group of slightly basic, high-molecular-weight proteins between 160 and 230 K, whose isotope ratios are about one-half that of the overall ratio for this material. Somewhat unexpectedly, the 44- to 49-K acidic proteins, the constituents of rapid axonal transport that increase so dramatically during regeneration, are turned on to a similar degree regardless of whether the tectum is present or not. Thus, the expression of these proteins may be regulated endogenously after axotomy in the retinal ganglion cells or may depend on extrinsic factors provided by the brain as a whole; however, interactions with the appropriate target field of the optic fibers, the tectum, are not a major regulatory factor.

The time course of the changes associated with target interactions was studied using double-labeling and one-dimensional protein separation methods. Results from these experiments are summarized in Figure 8, which shows the normalized ratios of the isotope used to label R + T animals relative to that used to label R − T animals (N = 2–7 per group for each time point); rapidly

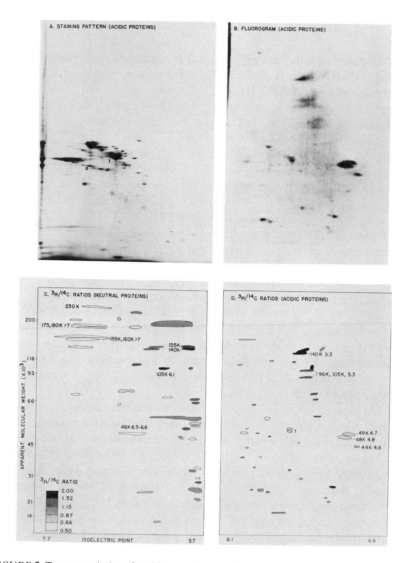

FIGURE 7. Target regulation of rapid axonal transport in the regenerating optic nerve: 2D gel analysis. Thirty-six days after surgery, retinas in 12 goldfish having both optic nerves crushed and the optic tecta left intact (R + T group) were labeled with [³H]proline; retinas of 12 goldfish regenerating for 36 days following bilateral optic nerve damage and the removal of both tecta (R − T group) were labeled with [¹⁴C]proline. Rapidly transported components present in the nerves of the two groups 5 hr after labeling were analyzed by 2DGE. (A) Coomassie brilliant blue staining pattern of the regenerating optic nerve (acidic proteins) includes tubulin (t) and actin (a). (B) Fluorogram of the same gel shows [³H]- and [¹⁴C]-labeled rapidly transported proteins in transit down the nerve. (C, D) Normalized [³H]/[¹⁴C] ratios for rapidly transported proteins having (C) neutral pIs (5.7–7.7) and (D) acidic pIs, as shown in A and B. Proteins on the far right end of C, the neutral two-dimensional gel, probably coincide with components that are well resolved in D, the acidic gel.

transported proteins that are relatively increased when the target is present are those that have ratios greater than one, whereas constituents that are relatively decreased when the tectum is present have a ratio below one. At the earliest times examined (10 and 15 days after surgery), no major differences appear between the R + T and R − T groups, a result that is not surprising in view of the fact that even in the R + T animals, regenerating optic fibers have barely begun to encounter the tectum. Beginning on day 24 and continuing through day 40, the R + T group shows a prominent increase between 120 and 160 K (Figure 8, middle). This presumably corresponds to the protein(s) around 140 K, pI 5.2–5.4, which was also shown in our 2DGE study (Figure 7) to increase nearly twofold when the tectum was encountered. It is also likely to correspond to the molecules of similar size that increase relative to controls at this time (Figure 2). The differential labeling of the 120 to 160-K proteins diminishes at times greter than 50 days and is not evident in the 5-month case shown on the bottom of Figure 8.

Another striking change associated with target interactions is the decreased labeling of constituents between 24 and 27 K in nerves that have been allowed to contact the optic tectum (also see Figure 2). This change can be seen in the 30-day case shown in the middle of Figure 8 and persists for months afterwards. These results indicate that the expression of the 24 to 27-K protein(s) increases at early stages of regeneration and decreases when the normal target is encountered but remains elevated for months when nerves are prevented from contacting the tectum. Other studies have shown that such optic nerves, when unable to contact the tectum, form widespread anomalous projections elsewhere in the brain, including to areas that had been denervated by removal of the tectum (Lo and Levine, 1981).

A variant of this experiment compared optic nerves regenerating with and without the optic tectum present within the same animal (Yoon *et al.*, in preparation). In this second series of experiments, both optic nerves were crushed, and only one optic tectum was removed; thus, one nerve was regenerating with the contralateral tectum present while the other nerve regenerated with its principal target tissue removed. One objective of these experiments was to distinguish whether the regulatory effects of the tectum seen in the previous series were mediated by trophic factors that may have been secreted from the tectum or by surface contact-related events instead. In the case in which comparisons had been made between two groups of animals, one having both tecta intact and the other having both removed, the differences in protein-labeling patterns seen between the R + T and R − T nerves could be attributed, *a priori,* to either type of regulation. In the second series, in which one tectum remains intact, although both nerves would have access to humoral factors that might be released by the tectum, only the nerve contralateral to the remaining tectum could benefit from surface contact-mediated phenomena. Thus, if the rapidly

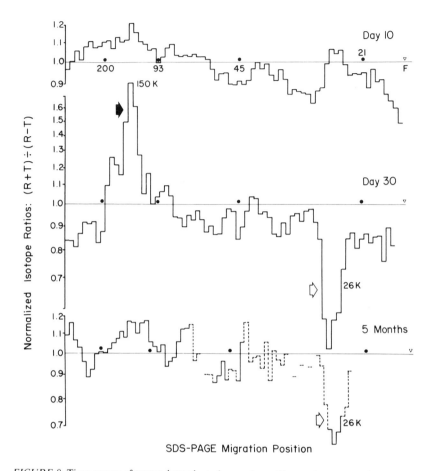

FIGURE 8. Time course of target-dependent changes in rapid axonal transport during regeneration. Retinal ganglion cells undergoing axonal regeneration with (R + T) and without (R − T) the contralateral tecta present were differentially labeled with [^{H}]- and [^{14}C]proline (N = 2–4 per group per time point). Rapidly transported proteins present in the R + T and R − T nerves after 5 hr were coelectrophoresed on SDS-polyacrylamide gels. A plot of the normalized isotope ratios in 1-mm slices shows little difference between the rapidly transported proteins in R + T and R − T nerves at early time points of regeneration (top); at 30 days (middle), coincident with the time of target innervation, nerves that are allowed to contact the tectum show an incresed transport for components between 120 and 160 K (dark arrow) and a decrease for proteins between 24 and 27 K (open arrow); enhanced labeling of the 24- 27-K components persists for 5 months in nerves that had been prevented from contacting the tectum (bottom). Solid lines indicate segments with S.E. of ratios ≤15%; dashed lines indicate SE ≤ 20%; open spaces indicate segments with SE > 20%; F, dye front.

transported proteins were found to be similar in the two nerves of these animals, the results would suggest that the regulatory effects of the tectum were mediated by humoral factors; if, on the other hand, the proteins on the two sides differed as in the previous set of experiments, then the results would argue that it is contact-mediated events between the nerve terminals and the tectum that are critical in regulating the pattern of transported proteins.

The results of the second series of experiments showed differences between the two nerves of single goldfish that were the same as those seen in the previous set of experiments. As before, differences between nerves regenerating with and without the tectum present were not apparent within the first 2–3 weeks of surgery, presumably because neither nerve had yet had any contact with the tectum. Differences between the two nerves appear by 3–4 weeks and then become more pronounced. At 5 weeks, the most prominent differences include an increased labeling of components between 120 and 160 K and a decreased labeling of low-molecular-weight components in nerves allowed to contact the contralateral tectum. With increasing time after surgery, optic fibers that fail to encounter their contralateral tectum recross to the intact ipsilateral tectum, where they compete for synaptic sites with the projections from the other retina (Lo and Levine, 1981). Presumably, this would cause the spectra of transported proteins in the two nerves to become similar to one another as time goes on, though this remains to be examined.

4. SUMMARY AND CONCLUSIONS

The changes in the molecular composition of the rapid phase of axonal transport demonstrated by these studies presumably correspond to the cell's successive requirements for constituents involved in such phenomena as motility of the growth cone, target recognition, adhesion, and the formation of synaptic specializations as regeneration proceeds. An early period of axonal outgrowth (8 days to 1 month) is marked by increases in rapidly transported proteins with apparent molecular weights of 210,000, 44–49,000 and 24–27,000. As visualized on two-dimensional gels, the change in the 44- to 49-K proteins is particularly striking. These proteins, which appear to be present in both the soluble and membrane fractions of the optic nerve terminals, increase more than 100-fold within the first 3 weeks of regeneration. The proteins incorporate considerably more proline than methionine, and when the former is used as a radiolabeled precursor, the proteins become among the most heavily labeled components of rapid axonal transport during regeneration. Other studies have confirmed the prominent increase of components with similar molecular weights during regeneration of the goldfish visual pathway (Heacock and Agranoff, 1982), in the regenerating retinotectal pathway of the toad (Skene and Willard, 1981*a*), in the developing rabbit visual pathway, and in regenerating rabbit peripheral nerve (Skene and Willard, 1981*b*). Regeneration of the toad visual pathway also involves increases in rapidly transported proteins with molecular masses of 50 K and 24 K (Skene and Willard, 1981*a*), the latter component possibly corresponding to the 24 to 27-K protein(s) found to be turned on at early stages of optic nerve regeneration in the goldfish in our one-dimensional gel study (Section 2.1, Figures 1, 2). Changes in proteins transported in other phases of axonal transport have also been described in the regenerating visual pathway of goldfish (Heacock and Agranoff, 1976, 1982; Giulian *et al.*, 1980; Quitschke *et al.*, 1980), to be described elsewhere in this volume.

Within the first 2 weeks of regeneration, the pattern of rapidly transported proteins does not depend on the optic tectum *per se*, though it could require trophic factors deriving from brain tissue in general (Schwartz *et al.*, 1982*a,b*). The neurotrophic protein nerve growth factor (NGF) has been shown to influence the regeneration of the optic nerve in lower vertebrates (Turner *et al.*, 1981, 1982; Yip and Grafstein, 1982), and appreciable amounts of this protein are in fact present in glial cells of the goldfish brain (Benowitz and Shashoua, 1979; Benowitz and Greene, 1979). Alternatively, the axotomy could lead to a shift in the retinal ganglion cells' program of protein metabolism and transport by removing a factor that is normally provided to these cells when they establish stable synapses (Varon and Bunge, 1980).

When outgrowing optic fibers begin interacting with the tectum at about 3–4 weeks after surgery, the pattern of rapidly transported proteins in the nerve shifts. A decline of at least 50% is seen in the labeling of components between 24 and 27 K and in the labeling of a group of neutral proteins between 155 and 230 K; at the same time, the labeling of components between 120 and 160 K, pI 5.2–5.3, nearly doubles. Surprisingly, target interactions do not seem to affect the expression of the acidic 44- to 48-K proteins; the decline in the labeling of these proteins with time occurs to a similar degree whether or not the tectum is present.

Thus, from these studies we can distinguish two types of changes in membrane protein transport during the regenerative process, one occurring early following axotomy and the other occurring when the growing fibers encounter the optic tectum. In terms of changes in specific proteins, we observe:

1. Proteins whose increase is initiated by axotomy but whose regulation appears to be independent of the optic tectum. The 44- to 49-K acidic proteins are the most prominent examples of this type. These components may be related to such early events as axon elongation or growth cone motility.
2. Proteins that increase following axotomy but decline when the appropriate target cells are encountered. In the range of 24 to 27 K, we find

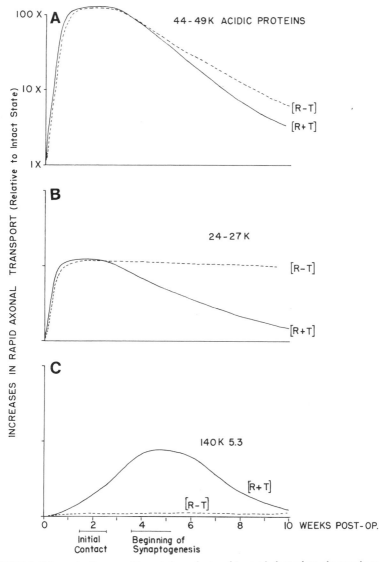

FIGURE 9. Schematic diagram of target-dependent and target-independent changes in rapidly transported proteins during optic nerve regeneration. (A) The group of acidic proteins with molecular masses of 44–49 K increases ~100-fold at early stages of regeneration and then declines regardless of whether the optic tectum is present (solid line) or absent (dashed line). (B) Components between 24 and 27 K increase severalfold during early stages of regeneration and then decline when the tectum is encountered (solid line); they remain turned on for months, however, in nerves prevented from interacting with their appropriate target tissue (dashed line). (C) The 140-K pI 5.3 protein increases at the time of contact between the optic fibers and the tectum (solid line).

proteins whose increase is striking at early time points but that then decline when the tectum is encountered; in nerves that are surgically prevented from interacting with the tectum, levels of these components remain elevated for months. Thus, the increased expression of the 24- to 27-K proteins seems to correspond with a growth stage in which axons have not yet finalized synaptic relationships with appropriate target cells.

3. Proteins that increase only when the appropriate target cells are encountered. The most prominent instance of this type is the protein that migrates at 140,000 daltons, pI 5.2–5.4. This protein increases for only a limited amount of time after innervation begins at about 25 days, continuing through the next 2–3 weeks. Retinal ganglion cells whose axons fail to encounter the tectum do not show a similar increase in these proteins. The appearance of these components may be related to the process of synaptogenesis *per se.*

Figure 9 schematically illustrates the time course of the changes for various rapidly transported components during reestablishment of retinotectal projections, as suggested by these studies. The obvious next steps will be to examine the generality of these observations to other instances of growth and plasticity in the vertebrate CNS, to identify the factors that regulate the changes in the expression of these components, and, finally, to gain some understanding of the biochemistry, localization, and physiological significance of the various molecular species visualized here. Progress along these lines will undoubtedly help to bring us closer to understanding the phenomena of neural development and regeneration at a molecular level and perhaps also to provide insights into how these processes might be controlled clinically.

ACKNOWLEDGMENTS

This chapter is dedicated to Professor Roger W. Sperry on the occasion of his 70th birthday. Portions of this work were done in collaboration with Drs. M. G. Yoon, E. R. Lewis, and V. E. Shashoua and with K. Padda. Figures 1, 2, and 4–6 are reproduced from the *Journal of Neuroscience* with permission from the Williams & Wilkins Company, and Figure 8 is from *Science* courtesy of the American Association for the Advancement of Science. Research support was provided by NINCDS Grant R01 NS16943 and by an Alfred P. Sloan Foundation Fellowship.

5. REFERENCES

Attardi, D. G., and Sperry, R. W., 1963, Preferential selection of central pathways by regenerating optic fibers, *Exp. Neurol.* 7:46–64.
Barondes, S. H., 1970, Brain glycomacromolecules and interneuronal recognition, in *The Neu-*

rosciences Second Study Program (F. O. Schmitt, ed.), pp. 747–760, Rockefeller University Press, New York.

Barondes, S. (ed), 1976, *Neuronal Recognition,* Plenum Press, New York.

Bennett, G., DiGiamberardino, L. Koenig, H. L., and Droz, B., 1973, Axonal migration of protein and glycoprotein to nerve endings. II. Radioautographic analysis of the renewal of glycoproteins in nerve endings of chicken ciliary ganglion after intracerebral injection of [³H]fucose and [³H]glucosamine, *Brain Res.* **60:**129–146.

Benowitz, L. I., and Greene, L. A., 1979, Nerve growth factor in the goldfish brain: Biological assay studies using pheochromocytoma cells, *Brain Res.* **162:**164–168.

Benowitz, L. I., and Lewis, E. R., 1982, *De novo* appearance of an acidic 46K protein in regenerating optic nerves, *Trans. Am. Soc. Neurochem.* **13**(1):318.

Benowitz, L. I., and Lewis, E. R., 1983, Increased transport of 44–49,000 dalton acidic proteins during optic nerve regeneration in the goldfish: A 2-D gel analysis, *J. Neurosci.* **3:**2153–2163.

Benowitz, L., and Padda, K., 1981, Molecular changes in regenerating retinotectal nerve terminals, *Neurosci. Abstr.* **7:**678.

Benowitz, L. I., and Shashoua, V. E., 1979, Immunoreactive sites for nerve growth factor (NGF) in the goldfish brain, *Brain Res.* **172:**561–565.

Benowitz, L. I., Shashoua, V. E., and Yoon, M. G., 1981, Specific changes in rapidly-transported proteins during regeneration of the goldfish optic nerve, *J. Neurosci.* **1:**300–307.

Benowitz, L. I., Yoon, M. G., and Lewis, E. R., 1983, Transported proteins in the regenerating optic nerve: Regulation by interactions with the optic tectum, *Science* **222:**185–188.

Bray, D., 1973, Model for membrane movements in the neural growth cone, *Nature* **244:**93–96.

Droz, B., Rambourg, A., and Koenig, H. L., 1975, The smooth endoplasmic reticulum: Structure and role in the renewal of axonal membrane and synaptic vesicles by fast axonal transport, *Brain Res.* **93:**1–13.

Feldman, E. L., Axelrod, D., Schwartz, M., and Agranoff, B. W., 1979, New neurite membrane is added at the growing tip, *Neurosci. Abstr.* **5:**303.

Forman, D. S., McEwen, B. S., and Grafstein, B., 1971, Rapid transport of radioactivity in goldfish optic nerve following injections of labeled glucosamine, *Brain Res.* **28:**119–130.

Giulian, D., Des Ruisseaux, H., and Cowburn, D., 1980, Biosynthesis and intraaxonal transport of proteins during neuronal regeneration, *J. Biol. Chem.* **255:**6494–6501.

Grafstein, B., 1975, The nerve cell body response to axotomy, *Exp. Neurol.* **48:**32–51.

Grafstein, B., and Forman, D. S., 1980, Intracellular transport in neurons, *Physiol. Rev.* **60:**1167–1283.

Grafstein, B., and Murray, M., 1969, Transport of protein in goldfish optic nerve during regeneration, *Exp. Neurol.* **25:**494–508.

Grafstein, B., Forman, D.S., and McEwen, B. S., 1972, Effects of temperature on axonal transport and turnover of protein in the goldfish visual system, *Exp. Neurol.* **34:**158–170.

Hammerschlag, R., and Stone, G. C., 1982, Membrane delivery by fast axonal transport, *Trends Neurosci.* **5:**12–15.

Heacock, A. M., and Agranoff, B. W., 1976, Enhanced labeling of a retinal protein during regeneration of optic nerve in goldfish, *Proc. Natl. Acad. Sci. U.S.A.* **73:**828–832.

Heacock, A. M., and Agranoff, B. W., 1982, Protein synthesis and transport in the regenerating goldfish visual system, *Neurochem. Res.* **7:**771–788.

Heacock, A. M., Klinger, P. D., Seguin, E. B., and Agranoff, B. W., 1982, Cholesterol synthesis and nerve regeneration, *Neurosci. Abstr.* **8:**761.

Ingoglia, N. A., and Tuliszewski, R., 1976, Transfer RNA may be axonally transported during regeneration of goldfish optic nerves, *Brain Res.* **112:**371–381.

Jacobson, M., 1978, *Developmental Neurobiology,* Second Edition, pp. 345–422, Plenum Press, New York.

Lo, R. Y. S., and Levine, R. L., 1981, Anatomical evidence for the influence of degenerating pathways on regenerating optic fibers following surgical manipulations in the visual system of the goldfish, *Brain Res.* **210**:61–81.

Lorenz, T., and Willard, M., 1978, Subcellular fractionation of intra-axonally transported polypeptides in the rabbit visual system, *Proc. Natl. Acad. Sci. U.S.A.* **75**:505–509.

Marotte, L. R., and Mark, R. F., 1975, Ultrastructural localization of synaptic input to the optic lobe of carp, *Exp. Neurol.* **49**:772–789.

McEwen, B. S., and Grafstein, B., 1968, Fast and slow components in axonal transport of protein, *J. Cell Biol.* **38**:494–508.

McQuarrie, I. G. and Grafstein, B., 1982, Protein synthesis and fast axonal transport in regenerating goldfish retinal ganglion cells, *Brain Res.* **235**:213–223.

Meyer, R. L., 1980, "Extra" optic fibers exclude normal fibers from tectal regions in the goldfish, *J. Comp. Neurol.* **183**:883–902.

Murray, M., 1973, ^{3}H-uridine incorporation by regenerating retinal ganglion cells of goldfish, *Exp. Neurol.* **39**:489–497.

Murray, M., 1976, Regeneration of retinal axons into the goldfish optic tectum, *J. Comp. Neurol.* **168**:175–195.

Murray, M., 1982, A quantitative study of regenerative sprouting by optic axons in goldfish, *J. Comp. Neurol.* **209**:352–362.

Murray, M., and Edwards, M. A., 1982, A quantitative study of the reinnervation of the goldfish optic tectum following optic nerve crush, *J. Comp. Neurol.* **209**:363–373.

Murray, M., and Forman, D. S., 1971, Fine structural changes in goldfish retinal ganglion cells during axonal regeneration, *Brain Res.* **32**:287–298.

Murray, M., and Grafstein, B., 1969, Changes in the morphology and amino acid incorporation of regenerating goldfish optic neurons, *Exp. Neurol.* **23**:544–560.

Nixon, R. A., 1980, Protein degradation in the mouse visual system. I. Degradation of axonally transported and retinal proteins, *Brain Res.* **200**:69–83.

Oakley, B. R. Kirsch, D. R., and Morris, N. R., 1980, A simplified ultrasensitive silver stain for detecting proteins in polyacrylamide gels, *Anal. Biochem.* **105**:361–363.

O'Farrell, P. H., 1975, High resolution two-dimensional electrophoresis of proteins, *J. Biol. Chem.* **250**:4007–4021.

Quitschke, W., Francis, S., and Schechter, N., 1980, Electrophoretic analysis of specific proteins in the regenerating goldfish retinotectal pathway, *Brain Res.* **201**:347–360.

Roth, S., and Marchase, R. B., 1976, An *in vitro* assay for retinotectal specificity, in: *Neuronal Recognition* (S. H. Barondes, ed.), pp. 227–247, Plenum Press, New York.

Schwartz, J. H., 1979, Axonal transport: Components, mechanisms, and specificity, *Annu. Rev. Neurosci.* **2**:467–504.

Schwartz, M., Mizrachi, Y., and Kimhi, Y., 1982a, Regenerating goldfish retinal explants: Induction and maintenance of neurites by conditioned medium from cells originating in the N.S., *Dev. Brain Res.* **3**:21–28.

Schwartz, M., Mizrachi, Y., and Eschhar, N., 1982b, Factors in goldfish brain induce neuritic outgrowth from explanted regenerating retinas, *Dev. Brain Res.* **3**:29–35.

Sharma, S. C., 1972, Reformation of retinotectal projections after various tectal ablations in adult goldfish, *Exp. Neurol.* **34**:171–182.

Skene, J. H. P., and Willard, M., 1981a, Changes in axonally transported proteins during axon regeneration in toad retinal ganglion cells, *J. Cell Biol.* **89**:86–95.

Skene, J. H. P., and Willard, M., 1981b, Axonally transported proteins associated with axon growth in rabbit central and peripheral nervous system, *J. Cell Biol.* **89**:96–103.

Skene, J. H. P., and Willard, M., 1981c, Characteristics of growth-associated polypeptides in regenerating toad retinal ganglion cell axons, *J. Neurosci.* **1**:419–426.

Sperry, R. W., 1943, Visuomotor coordination in the newt *(Triturus viridescens)* after regeneration of the optic nerves, *J. Comp. Neurol.* **79**:33–55.

Sperry, R. W., 1948, Patterning of central synapses in regeneration of the optic nerve in teleosts, *Physiol. Zool.* **21**:351–361.

Sperry, R. W., 1963, Chemoaffinity in the orderly growth of nerve fiber patterns and connections, *Proc. Natl. Acad. Sci. U.S.A.* **50**:703–710.

Springer, A. D., and Agranoff, B., 1977, Effect of temperature on rate of goldfish optic nerve regeneration: A Radioautographic and behavioral study, *Brain Res.* **128**:405–415.

Springer, A. D., Easter, S. S., and Agranoff, B. W., 1977, The role of the optic tectum in various visually mediated behaviors of goldfish, *Brain Res.* **128**:393–404.

Turner, J. E., Delaney, R. K., and Johnson, J. E., 1981, Retinal ganglion cell response to axotomy and nerve growth factor antiserum treatment in the regenerating visual system of the goldfish *(Carassius auratus)*, *Brain Res.* **204**:283–294.

Turner, J. E., Schwab, M. E., and Thoenen, H., 1982, Nerve growth factor stimulates neurite outgrowth from goldfish retinal explants: The influence of a prior lesion, *Dev. Brain Res.* **4**:59–66.

Varon, S., and Bunge, R. P., 1978, Trophic mechanisms in the peripheral nervous system, *Annu. Rev. Neurosci.* **1**:327–361.

Whittaker, V. P., and Greengard, P., 1971, The isolation of synaptosomes from the brain of a teleost fish, centriopristes striatus, *J. Neurochem.* **18**:173–176.

Yip, H. K., and Grafstein, B., 1982, Effect of nerve growth factor on regeneration of goldfish optic axons, *Brain Res.* **238**:329–339.

Yoon, M., 1971, Reorganization of retinotectal projection following surgical operations on the optic tectum of goldfish, *Exp. Neurol.* **33**:395–411.

Yoon, M. G., 1975, Readjustment of retinotectal projection following reimplantation of a rotated or inverted tectal tissue in adult goldfish, *J. Physiol. (Lond.)* **252**:137–158.

Yoon, M. G., Benowitz, L. I., and Baker, F. A., 1984, Interactions between regenerating optic fibers and the optic tectum regulate the pattern of proteins transported from the retina in goldfish. Submitted.

CHAPTER 11

REGULATION OF AXON GROWTH AND CYTOSKELETAL DEVELOPMENT

MARK WILLARD, J. H. PATE SKENE,
CAROLYN SIMON, KARINA MEIRI,
NOBUTAKA HIROKAWA, and
MARCIE GLICKSMAN

1. INTRODUCTION

The mature, steady-state axon is a temporally ephemeral collection of matter whose apparent constancy reflects a delicate balance between the continuous introduction of materials from the cell body by the process of axonal transport and their exit. At a given instant, the major morphological manifestations of

MARK WILLARD, CAROLYN SIMON, KARINA MEIRI, and MARCIE GLICKSMAN ●
Department of Anatomy and Neurobiology, Washington University School of Medicine, St.
Louis, Missouri 63110   NOBUTAKA HIROKAWA ● *Department of Anatomy, Faculty of*
Medicine, University of Tokyo, Hongo, Tokyo, 113 Japan   J. H. PATE SKENE ● *Depart-*
ment of Neurobiology, Stanford University, Palo Alto, California 94305

this steady state are the arrays of neurofilaments, microtubules, a variety of membrane bounded organelles, and the plasma membrane; these elements communicate with each other by a complex lattice of crosslinkers.

It is a wonder that a structure of such complexity can ever be reconstructed after it is injured. Yet most neurons of fish and amphibians and the neurons of the peripheral nervous system of mammals can successfully regenerate an injured axon. Even certain neurons of the mammalian central nervous system, which do not normally regrow an injured axon, have the potential to do so. This potential is illustrated by their ability to extend axons for several centimeters when they are provided with a graft of tissue from the peripheral nervous system (Aguayo, *et. al.*, 1982).

Because the mature axon represents the steady state of a system in rapid flux, axon growth can be viewed as a perturbation of this flux from the steady state. Here we consider mechanisms for the regulation of axon growth that involve changes in the expression of neuronal genes. In particular, we examine the evidence that special proteins are involved in axon growth and that the production of these proteins may be a critical factor in determining whether an axon will grow. Second, we consider evidence that special mechanisms (different from those later used in axon maintenance) may be required to generate the neurofilamentous cytoskeleton during maturation of axons in the course of development. The time at which these mechanisms are employed raises the speculation that they may influence a transition from a state of relative plasticity to a state of relative stability of the axon.

2. GROWTH-ASSOCIATED PROTEINS AND AXON GROWTH

2.1. Characteristics of Growth-Associated Proteins

In a mature, steady-state axon, materials synthesized in the cell body enter the axon and move to their destinations by the process of axonal transport. Electrophoretic analyses of newly synthesized radiolabeled proteins has indicated that different collections of proteins move down the axon at different velocities (reviewed in Grafstein and Forman, 1980; Baitinger *et al.*, 1982). The most rapidly moving proteins (group I) include plasma membrane proteins such as the Na^+, K^+-ATPase. Mitochondria move more slowly and are components of group II. Groups III and IV include actin and two forms of myosin as well as many other cytoplasmic proteins; these groups may include the movement of force-generating machinery used to transport other organelles. The transport of proteins that compose the neurofilamentous–microtubular cytoskeleton give rise to group V, which may represent the progressive displacement down the axon of the intact cytoskeleton (Hoffman and Lasek, 1975; Lasek and Hoffman, 1976).

The introduction of proteins into the axon in this highly ordered sequence must be exactly balanced by their exit from an axon in the steady state. The fates of specific proteins are known in only a few instances; proteins may exit from axons by means of their release from axon terminals, by means of degradation, and by means of their return to the cell body. In many respects, the transport processes that normally supply the mature axons with new plasma membrane, cytoskeleton, and cytoplasm would appear to have the potential to fabricate new axon if the balance between delivery and exit of materials were altered appropriately (Lasek and Black, 1977; Willard and Skene, 1982). Indeed, neurons are able to carry out certain activities associated with axon growth [e.g., the formation of structures that morphologically resemble growth cones and the formation of limited, although abortive, sprouts (Ramon y Cajal, 1928)] without the benefit of new information from the cell body.

On the other hand, certain considerations lead to the anticipation that new, growth-specific materials must be supplied from the cell body in order to establish a productive state of axon growth. For example, if any of the axonal structures that are essential for axon growth are composed of proteins peculiar to the growth state, it might be expected that the supply of these proteins from the cell body would be essential for axon growth. The growth cone may be such a growth-specific structure with a unique molecular composition. For example, lectins (which bind to certain glycoproteins) label the growth cone differently than they label the rest of the neuron (Pfenninger and Maylie-Pfenninger, 1981). Furthermore, Pfenninger and co-workers have recently demonstrated that subcellular fractions that are enriched with respect to growth cones are also enriched with respect to certain proteins (Pfenninger *et al.*, 1983). If, in fact, these proteins are unique to the growth cone and are required for its proper function, the supply of these proteins by axonal transport would necessarily be a critical event in establishing a competent growth state.

Because of the potential importance of such growth-specific materials, we designed an assay to detect them (Skene and Willard, 1981*a*; Levine *et al.*, 1981). The assay relies on the prediction that certain growth-specific proteins would be synthesized and axonally transported at greatly increased levels in neurons with growing axons as compared to neurons with stationary axons. It should be noted that such growth-associated synthesis and transport are not unique or necessary criteria for a protein with a growth-specific function. On the one hand, not all proteins showing growth-associated synthesis need necessarily perform growth-specific functions. For example, a protein that played a structural role in the stationary axon would be expected to undergo a dramatic growth-associated increase in synthesis if it normally turned over very slowly (Skene and Willard, 1981a; Willard and Skene, 1982). This is because its rate of synthesis in the normal axon would need to be only great enough to balance its slow rate of decay. A large increase in synthetic rate would then be required to generate the extra protein required to elaborate this structure in the newly forming axon, even though this protein would not be performing a growth-specific function. On the other hand, a protein with a growth-specific function would not necessarily undergo a growth-associated increase in synthesis and transport. For example, a protein whose growth-specific functions were regulated at some metabolic level other than synthesis or transport (for example, by means of a posttranslational modification) might be synthesized and transported at high levels even in a steady-state neuron. Such growth-specific proteins would not be discovered by our assay, which would detect only those growth specific-proteins whose functions are regulated at the level of synthesis or transport.

With these features of proteins with growth-specific functions in mind, we studied changes in protein transport in regenerating neurons of the toad (Skene and Willard, 1981a). When the optic nerve of the toad *Bufo marinus* is crushed, the retinal ganglion cells regrow their axons and form functional synaptic connections in the optic tectum. Using a variety of electrophoretic techniques, we compared radiolabeled proteins transported into regenerating axons with proteins transported into uninjured control axons and observed the following differences (Skene and Willard, 1981a). (1) Most axonally transported polypeptides were radiolabeled to a higher degree in regenerating axons than in stationary axons. The average increase in labeling was about threefold in the case of group I polypeptides and tenfold in the case of group IV polypeptides. These changes most likely reflect the increases in synthesis of materials (e.g., plasma membrane components and cytoskeletal components) required in elaborating structures of the growing axon. (2) The labeling of a few polypeptides decreased during regeneration. It seems reasonable to suppose that these polypeptides may perform functions (e.g., related to neurotransmitter release) that are not required in the regenerating axon. (3) The labeling of a small number of proteins, which we designated growth-associated proteins, or GAPs, increased much more (as much as 100-fold absolute increase) than the average during regeneration. The increased labeling of GAPs followed a time course that roughly corresponded to the regenerative growth of axons; after lag periods of similar durations to the delay between axon injury and initial axon outgrowth, the labeling of GAPs increased to high levels that were maintained through the period of axon regeneration and returned to basal levels at about the time that functional synaptic connections were restored. This pattern of growth-associated induction suggested that the GAPs may perform functions that are unique to the growth state of the axon.

The three toad GAPs that we studied in greatest detail (GAP-50, -43, and -24, designated by their molecular masses in kilodaltons) were group I polypeptides with properties characteristic of integral plasma membrane proteins (Skene and Willard, 1981b). GAP-24 turned over very rapidly ($t_{1/2}$ is several hours), a property that together with its rapid rate of transport indicates that the function it performs could be rapidly initiated or terminated by the induction or cessation of its synthesis in the cell body. GAP-50 and GAP-43, which turn over more slowly ($t_{1/2}$ is several days), appear to be transported preferentially to axon tips. GAP-50 is a fucosylated glycoprotein.

In the mammalian nervous sytem (Skene and Willard, 1981c), the transport of a polypeptide with the same molecular weight and isoelectric point (pI = 4.3) as GAP-43 was induced when regeneration of a peripheral nerve (the hypoglossal nerve) was initiated after the nerve was crushed. GAP-43 was also transported in the retinal ganglion cells of neonatal rabbits during developmental periods of axon elongation, but its degree of labeling was much lower in older rabbits. Most significantly, GAP-43 was not reinduced when the optic nerve of an adult rabbit was crushed; these CNS neurons do not successfully regenerate their axons. Thus, elevated transport of GAP-43 is correlated with regenerative axon growth in the toad CNS and mammalian PNS and with developmental axon growth in the mammalian CNS.

A second rabbit polypeptide, GAP-23, bears certain physical similarities to toad GAP-24, although the two differ perceptibly in molecular weight and isoelectric point. As in the case of GAP-43, the elevated transport of GAP-23 was correlated with axonal growth during development of the rabbit CNS (optic nerve). Unlike GAP-43, it was labeled significantly in the adult rabbit hypoglossal nerve and was not further induced when the hypoglossal nerve was crushed and axon regeneration was initiated. One explanation for the behavior of GAP-23,24 would be that it performs a growth-related function that is ongoing in mammalian peripheral nerves, such as the remodeling of neuromuscular junctions. If so, the differential expression of GAP-23 and GAP-43 would illustrate that different aspects of the growth state (e.g., major axon elongation and synapse formation) can be regulated independently (Skene and Willard, 1981c). Proteins with certain behaviors and properties similar to these GAPs have also been observed in regenerating goldfish optic nerve (Benowitz *et al.,* 1981; see L. I. Benowitz, Chapter 10, this volume; Giulian *et al.,* 1980) and in rat spinal motor neurons (Theiler and McClure, 1978; Bisby, 1980).

The potential significance of the GAPs is that their growth-associated transport is consistent with their performing special growth-specific functions. To confirm this possibility, it will be necessary to determine the functions of the GAPs. Although no specific GAP function has yet been identified, certain properties of the GAPs serve to limit the possibilities. For example, as noted above, slowly-turning-over constituents of a normal axon would be expected to be transported in greatly elevated amounts into a growing axon. However, this does not appear to be the explanation for the increased transport of the GAPs because they turn over quite rapidly, with half-lives ranging from several hours to several days (Skene and Willard, 1981*b*). A second observation that may provide a clue to GAP functions is that GAP-43 has a molecular weight and isoelectric point similar to those of a major protein in a subcellular fraction enriched with respect to growth cones (K. Meiri, K. H. Pfenninger, L. Ellis, and M. Willard, unpublished observations). If GAP-43 should prove to be a protein that is unique to the growth cone, this would support the conclusion that its function is growth specific, and the induction of its transport would indeed be a prerequisite for axon growth.

What type of growth-specific functions might GAPs perform? With the reservation that we do not know how many growth-specific proteins may have escaped detection by our assay (which most sensitively detects the proteins that most rapidly incorporate methionine), the small number of growth-associated proteins that have been observed suggests that only a small number of growth-specific functions must be performed to convert an axon from a steady state to a growth state (Skene and Willard, 1981*a,b*; Willard and Skene, 1982). This consideration raises the conjecture that a GAP might perform a function with pleitropic consequences, such that numerous components of the cell would be influenced to reorganize in a mode appropriate for axon extension. A GAP might then act on a branch point where the metabolic pathways that lead to the steady state and to axon growth diverge.

There are several specific ways that a protein might perform such a pleiotropic switching function. For example, if a GAP were a component or regulator of a membrane channel in the growth cone, many of the elements of the cell (e.g., actin, myosin, neurofilaments, microtubules, and membrane-bound organelles) that were exposed to the altered cytoplasmic milieu created by the action of the GAP could respond by reorganizing into a growth mode. A second way in which a few GAPs could influence the behavior of many other molecules would be by posttranslational modification. For example, if a GAP were a specific protease, acetylase, sulfatase, kinase, etc., it might modify a number of proteins (e.g., actin, tubulin) or, by modifying a few key proteins, initiate a sequence of modifications (e.g., a kinase activating a lipase) that would result in the altered molecular configurations necessary for axon growth.

With regard to the possibility that a GAP is a kinase, it is interesting to note that certain growth factors (epidermal growth factor and platelet-derived growth factor) and the gene products of certain RNA tumor viruses that are responsible for neoplastic transformations (the *src* gene products) are tyrosine kinases or activate tyrosine kinases (reviewed in Skene, 1983). As we anticipate in the case of the GAPs, these proteins appear to promote aspects of cell growth by performing pleiotropic switching functions. With respect to other types of posttranslational modifications that might occur specifically in growing axons, it is interesting to note that the amount of aminoacyl-tRNA increases substantially during regeneration of the goldfish optic axons (Ingoglia, 1979; N. A. Ingoglia *et al.,* Chapter 8, this volume). The amino acid can be transferred from aminoacyl-tRNA to proteins in a reaction mediated by aminoacyl-RNA transferase. Although the function of protein modification by aminoacylation is not known, if such modifications contributed to the generation of a growth state, then certain elements of the system (e.g., the transferase) might be candidates for GAPs. Because there is more than one GAP, it is likely that they accomplish the conversion of an axon to a growth state by several such mechanisms as these, all of which are currently speculations awaiting experimental scrutiny.

2.2. Regulation of the Synthesis and Transport of GAPs

If there are proteins that are not transported into steady-state axons but whose functions are essential for axon growth, then understanding the mechanism by which the synthesis and transport of these proteins is controlled is critical for understanding how axon growth is regulated. In particular, it would be important to identify the step in the sequence of events that leads from axon injury to GAP induction that fails to be accomplished in the mammalian CNS, because circumventing this failure may be a prerequisite for regenerative recovery of these axons following injury. There are several known pathways for information transfer from the periphery of neurons to the cell body that could potentially be used to convey signals that would regulate GAP synthesis and, hence, axon growth (e.g., Grafstein and McQuarrie, 1978; Forman, 1981; Willard and Skene, 1982). Examples of three such pathways are as follows.

First, neurons have the capacity to take up certain substances at their terminals and to transport them retrogradely to the cell body where, in some cases, they can alter the expression of neuronal genes (see K. Kristensson, Chapter 3, this volume). This pathway is illustrated by the uptake and retrograde transport of nerve growth factor (NGF) in sympathetic neurons; NGF that reaches the cell body by this pathway can alter the synthesis of enzymes involved in neurotransmission. If a substance that repressed GAP synthesis were obtained from the periphery (e.g., the postsynaptic terminal) by this route, the supply of GAP repressor to the cell body would be interrupted if the axon were injured; this interruption would lead to the induction of GAP gene expression.

A second informational pathway that could regulate a GAP in a manner that would insure its induction only when communication between the neuron and target cell was interrupted would be the following. A repressor of GAP synthesis would itself be synthesized in an inactive form in the cell body and would be activated (by means of posttranslational modification) only after it had been transported anterogradely into a functional axon terminal. The return of the activated repressor to the cell body by means of retrograde axonal transport would serve to prevent the synthesis of the GAP in neurons with functional synapses. When this pathway was interrupted by injury to the axon, only inactive repressor would be present in the cell body; consequently, the GAP would be induced in preparation for axon growth.

Certain features of such a pathway are illustrated by an 18-kilodalton polypeptide that is a component of the group I axonally transported proteins in retinal ganglion cells and appears to become modified when it reaches the axon terminals, i.e., the optic tectum in the case of toad and the superior colliculus and lateral geniculate nucleus in the case of the rabbit (Skene *et al.*, 1982; Kelly *et al.*, 1980). The modification is manifested as an apparent decrease in net negative charge on the protein and could therefore result from loss of negatively charged moieties (such as phosphate) or the addition of positively charged moieties. Two observations support the conclusion that this modification requires an intact synaptic terminal (Skene *et al.*, 1982). First, the tectal form of the protein was not generated in the ends of the axons of a toad optic nerve that had been crushed. Second, a toad optic tectum that had previously been treated with α-bungarotoxin failed to convert the nerve form of the 18-K polypeptide to the tectal form. Retinal–tectal transmission in the toad is mediated by nicotinic acetylcholine receptors (Freeman *et al.*, 1980); apparently, the disruption of the synapse caused by the binding of α-bungarotoxin to these receptors (Freeman, 1977) is sufficient to disrupt the mechanism by which the 18-K protein is modified in the optic tectum.

We do not know whether the tectal form of the 18-K polypeptides returns to the cell body by retrograde transport (although many group I proteins appear to do so) or whether it could alter the expresion of GAP genes. However, this 18-K polypeptide illustrates the existence of certain aspects of a pathway whereby the cell body could monitor the state of the synaptic terminals and alter the neuron's state of growth accordingly. Posttranslational modification and retrograde transport of proteins in regenerating axons are discussed by D. L. Wilson in this volume (Chapter 9).

An interesting consequence of regulatory mechanisms that depend on intact synapses for repressors of GAPs is that the concentration of repressor in the cell body might be proportional to the number of intact synaptic connections. The neuron might be able to use such a feature to "count" its synapses and regulate the number formed during the course of developmental or regenerative growth (Willard and Skene, 1982). As increasing numbers of synapses were formed by the growing axon, the level of active repressor in the cell body would increase until the concentration was sufficient to terminate the expression of the relevant growth-related genes; at this point synapse formation and axon growth would cease.

A third mechanism that could insure that the expression of a neuronal growth-related gene would be responsive to axon injury would result if the expression of these genes were contingent on the release of factors by nonneuronal cells in response to injury to the axon. Such a factor, or a "second messenger" produced as a consequence of release of such factors, might then be transported retrogradely to the cell body where it would induce the expression of the growth-related gene. The observation (Skene and Shooter, 1983) that the synthesis and release of a 37-kilodalton polypeptide is induced in nonneuronal cells when a rat sciatic nerve is crushed illustrates the potential of nonneuronal cells to respond to axotomy of neurons; the observation (e.g., Kristensson and Olsson, 1976; K. Kristensson, Chapter 3, this volume) that molecules supplied exogenously at a site of axon injury can be transported retrogradely to the cell body illustrates the availability of a retrograde pathway that could convey such an exogenously synthesized inducer to the cell body.

There is a particularly compelling reason to believe that growth-associated genes are in fact regulated by exogenously supplied inducers from nonneuronal cells. Certain neurons of the mammalian CNS that would not normally regenerate an injured axon can accomplish dramatic axon elongation when they are provided with a tissue graft from a mammalian peripheral nerve (Aguayo, *et al.*, 1982). These experiments demonstrate that a mature mammalian CNS neuron has the potential to regenerate its axon and, moreover, that information supplied by nonneuronal peripheral nerve cells is sufficient to allow the expression of this potential. Therefore, if alterations in neuronal gene expression are required to achieve a competent growth state, the factors necessary to acccomplish this regulation must be provided by the nonneuronal cells of peripheral nerve. This conclusion would not be valid if neurons that grow axons into the peripheral nerve grafts were a special class of neurons that were already producing growth-specific proteins before they had access to the PNS graft; in this case, the graft would supply some other prerequisite for axon growth such as a suitable substrate over which to grow.

These different hypothetical pathways for regulating the expression of growth-related genes are not mutually exclusive. In fact, the conclusion that different modes of axon growth (e.g., limited sprouting and axon elongation) require different combinations of neuronal gene products (e.g., GAP-23/24 and GAP-43, respectively) suggests that several different regulatory pathways are required to regulate independently the expression of different growth-related genes (Skene and Willard, 1981c).

3. REGULATION OF THE NEUROFILAMENT CROSS-LINKING POLYPEPTIDE DURING NEURONAL DEVELOPMENT

The behavior of the neurofilament proteins during the neonatal development of the rabbit visual system suggests that a special sequence of events, produced by a special choreography of neuronal gene expression, is initially employed to elaborate the neurofilamentous–microtubular cytoskeleton. Mammalian neurofilaments comprise three polypeptides (e.g., Hoffman and Lasek, 1975): a high-molecular-weight polypeptide (H, 195 K), a medium-molecular-weight polypeptide (M, 145 K), and a low-molecular-weight polypeptide (L, 73 K). L composes the core of the filament, whereas H is a component of the cross bridges between filaments (e.g., Willard and Simon, 1981; Hirokawa *et al.*, 1984). In the mature neuron, the H cross-bridging function is a specialization of the axon; the cell body and dendrites contain mostly M and L (Shaw *et al.*, 1981; Hirokawa *et al.*, 1984).

During development of the rabbit retinal ganglion cells, the three neurofilament polypeptides appear in a programmed sequence: M and L are present (albeit in low amounts) in the rabbit optic nerve from the time of birth, whereas H does not accumulate to detectable levels until 8 to 12 days after birth (Levine *et al.*, 1982; Willard and Simon, 1983). Thus, the neonatal axon resembles a dendrite with respect to its content of H and differentiates to the H phenotype of the adult axon only late during development. A similar sequence of appearance of neurofilament proteins has been observed in the rat cerebral cortex (Shaw and Weber, 1982) and in the rat optic nerve (Pachter and Liem, 1981). In the latter case, the appearance of M has been reported to precede the appearance of L; as in the rabbit, both polypeptides appear before H.

During the period after H first appears in the axon, the apparent velocities of axonal transport of the filament polypeptides change in rabbit retinal ganglion cells (Willard and Simon, 1983). The velocity of M and L decreases from about 9 mm per day in the 6-day-old rabbit to about 1 mm per day in the adult. Although the two events are not necessarily related, their temporal correspondence suggests that the reduction in the transport velocity of the filament polypeptides could be a consequence of the introduction of H into the axon. For example, if un-cross-linked neurofilaments composed of M and L are transported into the axon during the initial stages of neuronal development, then the introduction of the H cross-linking function might precipitate a "phase transition" from a state of independent neurofilamentous elements to a state characterized by the highly cross-linked matrix that composes the adult cytoskeleton. The cross-linked matrix might then be more difficult to translocate down the axon than its independent elements, and this would then account for the ninefold decrease in the transport velocity of the neurofilament proteins.

During approximately the same period that the velocity of the group V neurofilament polypeptides decreases, the velocity of the group IV polypeptides (actin and myosin, etc.) decreases about twofold. This reduction could also be a consequence of the advent of the H cross-linking function. For example, perhaps the additional cross links provided by H retard the passage of group IV material. Alternatively, if group IV and group V are partially coupled to each other, as would be the case if group IV provided the motive force for the transport of group V (Levine *et al.,* 1982; Levine and Willard, 1983), the drag produced on the group IV transport motor by the cross-linked cytoskeleton might result in a twofold reduction in the rate of movement of this group IV transport machinery.

What function could be served by the sequential introduction of the neurofilament proteins into the developing axons? The delayed appearance of the cross-linking polypeptide H compared to the core polypeptide L and the M polypeptide suggests that the cross-linking function of H is not needed or cannot be tolerated until late in development. One speculation as to why this might be so is that the appearance of H marks a transition from a state of growth to a state of stability. For example, suppose the cross linking of cytoskeleton functions by H serves to stabilize the axon in the configuration that prevails at the time of the introduction of H into the axon. Then it would be beneficial for the neuron to await a sign that the proper configuration had been attained before it initiated the transport of H. If this signal were provided only by a correctly contacted postsynaptic cell, then the induction of H by this signal after it was conveyed to the neuronal cell body would insure that only axons with proper synaptic connections would be stabilized by the cross-linking function of H. It is interesting to note that if such a hypothetical transition from the plastic state to the stable state of the axon were irreversible, the induction of the H cross-linking function would provide the molecular basis for a critical period after which the plastic functions that were terminated when H was induced could no longer be accomplished.

Although these conjectures are the result of nested speculations that await experimental examination, the staggered appearance of the different neurofilament proteins during development provides an opportunity to study the programmed regulation of expression of neuronal genes during development of the axon. Such studies should reveal how a neuronal gene can be differentially activated late in development and, in particular, should reveal the level of regulation of the H gene expression, the nature of the regulatory signal, how the proper timing of the supply of the signal is achieved, and what developmental events trigger the formation of the signal.

A<small>CKNOWLEDGMENTS</small>

We thank C. Baitinger, D. Clements, and R. Cheney for discussion, and Jan Hoffmann for typing. This work was supported by Grant EY02682 and a Neuromuscular Research Center Grant.

4. REFERENCES

Aguayo. A. J., Richardson, P. M., David, S., and Benfy, M., 1982, Transplantation of neurons and sheath cells—a tool for the study of regeneration, in: *Repair and Regeneration of the Nervous System* (J. G. Nichols, ed.) pp. 91–105, Springer Verlag, Berlin, Heidelberg, New York.

Baitinger, C., Levine, J., Lorenz, T., Simon, C., Skene, P., and Willard, M., 1982, Characteristics of axonally transported proteins, in: *Axoplasmic Transport* (D. G. Weiss, ed.), pp. 111–120, Springer-Verlag, Berlin, Heidelberg, New York.

Benowitz, L. I., Shashoua, V. E., and Yoon, M. G,. 1981, Specific changes in rapidly transported proteins during regeneration of the goldfish optic nerve, *J. Neurosci.* **1:**300–307.

Bisby, M. A., 1980, Changes in the composition of labeled protein transported in motor axons during their regeneration, *J. Neurobiol.* **11:**435–445.

Forman, D. S. 1983, Axonal transport and nerve regeneration: A review, in: *Spinal Cord Reconstruction* (C. C. Kao, R. P. Bunge, and P. J. Reir, eds.), pp. 75–86, Raven Press, New York.

Freeman, J. A., 1977, Possible regulatory function of acetylcholine receptor in maintenance of retinotectal synapses, *Nature* **269:**218–222.

Freeman, J. A., Schmidt, J. T., and Oswald, R. E., 1980, Effect of alpha-bungarotoxin on retinotectal synaptic transmission in the goldfish and the toad, *Neuroscience* **5:**929–942.

Giulian, D., des Ruisseaux, H., and Cowburn, D., 1980, Biosynthesis and intra-axonal transport during neuronal regeneration, *J. Biol. Chem.* **255:**6494–6501.

Grafstein, B., and Forman, D. S., 1980, Intracellular transport in neurons, *Physiol. Rev.* **60:**1167–1283.

Grafstein, B., and McQuarrie, I. G., 1978, The role of the nerve cell body in axon regneration, in: *Neuronal Plasticity* (C. Cotman, ed.), pp. 155–195, Raven Press, New York.

Hirokawa, N., Glicksman, M. A., and Willard, M. B., 1984, Organization of mammalian neurofilament polypeptides within the neuronal cytoskeleton, *J. Cell Biol.* **98:**1523–1536.

Hoffman, P. N., and Lasek, R. J., 1975, The slow component of axonal transport: Identification of major structural polypeptides of the axon and their generality among mammalian neurons, *J. Cell Biol.* **66:**351–356.

Ingoglia, N. A., 1979, 4S RNA is present in regenerating optic axons of goldfish, *Science* **206:**73–75.

Kelly, A. S., Wagner, J. A., and Kelly, R. B., 1980, Properties of individual nerve terminal proteins identified by two-dimensional gel electgrophoresis, *Brain Res.* **185:**192–197.

Kristensson, K., and Olsson, Y., 1976, Retrograde transport of horseradish peroxidase into transected axons. 3. Entry into injured axons and subsequent localization in perikaryon, *Brain Res.* **115:**201–213.

Lasek, R. J.,and Black, M. M., 1977, How do axons stop growing? Some clues from the metabolism of the proteins in the slow component of axonal transport, in: *Mechanisms, Regulation and Special Functions of Protein Synthesis in the Brain* (S. Roberts, eds.), pp. 161–169, Elsevier, Amsterdam.

Lasek, R. J., and Hoffman, P. N., 1976, The neuronal cytoskeleton, axonal transport and axonal growth, in: *Cell Motility,* Volume 3, (R. Goldman, T. Pollard, and J. Rosenbaum, eds.), pp. 1021–1049, Cold Spring Harbor Conferences on Cell Proliferation, Cold Spring Harbor Laboratory, New York.

Levine, J., and Willard, M., 1983, Redistribution of fodrin (a component of the cortical cytoplasm) accompanying capping of cell surface molecules, *Proc. Natl. Acad. Sci. U.S.A.* **80:**191–195.

Levine, J., Skene, P., and Willard, M., 1981, GAPs and fodrin: Novel axonally transported proteins, *Trends Neurosci.* **4:**273–277.

Levine, J., Simon, C., and Willard, M., 1982, Mechanistic implications of the behavior of axonally transported proteins, in: *Axoplasmic Transport* (D. G. Weiss, ed.), pp. 275–278, Springer-Verlag, Berlin, Heidelberg, New York.

Pachter, J. S., and Liem, R. K. H., 1984, Differential appearance of neurofilament triplet polypeptides in the developing rat optic nerve, *Devel. Biol.* **103:**200–210.

Pfenninger, K.H., and Maylie-Pfenninger, M. F., 1981, Lectin labeling of sprouting neurons. II. Relative movement and appearance of glycoconjugates during plasmalemma expansion, *J. Cell Biol.* **89:**547–559.

Pfenninger, K. H., Ellis, L., Johnson, M. P., Friedman, L. B., and Somlo, S., 1983, Nerve growth cones isolated from fetal rat brain: Subcellular fractionation and characterization, *Cell* **35:**573–584.

Ramon y Cajal, S., 1928, *Degeneration and Regeneration of the Nervous System,* Volume 2, Oxford University Press, Oxford.

Shaw, G., and Weber, K., 1982, Differential expression of neurofilament triplet proteins in brain development. *Nature* **298:**277–279.

Shaw, G., Osborn, M., and Weber, K., 1981, An immunofluorescence microscopical study of the neurofilament triplet proteins, vimentin, and glial fibrillary acidic protein within the adult rat brain, *Eur. J. Cell Biol.* **26:**68–82.

Skene, J. H. P., 1983, An oncogene abounds in brains, *Trends Neurosci.* **6:**353–354.

Skene, J. H. P, and Shooter, E., 1983, Denervated sheath cells secrete a new protein after nerve injury, *Proc. Natl. Acad. Sci. U.S.A.* **80:**4119–4173.

Skene, J. H. P, and Willard, M., 1981*a*, Changes in axonally transported proteins during axon regeneration in toad retinal ganglion cells, *J. Cell Biol.* **89:**86–95.

Skene, J. H. P., and Willard, M., 1981*b*, Characteristics of growth-associated proteins (GAPs) in regenerating toad retinal ganglion cells, *J. Neurosci.* **1:**419–426.

Skene, J. H. P., and Willard, M., 1981*c*, Axonally transported proteins associated with axon growth in rabbit central and peripheral nervous systems, *J. Cell Biol.* **89:**96–103.

Skene, J. H. P., Willard, M., and Freeman, J. A., 1982, Modification of an axonally transported protein in toad retinotectal terminals, *Soc. Neurosci. Abstr.* **9:**247.

Theiler, R. F., and McClure, W. O., 1978, Rapid axoplasmic transport of proteins in regenerating sensory nerve fibers, *J. Neurochem.* **31:**433–447.

Willard, M., and Simon, C., 1981, Antibody decoration of neurofilaments, *J. Cell Biol.* **89:**198–205.

Willard, M., and Simon, C., 1983, Modulations of neurofilament axonal transport during development of rabbit retinal ganglion cells, *Cell* (in press).

Willard, M., and Skene, J. H. P., 1982, Molecular events in axonal regeneration, in: *Repair and Regeneration of the Nervous System* (J. G. Nicholls, ed.), pp. 71–89, Springer-Verlag, Berlin, Heidelberg, New York.

EFFECT OF A CONDITIONING LESION ON AXONAL TRANSPORT DURING REGENERATION
The Role of Slow Transport

IRVINE G. MCQUARRIE

1. INTRODUCTION

The term "conditioning lesion effect" refers to the earlier formation and/or accelerated outgrowth of axonal sprouts in response to a second growth stimulus as compared to a single growth stimulus. Although the first (conditioning) stimulus can be a direct axotomy or partial denervation of an end organ (to produce collateral sprouting), it is important that the second (testing) stimulus be a direct axotomy. It is preferable to locate the testing axotomy far enough proximal to the conditioning axotomy that the intervening segment of nerve is sufficiently long to permit measuring the outgrowth rate.

IRVINE G. MCQUARRIE ● *Veterans Administration Medical Center and Department of Anatomy and Developmental Genetics, Case Western Reserve University School of Medicine, Cleveland, Ohio 44106*

In recent years it has become possible to analyze the conditioning lesion effect by relating the synthesis of proteins at the nerve cell body and their transport through the axon to changes in the growth state of the neuron. This method depends on labeling newly synthesized proteins at the nerve cell body by a local injection of radioactive amino acids and allowing sufficient time for these proteins to enter the axon. The growth state of the neuron is altered by using the conditioning lesion paradigm, and isotope injections are timed so that pulse-labeled proteins can be captured within the axon at various intervals after either the conditioning or testing stimulus. Both the conditioning lesion effect and axonal transport during regeneration are topics that need to be considered in some detail before axonal transport data from a conditioning lesion experiment can be discussed.

1.1. The Conditioning Lesion Effect

This subject has been reviewed by Grafstein and McQuarrie (1978) and by Forman et al. (1981). However, new conditioning events have since been described, and progress has been made toward understanding the signal that initiates the conditioning lesion effect. These developments necessitate an in-depth review at this time.

1.1.1. Measurement of the Effect

Following an axotomizing lesion, new sprouts (daughter axons) arise from the parent axon stumps that remain attached to the nerve cell bodies. If this "crop" of sprouts is removed after a suitable interval, the second crop almost invariably forms more rapidly and/or elongates more rapidly than the first. This "conditioning lesion effect" (McQuarrie et al., 1977) is defined in terms of time factors. These include (1) the "conditioning interval" (Forman et al., 1980) or time between the conditioning and testing lesions, (2) the "initial delay" (Forman et al., 1979) or time between the testing lesion and the onset of sprout formation; (3) the "rate of outgrowth" (McQuarrie and Grafstein, 1973) or the mean distance per day that a defined subpopulation of sprouts advances through the distal nerve stump, and (4) the "latent period" (Gutmann, 1942) or time between the testing lesion and the onset of functional recovery. Thus, the conditioning lesion effect in a particular neuron is best characterized by measuring the initial delay, outgrowth rate, and latent period after testing lesions that have been preceded by different conditioning intervals. This has been done only for goldfish optic axons (Table 1) and rat sciatic sensory axons (Table 2).

TABLE 1.   The Conditioning Lesion Effect in Goldfish Retinal Ganglion Cells[a]

Conditioning interval	Initial delay	Outgrowth rate	Latent period	Reference
14 days	50% less	—	—	Lanners and Grafstein (1980a,b)
14 days	43% less	95% faster	56% less	McQuarrie and Grafstein (1981)
7 days	—	—	34% less	Edwards et al. (1981)
14 days	—	—	56% less	Edwards et al. (1981)
21 days	—	—	10% less	Edwards et al. (1981)

[a] With conditioning and testing lesions less than 1 mm apart.

1.1.2.   Generality of the Effect in Specific Types of Neurons

1.1.2a.   Studies in the CNS.   The standard models for CNS regeneration (the optic nerves of fish and amphibia) have been examined for conditioning lesion effects. The most marked effect is seen in goldfish optic axons (Table 1), where a variety of criteria indicate that regeneration is up to 100% faster. These include measurement of axonal outgrowth from retinal explants (Landreth and Agranoff, 1976), determination of the initial delay by standard histology (McQuarrie and Grafstein, 1981) or electron microscopy (Lanners and Grafstein, 1980a), determination of the outgrowth rate by histological and axonal transport methods (McQuarrie and Grafstein, 1981), and determination of the latent period by timing the arrival of labeled axons at the optic tectum (McQuarrie and Grafstein, 1981) or the return of vision (Edwards et al., 1981). Robust effects have also been described in the optic axons of salamanders by using standard histological methods (Brock and Turner, 1978, 1982) and in frogs by measuring outgrowth from retinal explants (Agranoff et al., 1976).

TABLE 2.   The Conditioning Lesion Effect in Sensory Neurons of the Rat Sciatic Nerve[a]

Conditioning interval	Initial delay	Outgrowth rate	Latent period	Reference
7 days	33% less	—	—	Forman et al. (1980)
14 days	47% less	—	—	Forman et al. (1980)
28 days	40% less	—	—	Forman et al. (1980)
14 days	—	23% faster	—	McQuarrie et al. (1977)
14 days	—	25% faster	—	Oblinger and Lasek (1983a)
14 days	—	40% faster	—	Carlsen (1982)
7 days	—	43% faster	—	Bisby and Pollock (1983)
14 days	—	—	12% less	M. A. Bisby (personal communication)

[a] With the conditioning lesion located 20–50 mm distal to the testing lesion.

1.1.2b. Studies in Peripheral Nerves. The length of peripheral axons permits the conditioning and testing lesions to be widely separated, thereby eliminating the possibility that axons elongating from a testing lesion will be influenced by the prior nerve degeneration that has been caused by the conditioning lesion. The disadvantage is that the nerve cell bodies are located in the spinal column or cranium, necessitating a laminectomy or craniotomy to carry out axonal transport studies (Frizell and Sjostrand, 1974; Bisby, 1978) or to measure outgrowth distances by labeling of growing fibers through axonal transport (Frizell and Sjostrand, 1974; Griffin *et al.,* 1976; Forman and Berenberg, 1978). This disadvantage is minimized somewhat because the outgrowth distance for leading sensory axons can be determined by using a simple nerve pinch test (Young and Medawar, 1940) that depends on the increased sensitivity of outgrowing sensory axon tips to mechanical stimuli (Konorski and Lubinska, 1946). Although this method for locating leading axons is not as accurate as the axonal transport method (McQuarrie, 1978), in most instances where it has been combined with conditioning lesions (Table 2), the pinch test has revealed a shortened initial delay and a 20–40% acceleration of outgrowth in the rat sciatic nerve (McQuarrie *et al.,* 1977; Forman *et al.,* 1980; Carlsen, 1982; Bisby and Pollock, 1983), findings that have been confirmed by the axonal transport method (Oblinger and Lasek, 1983*a;* Bisby and Pollock, 1983). In the frog sciatic nerve, after a conditioning interval of 14 days, the pinch test shows a 12% decrease in the initial delay and a 12% increase in the outgrowth rate (Carlsen, 1983).

In motor axons of the rat sciatic nerve, the axonal transport method shows that the majority of conditioned axons advance 35–40% faster than controls (McQuarrie, 1978; Sparrow and Grafstein, 1983). In line with this acceleration, the latent period for recovery of motor reflexes is shortened by 27%, provided that the neuromuscular junctions are preserved by use of electrical stimulation (Sebille and Bondoux-Jahan, 1980). Even if electrical stimulation is not used, the latent period to motor reflex recovery in the rabbit sciatic nerve is reduced by 10% (Gutmann, 1942). Using the most reliable but cumbersome methods—light microscopy of silver-stained axons and electron microscopy of myelinated axons—a number of workers have confirmed the conditioning lesion effect on peripheral axons. Lubinska (1952) found a 59% decrease in the initial delay but no change in outgrowth rate for sciatic nerve axons of the frog when a 5-day conditioning interval was used. In the mouse sciatic nerve examined by light microscopy (McQuarrie, 1979) and in the rat sciatic nerve examined by electron microscopy (McQuarrie, 1983*a*) or light microscopy (Wells and Bernstein, 1978), the initial delay is significantly shortened by a 14-day conditioning interval. Another exacting method—electrophysiological detection of motor end-plate reinnervation—has been used to detect the conditioning lesion effect on mouse motor axons after a conditioning interval of 4 days (Brown and Hopkins, 1981).

1.1.2c. Detrimental or Indifferent Effects of Conditioning Lesions. To date, there is limited evidence that conditioning intervals in the range of 2 to 28 days can have detrimental or indifferent effects on outgrowth. The only example of indifference is found in the L5 dorsal root axons of the rat (Oblinger and Lasek, 1983*b*). In regard to negative effects, the postganglionic sympathetic axons of the rat sciatic nerve show a reduced outgrowth rate, even though the initial delay is shortened substantially (McQuarrie *et al.,* 1978). This suggests that the conditioning lesion paradigm may have induced neuronal death, even though counts of parent axons after a testing lesions alone are no greater than counts after a testing lesion preceded by a conditioning lesion. Arvidsson and Aldskogius (1982) report a 26% reduction in the numbers of neurons in the rat hypoglossal nucleus with conditioning intervals of 10–20 days compared to no reduction after a testing lesion alone.

1.1.3. Suitable Conditioning Intervals

Two studies have attempted to define the optimum conditioning interval in systems showing a positive conditioning effect, one by measuring the latent period for recovery of vision in goldfish (Edwards *et al.,* 1981), the other by measuring the outgrowth rate of sensory axons in the rat sciatic nerve (Forman *et al.,* 1980). Both studies indicate that the optimum interval is 2 weeks and that the minimum effective interval is 2 days.

1.1.4. Effective Conditioning Events

1.1.4a. Direct Axotomy as a Conditioning Event. In all of the early descriptions of the conditioning lesion effect, the conditioning event involved direct axotomy of the nerve in question (Gutmann, 1942; Lubinska, 1952; Ducker *et al.,* 1969; McQuarrie and Grafstein, 1973). More recently, it has become apparent that the conditioning event need not damage the axon. Rather, the important requirement is that axonal growth occur. Aside from direct axotomy, the collateral sprouting that follows partial denervation of an end organ is an effective conditioning event. Finally, it is now worthwhile to view embryonic axonal outgrowth as a special kind of conditioning event.

1.1.4b. Collateral Sprout Formation as a Conditioning Event. Sparrow and Grafstein (1983) have stimulated collateral sprout formation in the leg muscles of rats by a standard method: ligating and dividing the L4 and L6 spinal nerves so as to isolate the L5 motor axons. Within 3 days, the L5 motor axons begin to form collateral sprouts to the vacated L4 and L6 motor end plates in muscles that had originally received a joint innervation from either the L4 and L5 spinal nerves or the L5 and L6 spinal nerves. One week after the conditioning event, a testing lesion is carried out by crushing the sciatic nerve, and, after 8 days, the outgrowth distance is 39% greater than after a testing lesion preceded by a sham conditioning lesion. This effect is essentially identical to the 35% increase that is found when the conditioning lesion is a direct axotomy of the same motor axons (McQuarrie, 1978).

Collateral sprout formation is also an effective conditioning event in the goldfish optic system. When the cerebral hemispheres are removed to permit a conditioning axotomy of one optic tract (McQuarrie and Grafstein, 1982*b*), any axons of the contralateral tract that project to tectal neurons receiving afferents from the cerebral hemispheres may be stimulated to form collateral sprouts. Since the tectal targets of the optic axons include neurons of the stratum griseum centrale (Schmidt, 1979; Springer and Gaffney, 1981) that also receive afferents from the area dorsalis pars centralis of each cerebral hemisphere (Luiten, 1981; Vanegas and Ebbesson, 1976; Northcutt, 1981), optic axon terminals are likely to form collateral sprouts (if the telencephalic afferents and retinal afferents form adjacent or overlapping synaptic fields on the tectal neurons). This apparently occurs, since removal of the cerebral hemispheres has a conditioning lesion effect (McQuarrie and Grafstein, 1982*b*). In light of the strong evidence that collateral sprout formation can be a conditioning event (Sparrow and Grafstein, 1983), other possible explanations for this effect must be considered speculative.

1.1.4c. Embryonic Axonal Outgrowth: A Special Type of Conditioning Event. Collins and Lee (1982) find that single dissociated neurons of the chicken ciliary ganglion are able to extend neurites in culture if they are plated at embryonic stage 35 (a time when they are still extending axons), whereas if ganglion removal and neuronal plating are delayed until stage 40 (after ciliary axons have formed end-organ connections), the dissociated neurons fail to extend neurites. They suggest that stage 35 ciliary neurons are naturally conditioned in the sense that a conditioning axotomy of older neurons induces dedifferentiation to a "state resembling that which they possessed embryonically before forming functional synapses." They point out that a standard conditioning lesion effect can be induced at stage 40 by explanting whole segments of ganglion, waiting a 3- to 4-day conditioning interval to allow the growth state to be recalled, and providing testing axotomies by dissociating the cells for secondary culture. Thus, embryonic neurons that have not yet formed synapses are already in a growth state, a state that may be recalled in more mature neurons by applying a conditioning lesion. This developmental growth state apparently accounts for the ability of some CNS neurons to regenerate axons in neonatal mammals (Schneider, 1981; Iacovitti *et al.,* 1981; Kalil and Reh, 1982).

For *in vivo* confirmation of the Collins and Lee hypothesis, one must completely transect a CNS tract containing axons that have not yet formed connections, at a time when axons are no longer being added to the tract at the level of transection. If the divided axons form sprouts, and these sprouts either traverse or bypass the lesion to reach their appropriate targets, then the *in vitro* experiment of Collins and Lee (1982) will have been replicated *in vivo,* provided that outgrowth does not occur if the tract is divided after synaptogenesis. Kalil and Reh (1982) have done so, and found (1) that the hamster pyramidal tract is suitable for studying this possibility, (2) that its axons exhibit impressive regeneration around the lesion site only if they are lesioned prior to synaptogenesis, and (3) that the daughter axons innervate appropriate targets in the spinal cord to produce behaviors that depend on intact corticospinal pathways (Reh and Kalil, 1982). It must be understood that when a testing lesion is carried out on outgrowing axons in the mammalian CNS, the end point for the "conditioning lesion effect" is axonal outgrowth, however slow, in place of the failure of outgrowth that occurs after synapse formation. Finally, the concept of a conditioning interval becomes moot because the neuron is already in a growth state—one need not wait for that state to be recalled.

1.1.5. Origin and Action of the Conditioning Event

1.1.5a. Chemical Signalling versus Physical Facilitation. The conditioning events of axotomy and partial end-organ denervation have different effects on the tissues through which regenerating axons must grow after the testing axotomy. A conditioning axotomy causes Wallerian degeneration of the distal axons as well as the atrophy of sensory receptors, myoneural junctions, and muscle fibers, whereas partial end-organ denervation does not cause any degenerative alterations of the axons to be affected by testing axotomies. Those axons will, however, form collateral sprouts prior to the testing axotomies, apparently as a result of sprouting factors released by the nearby degenerating motor end plates (or their atrophying muscle fibers) and taken up by axon terminals (Cotman *et al.,* 1981). Similar factors might be released by degenerating axons or reactive glial cells when a conditioning axotomy is employed (see discussion below). These "conditioning signals" would then be retrogradely transported to the nerve cell body (Kristensson and Olsson, 1975; Singer *et al.,* 1982) to induce the metabolic response to axotomy (Grafstein and McQuarrie, 1978) or partial end-organ denervation (Watson, 1973; McQuarrie and Grafstein, 1982*b*).

An increased magnitude of the nerve cell body reaction has long been known to follow successive axotomies (Howe and Bodian, 1941; Romanes,

1951), and the hypothesis that this is related to accelerated axonal outgrowth was first advanced by Ducker *et al.* (1969). Recently, Carlsen (1983) has offered direct evidence supporting this hypothesis, finding that a testing lesion of the sciatic nerve in frogs cooled to 15°C results in a failure of the cell body reaction to develop and abortive axonal outgrowth, whereas a testing lesion preceded by a conditioning lesion results in the development of a cell body reaction and successful axonal outgrowth.

Although the hypothesis that a conditioning event induces a growth state in the neuron may now appear reasonable, it has only recently superseded the notion that the predegenerated nerve physically favors axonal outgrowth. Since Gutmann's (1942) original description of a shortened latent period after the second of two successive nerve lesions, the conditioning lesion effect has been attributed to particular aspects of Wallerian degeneration, with Schwann cell proliferation and the removal of axonal debris being mentioned most often. Gutmann introduces this idea by suggesting that "there is an excess of Schwann bands in the peripheral trunk, and in the muscle itself the new fibres have a greater chance of finding suitable pathways." Subsequently, Thomas (1970) confirmed that each successive axotomy causes a 60–70% increase in the number of Schwann cells within the distal nerve stump. However, there is no evidence that the additional Schwann cells are responsible for accelerated outgrowth. Lubinska (1952), and more recently Brown and Hopkins (1981), have suggested that the removal of axonal debris from the degenerated nerve stump is the feature of the conditioning lesion that promotes accelerated outgrowth from a subsequent testing lesion. This hypothesis has also proven difficult to substantiate, even though the physical properies of the substratum over which an axon advances are known to have an important influence on the direction and speed of outgrowth (Letourneau, 1982).

These speculations on the physical role of a predegenerated nerve become moot when the conditioning event is partial end-organ degeneration. Even when the conditioning event is an axotomy, they are further weakened by the observation that the conditioning lesion effect occurs when the testing lesion removes a section of nerve proximal to the conditioning lesion, forcing axons to grow through a fresh connective tissue wound (McQuarrie and Grafstein, 1973). Accelerated outgrowth is also seen when the testing axotomy is a nerve crush located 50 mm proximal to the conditioning lesion, forcing axons to grow through a freshly degenerating nerve segment rather than the predegenerated segment (McQuarrie *et al.*, 1977).

1.1.5b. Role of Glial Cells. Having established that the conditioning lesion effect is based on alterations in neuronal metabolism, we must now consider the possibility that the glial cells that support degenerating axons are the source of the conditioning agent(s) that trigger the cell body reaction. Four arguments support this hypothesis. (1) Making the conditioning and testing lesions at the same locus on the nerve, causing growth to occur in a predege-nerating segment, evokes a more marked acceleration of outgrowth than when the testing lesion is located some distance proximal to the conditioning lesion (Bisby and Pollock, 1983). (2) In all cases, axons growing out from a testing lesion immediately encouter a degenerating nerve, even when the testing lesion is placed proximal to the conditioning lesion. (3) There is compelling evidence that the nerve cell body reaction is triggered by materials that are conveyed to it from the lesion site via retrograde axonal transport (Kristensson and Olsson, 1975; Singer *et al.,* 1982). (4) The retrogradely transported signal is appar-ently not only axonal in origin, since increasing degrees of extraaxonal nerve damage during axotomy produce increasing degrees of cell body reaction (Tor-vik and Skjorten, 1971; Cheah and Geffen, 1973). This feature cannot be accounted for by the other possible retrograde signals (Forman, 1982): an ear-lier and more abundant return of anterogradely transported materials or a fail-ure of retrogradely transported trophic materials (produced by the end organ) to arrive at the nerve cell body. The operative glial factor(s) are apparently acting to control the magnitude of the cell body reaction rather than to align or lure outgrowing axons: outgrowth rates do not fluctuate in transit, whereas the numbers of glial cells and the concentrations of the putative neurotrophic substances that they release into the extracellular fluid change almost daily and vary with distance from the lesion site (Bradley and Asbury, 1970; Forman *et al.,* 1979; Richardson and Ebendal, 1982; Bisby and Pollock, 1983).

1.1.5c. Role of Degenerating Axons and Atrophying End Organs. Both types of conditioning events involve degenerating axons and atrophying end organs. Either of these, as well as glial cells, may be the source of the condi-tioning agent(s) that are taken up by the parent axon and returned to the nerve cell body via retrograde axonal transport, there to trigger the cell body response. Although neither would account for the magnification of the cell body response that occurs when the degree of trauma to a nerve is increased (Torvik and Skjorten, 1971; Cheah and Geffen, 1973), they may be supple-mentary sources of the putative neuron-stimulating (neuronotrophic) agent. Axon-guiding (neurotropic) influences are also released by denervated tissues, and these often have neuronotrophic actions as well. Clearly, it is important to bring these agents into focus, since one or more of them apparently serve to trigger the cell body response.

1.1.5d. Neurotropic and Neuronotrophic Aspects of Denervation. Since the investigations of Forssman in 1898, which Ramon y Cajal (1928) has sum-marized, it has been recognized that peripheral nerves undergoing Wallerian degeneration release neurotropic substances. In one of Forssman's experiments, the sciatic nerve is transected where it branches into peroneal and tibial nerves, and these branches are capped with collodion. Axonal sprouts eventually cir-cumvent the hard collodion caps to enter the distal stumps after "describing very complicated turns." This led Forssman to a more definitive experiment wherein outgrowing sprouts are confronted with a choice between two entubulated lures of minced tissues, one containing nervous tissue and the other containing parenchymal tissue from various other organs: axonal sprouts invariably choose to enter the tube containing nervous tissue.

Having been able to confirm and extend these observations, Ramon y Cajal (1928) finds that "the active substances are elaborated by the cells of Schwann" and that their release is greatest "during the second and third week after the nerve section." While concluding that other factors are also important for insuring successful regeneration, these being "the mechanical guidance of the sprouts along the old sheaths" and "the superproduction of fibres," he suggests that the release of neurotropic substances from the distal nerve stumps (and the denervated end organs) is the most important factor.

Weiss and Taylor (1944) have tested this hypothesis by using a Y-shaped arterial sleeve to provide outgrowing axons with a decision between nerve grafts and nonnervous tissues (tendon, blood clot, tissue exudates). They find that an approximately equal number of axons enter each branch of the arterial sleeve and discount any neurotropic influence in favor of mechanical guidance. This view, however, has recently been challenged by *in vitro* studies indicating that neurites selectively innervate their appropriate end organs when confronted with a choice (Chamley *et al.,* 1973; Coughlin, 1975; Ebendal and Jacobson, 1977), so it has again become necessary to repeat the Forssman experiment.

With modern techniques, including the use of an acellular and impermeable material (silastic) for the Y-shaped sleeve and the combined use of morphometric and axonal transport methods to quantitate axonal outgrowth, Politis *et al.* (1982) have presented axonal sprouts with a choice between a distal degenerating nerve stump and a distal nerve stump treated to prevent cell division and protein synthesis. They found that sprouts enter untreated distal stumps two to ten times more frequently than they enter stumps in which degeneration has been arrested. Nuclepore® filters (0.2 μm) and interstump separation distances of up to 5 mm do not alter the response, indicating that the neurotropic agent is soluble rather than cell bound. Ramon y Cajal's observation that distal stumps that have become enriched in Schwann cells, by virtue of prolonged denervation, are a better neurotropic lure than freshly-denervated stumps is also confirmed by Politis *et al.* (1982): twice as many proximal stump axons innervate distal stumps that had been degenerating for 8 weeks as innervate stumps that had been freshly denervated. Thus, during Wallerian degeneration, Schwann cells release a neurotropic substance approximately in proportion to their numbers.

1.1.5e. Relationship of the Schwann Cell Neurotropic Factor to NGF. The Schwann cell neurotropic factor differs from Nerve Growth Factor (NGF), the traditional neurotropic substance (Gundersen and Barrett, 1980; Greene and Shooter, 1980), because motor and sensory axons are affected equally (Politis *et al.*, 1982). Nonetheless, Schwann cells *in vitro* are known to produce a factor with NGF-like neurotropic activity (Burnham *et al.*, 1972; Richardson and Ebendal, 1982). However, its activity is blocked to only a minimal extent by anti-NGF (Varon *et al.*, 1981; Lundborg *et al.*, 1982; Richardson and Ebendal, 1982), indicating that the Schwann cell neurotropic factor is chemically different from NGF. This is in line with evidence indicating that the Schwann cell neurotropic factor is capable of directing neurite elongation in cholinergic neurons, which are unresponsive to NGF (Adler and Varon, 1981; Richardson and Ebendal, 1982).

1.1.5f. Neuronotrophic Effects of Schwann Cells. Although it is now clear that Schwann cells in degenerating nerves elaborate one or more neurotropic factors, the evidence that these same factors are neuronotrophic is circumstantial. The indirect evidence, however, is persuasive: peripheral nerve grafts placed into or adjacent to the CNS stimulate the outgrowth of intrinsic CNS axons over distances of several centimeters (Richardson *et al.*, 1980, 1982; David and Aguayo, 1981). This is especially impressive because these axons cease to elongate on reentering the CNS. In addition, the converse paradigm—confronting peripheral axons with central glia—produces adversive behavior in the peripheral axons: the few that enter the CNS graft grow poorly, and the majority circumvent it (Aguayo *et al.*, 1978; Weinberg and Spencer, 1979). Finally, it is important to note that even though the neurotropic/neuronotrophic factor(s) elaborated by the Schwann cell are apparently more potent than analogous CNS factors, analogous CNS factors clearly exist (Banker, 1980; Schwartz *et al.*, 1982; Nieto-Sampedro *et al.*, 1982).

1.2. Axonal Transport of Proteins during Regeneration

This subject has recently been reviewed in depth (Forman, 1982; McQuarrie, 1983*b*), as has the broader subject of intraneuronal protein transport (Grafstein and Forman, 1980; Brady and Lasek, 1982). The new observations and ideas that have subsequently appeared are reviewed elsewhere in this volume. Since the influence of the conditioning lesion paradigm on axonal transport has only been examined in goldfish optic axons, the principles of axonal transport can briefly be summarized in the course of describing the background and methodology for these experiments. Protein transport is emphasized because growing axons require a source of protein but have none of the machinery that is needed to make it, including ribosomes (Zelena, 1972) and ribosomal RNA (Edstrom *et al.*, 1973; Black and Lasek, 1977). Axonal growth depends, therefore, on a system for transferring proteins from the site of synthesis (the nerve cell body) to the site of growth (the axon tip).

1.2.1.   The Rate Components of Axonal Transport in Goldfish Retinal Ganglion Cells

In the optic axons of goldfish, three rate components of anterograde protein transport have been described (Table 3): (1) fast component, (2) slow component a (SCa), and (3) slow component b (SCb). These rate components are universal features of axons and have a number of properties in common, even though the rates themselves vary with body temperature (Grafstein and Forman, 1980; Brady and Lasek, 1982). The fast component conveys proteins that are known to associate with membranous elements of the axon (axolemma, smooth endoplasmic reticulum) as well as tubulovesicular organelles.

Accordingly, when the fast component is pulse labeled by injecting radioactive amino acids near a nucleus of nerve cell bodies and sacrificing the animal after an appropriate interval, most of the labeled protein is insoluble in aqueous buffers (McEwen and Grafstein, 1968). The slow components, moving two to three orders of magnitude more slowly, differ in that approximately half of the labeled proteins are soluble—apparently because the predominant polypeptides (tubulin, actin) are found in readily depolymerized macromolecules.

There are also fast and slow rate components of retrograde transport (Table 3). Fast retrograde transport is largely composed of materials originally conveyed into the axons by fast anterograde transport. Apparently, a small fraction of all anterogradely fast-transported materials return to the nerve cell body via fast retrograde transport. There, they may have a negative feedback influence on protein synthesis or affect the fraction of newly synthesized protein that is diverted to the axonal transport channel. Materials extrinsic to the neuron, including small proteins (e.g., horseradish peroxidase) and those internalized via specific receptors (nerve growth factor, tetanus toxin, various viruses), are also carried to the cell body via retrograde transport. Bisby (1980) has recently published a review of these and other aspects of retrograde transport (see M. A. Bisby, Chapter 4, this volume).

1.2.2.   Axonal Transport during Goldfish Optic Nerve Regeneration

Axonal protein transport provides the "life blood" needed for axonal outgrowth. When protein synthesis in retinal ganglion cells is depressed by doses of acetoxycycloheximide that are not lethal to neurons, axonal outgrowth is dramatically retarded (McQuarrie and Grafstein, 1983). Similar results are obtained when the axonal transport mechanism is disrupted by colchicine (Grafstein, 1971) or dibutyryl cyclic AMP (McQuarrie and Grafstein, 1983). This dependence of axonal growth on protein transport suggests that axonal transport might increase during outgrowth and that axonal transport might increase more markedly during accelerated outgrowth. Both predictions prove to be true in the only neurons in which both have been tested—the retinal

TABLE 3.   The Rate Components of Axonal Transport in Goldfish Retinal
Ganglion Cells

Rate component	Rate (mm/day)	Materials transported	Reference
Anterograde			
Fast	40–100	Membrane-bound proteins and lipids	McEwen and Grafstein (1968); Elam and Agranoff (1971); Forman et al. (1972); Currie et al. (1978); McQuarrie and Grafstein (1982a)
Slow, a	0.02	Neurofilament polypeptides	McQuarrie and Lasek (1981); McQuarrie et al. (1984)
Slow, b	0.2–0.4	Tubulin, actin	Grafstein and Murray (1969); Grafstein et al. (1970); Giulian et al. (1980); McQuarrie and Lasek (1981)
Retrograde			
Fast	36–80	Glycoproteins	Whitnall et al. (1982)
Slow	0.6–4.0	46-kilodalton polypeptide	Williams and Agranoff (1983)

ganglion cells of goldfish. The changes seen with normal outgrowth are presented here as an introduction to the changes seen with accelerated outgrowth.

    1.2.2a.   Changes in Protein Synthesis.   Following axotomy, the incorporation of intraocularly injected [^{3}H]amino acids into protein has been studied morphologically (using autoradiography) and biochemically (using gel electrophoresis in combination with fluorography) (see B. W. Agranoff and T. S. Ford-Holevinski, Chapter 5, this volume). With light microscopic autoradiography, amino acid incorporation is seen to increase twofold by 10 days after axotomy (McQuarrie and Grafstein, 1982a). With the arrival of optic axons at the tectum, beginning 10–15 days after axotomy (McQuarrie and Grafstein, 1981; Heacock and Agranoff, 1982), there is a further sharp increase to 500% of normal followed by a gradual decrease. These observations confirm and extend earlier observations made by Murray and Grafstein (1969). At the electron microscopic level, the peak at 2 weeks after axotomy is seen to involve a preferential labeling of the Golgi apparatus and plasma membrane (Whitnall and Grafstein, 1982) in line with the observation that the plasma membranes of regenerating neurons (even at sites distant from sprout formation), and other growing cells, have a high turnover rate (Bunge, 1977;

Tessler *et al.,* 1980; Black, 1980). Preferential labeling of the nucleus and nucleolus also occurs (Whitnall and Grafstein, 1982), suggesting either a high turnover rate for RNAs or an increased demand. This is consistent with the repeated observation that the number and size of nucleoli increase markedly after axotomy (Murray and Grafstein, 1969; McQuarrie and Grafstein, 1982*b*), and an autoradiographic study showing a twofold increase in the incorporation of [^{3}H]uridine into RNA over the 3- to 28-day interval after axotomy (Murray, 1973).

Biochemical studies of goldfish retinas after the injection of labeled RNA precursors show that the turnover of messenger RNA increases (i.e., there is an increased delivery of poly(A)-containing RNA into the cytoplasm at 10–14 days after axotomy) and that the labeling of free ribosomes increases to reach a peak 140% increase at 8 days (Burrell *et al.,* 1978). One would, of course, like to know which proteins are being synthesized so aggressively. Work done on a number of regenerating neurons indicates that the synthesis of neurotransmitter-related proteins is markedly decreased soon after axotomy (Forman, 1982), and biochemical studies of labeled goldfish retinas show that actin and tubulin, normally the most abundantly synthesized proteins, exhibit a disproportionate increase in synthesis during regeneration (Giulian *et al.,* 1980; Heacock and Agranoff, 1982). Other polypeptides, which have yet to be identified, increase disproportionately. These are mentioned when I describe the rate components with which they travel in the axon.

1.2.2b. Changes in Fast Transport. The time course of change in the amount of labeled fast-transported protein corresponds to the time course of change in protein synthesis, with a peak fivefold increase being seen at 15 days after axotomy (McQuarrie and Grafstein, 1982*a*). However, the rate at which the labeled wave advances is also seen to double, so that the fraction of newly synthesized protein that is directed to the fast transport route must have doubled as well. Retrograde fast transport, as might be predicted, increases proportionately (Whitnall *et al.,* 1982). The particular polypeptides that increase have been characterized by using gel electrophoresis in combination with measurements of radioactivity in 1-mm slices of gel tracks (Giulian *et al.,* 1980; Benowitz *et al.,* 1981; L. I. Benowitz, Chapter 10, this volume). These studies show that different polypeptides increase disproportionately at different stages of regeneration. The most dramatically increased polypeptides at 8 days after axotomy show little or no increase by 39 days, and the polypeptides that have become prominent by 39 days had shown little increase by 21 days after axotomy. A 44- to 49-kilodalton polypeptide shows the most dramatic increase, beginning at 8 days and lasting through 29 days (Benowitz *et al.,* 1981; Heacock and Agranoff, 1982). A less prominent increase of a polypeptide with a molecular mass of 155 kilodaltons has also been reported by two laboratories (Giulian *et al.,* 1980; Benowitz *et al.,* 1981).

1.2.2c. Changes in Slow Transport. When the labeled slow transport wave enters a normal optic nerve, the peak passes the point 1 mm behind the eye at 8–10 days after injection, whereas in nerves that had been cut 4 days prior to injection, the peak passes that point at 4–5 days after injection (Grafstein and Murray, 1969). Further analysis shows that this change in transport rate begins 6 days after axotomy and increases to 300% of normal by 17 days (Grafstein and Murray, 1969; Grafstein, 1971); in addition, the level of radioactivity in the peak doubles during regeneration. Because this transport rate is on the order of 1 mm/day, it represents the faster of the two slow components, termed SCb (Table 3). Normally, this rate component carries the bulk of the labeled tubulin and actin (Grafstein *et al.,* 1971; Giulian *et al.,* 1980; Heacock and Agranoff, 1982). Even so, two studies note that these already abundant polypeptides show a disproportionate increase in labeling during axonal regeneration, with the increase in tubulin being an order of magnitude greater than the underlying two- to threefold increase in SCb (Giulian *et al.,* 1980; Heacock and Agranoff, 1982). Both studies also show a disproportionate increase for polypeptides with molecular masses of approximately 70 kilodaltons.

The changes in SCa, the rate component normally advancing at 0.02 mm/day, have yet to be evaluated in detail during regeneration. Nonetheless, preliminary studies suggest that the labeling of the neurofilament polypeptides moving with SCa does not increase and may even decrease (McQuarrie and Lasek, 1981) in line with observations made in regenerating sciatic motor axons of the rat (Hoffman and Lasek, 1980).

2. EFFECTS OF CONDITIONING LESIONS ON AXONAL TRANSPORT

2.1. Effect on Protein Synthesis

The method for estimating protein synthesis autoradiographically in retinal ganglion cells is based on (1) injection of labeled amino acids into the vitreous humor, (2) a short injection–sacrifice interval (2 hr), (3) correction for variation in the exposure of the retina to the precursor, and (4) use of a fixation procedure that washes out the unincorporated precursor. With these precautions, the sectional areas and silver grain densities for 55–70 cells per group are determined; the combined mean percentage change from normal represents the change in amino acid incorporation. With a 2-week conditioning interval, incorporation at 24 hr after the testing lesion is 450% of normal, which is approximately the same as the peak value seen at 15 days after a testing lesion alone (McQuarrie and Grafstein, 1982*b*). By 8 days, incorporation has increased to 750% of normal and remains at this level through 22 days.

2.2. Effect on Fast Transport

The method for evaluating fast transport in the goldfish optic system requires careful timing of the injection–sacrifice interval so that the labeled wave of protein is captured in the optic axons on the retinal side of any lesions (McQuarrie and Grafstein, 1982*a*). Because wave amplitudes vary more than the amplitudes of the trailing plateaus, the latter are used to estimate the amount of transported material. A 2-hr injection–sacrifice interval is employed to capture the advancing wave within the optic axons before they can accumulate at the lesion site. The time course of change in this plateau level is the same whether or not the testing lesion is preceded by a conditioning lesion with one exception: the level is 70% greater at 24 hr after the testing lesion (15 days after the conditioning lesion) than the level at 15 days after a testing lesion alone. This increase is remarkable because it is seen at a time when protein synthesis has not increased, suggesting that a larger fraction of newly synthesized protein enters the axon during the phase of sprout formation (McQuarrie and Grafstein, 1982*b*).

2.3. Effect on Slow Transport

Since the labeled slow transport wave is broader than the length of the optic axons, it is studied by using a 3-day injection–sacrifice interval and analyzing the leading shoulder of the wave that has entered the optic axons. When the logarithm of the radioactivity in consecutive 0.25-mm nerve segments is plotted (Grafstein and Murray, 1969; McQuarrie and Grafstein, 1982*b*), a linear regression of radioactivity on distance is obtained. The slope in degrees is given by the arctangent and is decreasingly negative until the peak of the wave enters the nerve. As the peak passes through the nerve, the slope becomes zero and then positive. Since the rate of transport is normally 0.4 mm/day, increasing to 1.2 mm/day after a testing lesion alone, the peak would not be expected to enter the nerve after an injection–sacrifice interval as short as 3 days (Grafstein and Murray, 1969). Nonetheless, the effect of a conditioning axotomy is such that by 8 days after the testing lesion the peak has largely passed through the nerve (McQuarrie and Grafstein, 1982*b*), indicating a transport rate of 1.5–2.0 mm/day. The amount of labeled protein conveyed by slow transport increases two- to threefold (over the level seen at 15 days after a testing lesion alone) by 24 hr after a testing lesion preceded by a conditioning lesion. This suggests that the cell responds to a second growth stimulus by diverting additional quantities of newly synthesized protein to the axon until a further increase in synthesis can meet the requirements of accelerated outgrowth.

2.4. Effect of Conditioning Events on Transport and Outgrowth

These experiments are internally controlled by confronting the contralateral optic axons with a different conditioning event, partial end-organ denervation, as opposed to direct axotomy (cf. Section 1.1). Two weeks later, both optic tracts are subjected to identical testing lesions by cutting the optic chiasma. After 8 days, the outgrowth distances for axons that have received a conditioning axotomy are 60% greater than those of axons that were subjected to partial end-organ denervation (McQuarrie and Grafstein, 1982*b*). In both instances, the outgrowth distances are greater than those seen after a testing lesion alone (Grafstein, 1971).

When a conditioning lesion is used, the period of axonal outgrowth extends from 2 to 21 days after the testing lesion, with axons beginning to reach their targets in the tectum during the second week (McQuarrie and Grafstein, 1981). One would expect the axonal transport events that are most closely associated with accelerated outgrowth to be most pronounced at this time. Interestingly, fast transport during the 2- to 21-day period proves to be no greater because of a conditioning lesion than it is after a testing lesion alone (McQuarrie and Grafstein, 1982*b*). On the other hand, slow transport at 8 days after the testing lesion shows a pattern of progressive augmentation in relation to the conditioning status, from a testing lesion alone through a testing lesion preceded by partial end-organ denervation to a testing lesion preceded by axotomy (McQuarrie and Grafstein, 1982*b*). Each step in the augmentation involves a significant increase in the rate at which the labeled slow transport wave advances, an increase that corresponds to the increase in maximum outgrowth rates. There is also a marked increase in the magnitude of slow transport labeling that corresponds to the increase in protein synthesis. These latter two changes, however, are no greater after conditioning by axotomy than after conditioning by end-organ denervation. Thus, it is the overall flux (amount passing a given point per unit time) of slowly transported materials that governs outgrowth.

3. DISCUSSION

From this study in goldfish optic axons, one can conclude that a conditioning event is responsible for specific departures from the response to a testing axotomy alone: an additional increase in protein synthesis beginning days after the testing lesion, an early but transient increase in fast transport, and an early as well as sustained increase in slow transport. The latter effect is the most impressive because it coincides with the outgrowth phase and is most pronounced when the conditioning event is an axotomy, associating the increase in slow transport with a greater magnitude of protein synthesis and greater outgrowth distances. The relevant subcomponent of slow transport appears to be SCb (McQuarrie and Grafstein, 1982b), so it is important to note that the principal proteins carried by SCb are the subunits that form microtubules and microfilaments upon polymerization. Since this rate component is apparently responsible for accelerated outgrowth, the rate of axonal elongation may well depend on the assembly conditions for these cytoskeletal polypeptides. This role for the cytoskeletal polypeptides is an extensive subject that is the topic of a separate review article (McQuarrie, 1983b).

Any explanation for the degree of fine tuning described above in response to conditioning events must postulate that the cell body keeps informed as to the progress of outgrowth (Watson, 1970; D. L. Wilson, Chapter 9, this volume). This may involve a cue that differs from the cue signaling the occurrence of an axotomy (cf. Section 1), since an exogenous cue is unlikely to provide the requisite information. The most attractive hypothesis is that a posttranslational modification of a fast-transported protein occurs at the outgrowing tip, as indicated by the observations of Benowitz et al. (1981), with the progressively more delayed return of this modified polypeptide to the cell body being the cue. A polypeptide that is anterogradely transported in greater amounts after axotomy would seem to be required for this role, since the optimum conditioning interval of 1–2 weeks requires a cue that is augmented in response to axotomy, thereby stimulating an augmented growth response. To date, the only fast-transported polypeptide that has been observed by more than one laboratory to increase after axotomy is in the 155-kilodalton molecular mass range (Giulian et al., 1980; Benowitz et al., 1981).

One would like to test these ideas in a simpler model system, one that reduces the extraneous factors to a minimum and focuses attention on the essential factors, which are a centralized capacity for protein synthesis and a peripheral axonlike extension of the cell that is capable of regeneration. The regeneration of bacterial flagellae appears to represent such a model (Silflow et al., 1982). In *Chlamydomonas,* flagellar regeneration begins 12–15 min after flagella are sheared off, and 85–90% of the full length of 12–13 μm is regained by 60 min after shearing (Randall et al., 1967; Weeks et al., 1977). The onset of flagellar outgrowth is preceded by the transcription of previously dormant tubulin genes to produce tubulin mRNA, so that newly synthesized tubulin is available to the cell even though it already contains sufficient tubulin to regenerate flagellae to 50% of their normal length (Rosenbaum et al., 1969; Silflow et al., 1982).

Consistent with this reflexive response to deflagellation, prevention of flagellar growth with colchicine has no effect on the magnitude or time course of tubulin synthesis (Lefebvre et al., 1978; Silflow et al., 1982). When the pool of monomeric tubulin in the cytoplasm is expanded by inducing flagellar resorption with PPi, discontinuance of the PPi results in accelerated flagellar regeneration compared to that seen after shearing alone (Lefebvre *et al.,* 1977). Similarly, the tubulin pool can be expanded in both sea urchins (Merlino *et al.,* 1978) and *Chlamydomonas* (J. Schloss and J. L. Rosenbaum, personal communication) by repeatedly shearing off the newly formed cilia or flagellae to produce additional tubulin mRNA. Thus, an acceleration of outgrowth is associated with an increase in the availability of monomeric tubulin just as accelerated axonal outgrowth is associated with an increased amplitude and rate of the slow transport wave that conveys tubulin (Hoffman and Lasek, 1980; Heacock and Agranoff, 1982; McQuarrie and Grafstein, 1982*b*; McQuarrie 1983*b,c*).

Flagellar regeneration therefore parallels axonal regeneration in several respects, even to the point of ruling out the possibility that changes in tubulin concentration are the signaling mechanism that initiates increased tubulin mRNA transcription (Silflow *et al.,* 1982).

ACKNOWLEDGMENTS

This study was supported by a Career Development Award from the Veterans Administration and by Grant NS-18975 from the U.S. Public Health Service.

4. REFERENCES

Adler, R., and Varon, S., 1981, Neuritic guidance by nonneuronal cells of ganglionic origin, *Dev. Biol.* **86**:69–80.

Agranoff, B. W., Field, P., and Gaze, R. M., 1976, Neurite outgrowth from explanted *Xenopus* retina: An effect of prior optic nerve section, *Brain Res.* **113**:225–234.

Aguayo, A. J., Dickson, R., Trecarten, J., Attiwell, M., Bray, G. M., and Richardson, P., 1978, Ensheathment and myelination of regenerating PNS fibres by transplanted optic nerve glia, *Neurosci. Lett.* **9**:97–104.

Arvidsson, J., and Aldskogius, H., 1982, Effect of repeated hypoglossal nerve lesions on the number of neurons in the hypoglossal nucleus of adult rats, *Exp. Neurol.* **75**:520–524.

Banker, G. A., 1980, Trophic interactions between astroglial cells and hippocampal neurons in culture, *Science* **209**:809–810.

Benowitz, L. I., Shashoua, V. E., and Yoon, M. G., 1981, Specific changes in rapidly transported proteins during regeneration of the goldfish optic nerve, *J. Neurosci.* **1**:300–307.

Bisby, M. A., 1978, Fast axonal transport of labeled protein in sensory axons during regeneration, *Exp. Neurol.* **61**:281–300.

Bisby, M. A., 1980, Retrograde axonal transport, *Adv. Cell Neurobiol.* **1**:69–117.

Bisby, M. A., and Pollock, B., 1983, Increased regeneration rate in peripheral nerve axons following double lesions: Enhancement of the conditioning lesion phenomenon, *J. Neurobiol.* **14**:467–472.

Black, M. M., and Lasek, R. J., 1977, The presence of transfer RNA in the axoplasm of the squid giant axon, *J. Neurobiol.* **8:**229–237.

Black, P. J., 1980, Shedding from the cell surface of normal and cancer cells, *Adv. Cancer Res.* **32:**75–199.

Bradley, W. G., and Asbury, A. K., 1970, Duration of synthesis phase in neurilemma cells in mouse sciatic nerve during regeneration, *Exp. Neurol.* **26:**275–282.

Brady, S. T., and Lasek, R. J., 1982, Axonal transport: A cell-biological method for studying proteins that associate with the cytoskeleton, *Methods Cell Biol.* **25:**365–398.

Brock, T. O., and Turner, J. E., 1978, The effect of repeated nerve injury on the retinal ganglion cell and axonal regeneration response in the optic nerve of the newt *(Triturus viridescens),* *Soc. Neurosci. Abstr.* **4:**529.

Brock, T. O., and Turner, J. E., 1982, Retinal ganglion cell body response to repeated axotomy in the regenerating visual system of newt *(Notophthalmus viridescens),* *Exp. Neurol.* **78:**316–330.

Brown, M. C., and Hopkins, W. G., 1981, Role of degenerating axon pathways in regeneration of mouse soleus motor axons, *J. Physiol. (Lond.)* **318:**365–373.

Bunge, M. B., 1977, Initial endocytosis of peroxidase or ferritin by growth cones of cultured nerve cells, *J. Neurocytol.* **6:**407–439.

Burnham, P. A., Raiborn, C., and Varon, S., 1972, Replacement of nerve growth factor by ganglionic non-neuronal cells for the survival in vitro of dissociated ganglionic neurons, *Proc. Natl. Acad. Sci. U.S.A.* **69:**3556–3560.

Burrell, H. R., Dokas, L. A., and Agranoff, B. W., 1978, RNA metabolism in the goldfish retina during optic nerve regeneration, *J. Neurochem.* **31:**289–298.

Carlsen, R. C., 1982, Comparison of adenylate-cyclase activity in segments of rat sciatic nerve with a condition–test or test lesion, *Exp. Neurol.* **77:**254–265.

Carlsen, R. C., 1983, Delayed induction of the cell body response and enhancement of regeneration following a condition/test lesion of frog peripheral nerve at 15°C, *Brain Res.* **279:**9–18.

Chamley, J. H., Goller, I., and Burnstock, G., 1973, Selective growth of sympathetic nerve fibers to explants of normally densely innervated autonomic effector organs in tissue culture, *Dev. Biol.* **31:**363–379.

Cheah, T. B., and Geffen, L. B., 1973, Effects of axonal injury on norepinephrine, tyrosine hydroxylase and monoamine oxidase levels in sympathetic ganglia, *J. Neurobiol.* **4:**443–452.

Collins, F., and Lee, M. R., 1982, A reversible developmental change in the ability of ciliary ganglion neurons to extend neurites in culture, *J. Neurosci.* **2:**424–430.

Cotman, C. W., Nieto-Sampedro, M., and Harris, E. W., 1981, Synapse replacement in the nervous system of adult vertebrates, *Physiol. Rev.* **61:**684–784.

Coughlin, M. D., 1975, Target organ stimulation of parasympathetic nerve growth in the developing mouse submandibular gland, *Dev. Biol.* **61:**131–139.

Currie, J. R., Grafstein, B., Whitnall, M. H., and Alpert, R., 1978, Axonal transport of lipid in goldfish optic axons, *Neurochem. Res.* **3:**479–492.

David, S., and Aguayo, A. J., 1981, Axonal elongation into peripheral nervous system "bridges" after central nervous system injury in adult rats, *Science* **214:**931–933.

Ducker, T. B., Kempe, L. G., and Hayes, G. J., 1969, The metabolic background for peripheral nerve surgery, *J. Neurosurg.* **30:**270–280.

Ebendal, T., and Jacobson, C. O., 1977, Tissue explants affecting extension and orientation of axons in cultures of chick ganglia, *Exp. Cell Res.* **105:**379–387.

Edstrom, A., Edstrom, J. -E., and Hokfelt, T., 1973, Sedimentation analysis of ribonucleic acid extracted from isolated Mauthner nerve fibre components, *J. Neurochem.* **16:**53–66.

Edwards, D. L., Alpert, R. M., and Grafstein, B., 1981, Recovery of vision in regeneration of goldfish optic axons: Enhancement of axonal outgrowth by a conditioning lesion, *Exp. Neurol.* **72**:672–686.

Elam, J. S., and Agranoff, B. W., 1971, Rapid transport of protein in the optic system of the goldfish, *J. Neurochem.* **18**:375–387.

Forman, D. S., 1982, Axonal transport and nerve regeneration: A review, in: *Spinal Cord Reconstruction* (C. C. Kao, R. P. Bunge, and P. Reier, eds.), pp. 75–86, Raven Press, New York.

Forman, D. S., and Berenberg, R. A., 1978, Regeneration of motor axons in the rat sciatic nerve studied by labeling with axonally transported radioactive protein, *Brain Res.* **156**:213–225.

Forman, D. S., Grafstein, B., and McEwen, B. S., 1972, Rapid axonal transport of (^{3}H)fucosyl glycoproteins in the goldfish optic system, *Brain Res.* **48**:327–342.

Forman, D. S., Wood, D. K., and DeSilva, S., 1979, Rate of regeneration of sensory axons in transected rat sciatic nerve repaired with epineurial sutures, *J. Neurol. Sci.* **44**:55–59.

Forman, D. S. McQuarrie, I. G., Labore, F. W., Wood, D. K., Stone, L. S., Braddock, C. H., and Fuchs, D. A., 1980, Time course of the conditioning lesion effect on axonal regeneration, *Brain Res.* **182**:180–185.

Forman, D. S., McQuarrie, I. G., Grafstein, B., and Edwards, D. L., 1981, Effect of a conditioning lesion on axonal regeneration and recovery of function, in: *Lesion-Induced Neuronal Plasticity in Sensorimotor Systems* (H. Flohr and W. Precht, eds.), pp. 103–113, Springer-Verlag, Berlin, Heidelberg, New York.

Frizell, M., and Sjostrand, J., 1974, The axonal transport of slowly migrating (^{3}H)leucine-labeled proteins and the regeneration rate in regenerating hypoglossal and vagus nerves of the rabbit, *Brain Res.* **81**:267–283.

Giulian, D., DesRuisseaux, H., and Cowburn, D., 1980, Biosynthesis and intra-axonal transport of proteins during neuronal regeneration, *J. Biol. Chem.* **255**:6494–6501.

Grafstein, B., 1971, Role of slow axonal transport in nerve regeneration, *Acta Neuropathol. (Berl.) [Suppl.]* **5**:144–152.

Grafstein, B., and Forman, D. S., 1980, Intracellular transport in neurons, *Physiol. Rev.* **60**:1167–1283.

Grafstein, B., and McQuarrie, I. G., 1978, Role of the nerve cell body in axonal regeneration, in: *Neuronal Plasticity* (C. W. Cotman, ed.), pp. 155–195, Raven Press, New York.

Grafstein, B., and Murray, M., 1969, Transport of protein in goldfish optic nerve during regeneration, *Exp. Neurol.* **25**:494–508.

Grafstein, B., McEwen, B. S., and Shelanski, M., 1970, Axonal transport of neurotubule protein, *Nature* **227**:289–290.

Greene, L. A., and Shooter, E. M., 1980, The nerve growth factor: Biochemistry, synthesis, and mechanism of action, *Annu. Rev. Neurosci.* **3**:353–402.

Griffin, J. W., Drachman, D. B., and Price, D. L., 1976, Fast axonal transport in motor nerve regeneration, *J. Neurobiol.* **7**:355–370.

Gundersen, R. W., and Barrett, J. N., 1980, Characterization of the turning response of dorsal root neurites toward nerve growth factor, *J. Cell Biol.* **87**:546–554.

Gutmann, E., 1942, Factors affecting recovery of motor function after nerve lesions, *J. Neurol. Neurosurg.* **5**:81–95.

Gutmann, E., Guttmann, L., Medawar, P. B., and Young, J. Z., 1942, The rate of regeneration of nerve, *J. Exp. Biol.* **19**:14–44.

Heacock, A. M., and Agranoff, B. W., 1982, Protein synthesis and transport in the regenerating goldfish visual system, *Neurochem. Res.* **7**:771–788.

Hoffman, P. N., and Lasek, R. J., 1980, Axonal transport of the cytoskeleton in regenerating motor neurons: Constancy and change, *Brain Res.* **202**:317–333.

Howe, H. A., and Bodian, D., 1941, Refractoriness of nerve cells to poliomyelitis virus after interruption of their axons, *Johns Hopkins Hosp. Bull.* **69**:92–103.

Iacovitti, L., Reis, D. J., and Joh, T. H., 1981, Reactive proliferation of brain stem noradrenergic nerves following neonatal cerebellectomy in rats: Role of target maturation on neuronal response to injury during development, *Dev. Brain Res.* **1**:3–24.

Kalil, K., and Reh, T., 1982, A light and electron microscopic study of regrowing pyramidal tract fibers, *J. Comp. Neurol.* **211**:265–275.

Konorski, J., and Lubinska, L., 1946, Mechanical excitability of regenerating nerve fibers, *Lancet* **1**:609–610.

Kristensson, K., and Olsson, Y., 1975, Retrograde transport of horseradish peroxidase in transected axons. II. Relations betwen rate of transfer from the site of injury to the perikaryon and onset of chromatolysis, *J. Neurocytol.* **4**:653–661.

Landreth, G. E., and Agranoff, B. W., 1976, Explant culture of adult goldfish retina: Effect of prior optic nerve crush, *Brain Res.* **118**:299–303.

Lanners, H. N., and Grafstein, B., 1980a, Effect of a conditioning lesion on regeneration of goldfish optic axons: Ultrastructural evidence of enhanced outgrowth and pinocytosis, *Brain Res.* **196**:547–553.

Lanners, H. N., and Grafstein, B., 1980b, Early stages of axonal regeneration in the goldfish optic tract; An electron microscopic study, *J. Neurocytol.* **9**:733–751.

LeFebvre, P. A., Nordstrom, S. A., Moulder, J. E., and Rosenbaum, J. L., 1978, Flagellar elongation and shortening in *Chlamydomonas*. IV. Effects of flagellar detachment, regeneration, and resorption on the induction of flagellar protein synthesis, *J. Cell Biol.* **78**:8–27.

Letourneau, P. C., 1982, Nerve fiber growth and its regulation by extrinsic factors, in: *Neuronal Development* (N. C. Spitzer, ed.) pp. 213–254, Plenum Press, New York.

Lubinska, L., 1952, The influence of the state of the peripheral stump on the early stages of nerve regeneration, *Acta Biol. Exp. (Warsaw)* **16**:55–63.

Luiten, P. G. M., 1981, Afferent and efferent connections of the optic tectum in the carp, *Brain Res.* **220**:51–66.

Lundborg, G., Longo, F. M., and Varon, S., 1982, Nerve regeneration model and trophic factors *in vivo, Brain Res.* **232**:157–161.

Manthorpe, M., Luyten, W., Longo, F. M., and Varon, S., 1983, Endogenous and exogenous factors support neuronal survival and choline acetyltransferase activity in embryonic spinal cord cultures, *Brain Res.* **267**:57–66.

McEwen, B. S., and Grafstein, B., 1968, Fast and slow components in axonal transport of protein, *J. Cell Biol.* **38**:494–508.

McQuarrie, I. G., 1978, The effect of a conditioning lesion on motor axons, *Brain Res.* **152**:597–602.

McQuarrie, I. G., 1979, Accelerated axonal sprouting after nerve transection, *Brain Res.* **167**:185–188.

McQuarrie, I. G., 1983a, Effect of a conditioning axotomy on axonal sprout formation at nodes of Ranvier following a testing axotomy, *Anat. Rec.* **205**:119A–120A.

McQuarrie, I. G., 1983b, Role of the axonal cytoskeleton in the regenerating nervous system, in: *Nerve, Organ and Tissue Regeneration: Research Perspectives* (F. J. Seil, ed.) pp. 51–88, Academic Press, New York.

McQuarrie, I. G., 1983c, Transport of cytoskeletal proteins in regenerating axons accelerated by a conditioning axotomy, *J. Cell Biol.* **99**:241a.

McQuarrie, I. G., and Grafstein, B., 1973, Axon outgrowth enhanced by a previous nerve injury, *Arch. Neurol.* **29**:53–55.

McQuarrie, I. G., and Grafstein, B., 1981, Effect of a conditioning lesion on optic nerve regeneration in goldfish, *Brain Res.* **216**:253–264.

McQuarrie, I. G., and Grafstein, B., 1982a, Protein synthesis and fast axonal transport in regenerating goldfish retinal ganglion cells, *Brain Res.* **235**:213–223.

McQuarrie, I. G., and Grafstein, B., 1982b, Protein synthesis and axonal transport in goldfish retinal ganglion cells during regeneration accelerated by a conditioning lesion, *Brain Res.* **251**:25–31.

McQuarrie, I. G., and Grafstein, B., 1983, Effect of acetoxycycloheximide and dibutyryl adenosine cyclic 3':5'-monophosphate on axonal regeneration in the goldfish optic nerve, *Brain Res.* **279**:377–381.

McQuarrie, I. G., and Lasek, R. J., 1981, Axonal transport of labeled neurofilament proteins in goldfish optic axons, *J. Cell Biol.* **91**:234a.

McQuarrie, I. G., Phillips, L. L., and Autilio-Gambetti, L., 1984, Axonal transport of neurofilament proteins in goldfish optic nerves, *Trans. Am. Soc. Neurochem.* **15**:136.

McQuarrie, I. G., Grafstein, B., and Gershon, M. D., 1977, Axonal regeneration in the rat sciatic nerve: Effect of a conditioning lesion and of dbcAMP, *Brain Res.* **132**:443–453.

McQuarrie, I. G., Grafstein, B., Dreyfus, C. F., and Gershon, M. D., 1978, Regeneration of adrenergic axons in rat sciatic nerve: Effect of a conditioning lesion, *Brain Res.* **141**:21–34.

Merlino, G. T., Chamberlain, J. P., and Kleinsmith, L. J., 1978, Effects of deciliation on tubulin messenger RNA activity in sea urchin embryos, *J. Biol. Chem.* **253**:7078–7085.

Murray, M., 1973, ^{3}H-uridine incorporation by regenerating retinal ganglion cells of goldfish, *Exp. Neurol.* **39**:489–497.

Murray, M., and Grafstein, B., 1969, Changes in the morphology and amino acid incorporation of regenerating goldfish optic neurons, *Exp. Neurol.* **23**:544–560.

Nieto-Sampedro, M., Lewis, E. R., Cotman, C. W., Manthrope, M., Skaper, S. D., Barbin, G., Longo, F. M., and Caron, S., 1982, Brain injury causes a time-dependent increase in neuronotrophic activity at the lesion site, *Science* **217**:860–861.

Northcutt, R. G., 1981, Evolution of the telencephalon in nonmammals, *Annu. Rev. Neurosci.* **4**:301–350.

Oblinger, M. M., and Lasek, R. J., 1983a, Effect of a conditioning lesion on the rate of regeneration of two branches of the dorsal root ganglion (DRG) cell, *Anat. Rec.* **205**:145A–146A.

Oblinger, M. M., and Lasek, R. J., 1983b, Central and peripheral axotomy of dorsal root ganglion (DRG) cells differentially affects slow axonal transport, *Soc. Neurosci. Abstr.* **9**:148.

Politis, M. J., Ederle, K., and Spencer, P. S., 1982, Tropism in nerve regeneration *in vivo*. Attraction of regenerating axons by diffusible factors derived from cells in distal nerve stumps of transected peripheral nerves, *Brain Res.* **253**:1–12.

Ramon y Cajal, S., 1928, (R. M. May, Trans.), *Degeneration and Regeneration of the Nervous System*, Vol. 1, pp. 329–375, (1968 facsimile of 1928 ed.), Hafner, London.

Randall, J., Cavalier-Smith, T., McVittie, A., Warr, M., and Hopkins, J., 1967, Developmental and control processes in the basal bodies and flagella of *Chlamydomonas reinhardii*, *Dev. Biol. [Suppl.]* **1**:43–83.

Reh, T., and Kalil, K., 1982, Functional role of regrowing pyramidal tract fibers, *J. Comp. Neurol.* **211**:276–283.

Richardson, P. M., and Ebendal, T., 1982, Nerve growth activities in rat peripheral nerve, *Brain Res.* **246**:57–64.

Richardson, P. M., McGuinness, U. M., and Aguayo, A. J., 1980, Axons from CBS neurones regenerate into PNS grafts, *Nature* **284**:264–265.

Richardson, P. M., McGuinness, U. M., and Aguayo, A. J., 1982, Peripheral nerve autografts to the rat spinal cord: Studies with axonal tracer methods, *Brain Res.* **237**:147–162.

Romanes, G. J., 1951, The motor cell columns of the lumbosacral spinal cord of the cat, *J. Comp. Neurol.* **94**:313–364.

Rosenbaum, J. L., Moulder, J. E., and Ringo, D. L., 1969, Flagellar elongation and shortening in *Chlamydomonas*. I. The use of cycloheximide and colchicine to study the synthesis and assemby of flagellar proteins, *J. Cell Biol.* **41**:600–619.

Schmidt, J. T., 1979, The laminar organization of optic nerve fibres in the tectum of goldfish, *Proc. Soc. Lond. [Biol.]* **205**:287–306.

Schneider, G. E., 1981, Early lesions and abnormal neuronal connections, *Trends Neurosci.* **4**:187–192.

Schwartz, M., Mizrachi, Y., and Eshhar, N., 1982, Factor(s) from goldfish brain induce neuritic outgrowth from enplanted regenerating retinas, *Dev. Brain Res.* **3**:29–35.

Sebille, A., and Bondoux-Jahan, M., 1980, Effects of electric stimulation and previous nerve injury on motor function recovery in rats, *Brain Res.* **192**:562–565.

Silflow, C. D., LeFebvre, P. A., McKeithan, T. W., Schloss, J. A., Keller, L. R., and Rosenbaum, J. L., 1982, Expression of flagellar protein genes during flagellar regeneration in *Chlamydomonas, Cold Spring Harbor Symp. Quant. Biol.* **46**(1):157–169.

Singer, P.A., Mehler, S., and Fernandez, H. L., 1982, Blockade of retrograde axonal transport delays the onset of metabolic and morphologic changes induced by axotomy, *J. Neurosci.* **2**:1299–1306.

Sparrow, J. R., and Grafstein, B., 1983, Prior collateral sprouting enhances axonal regeneration, *Brain Res.* **269**:133–136.

Springer, A. D., and Gaffney, J. S., 1981, Retinal projections in the goldfish: A study using cobaltous-lysine, *J. Comp. Neurol.* **203**:401–424.

Tessler, A., Autilio-Gambetti, L., and Gambetti, P., 1980, Axonal growth during regeneration: A quantitative autoradiographic study, *J. Cell biol.* **87**:197–203.

Thomas, P. K., 1970, The cellular response to nerve injury. 3. The effect of repeated crush, *J. Anat. (Lond.)* **106**:463–470.

Torvik, A., and Skjorten, F., 1971, Electron microscope observations on nerve cell regeneration and degeneration after axon lesions. I. Changes in the nerve cell cytoplasm, *Acta Neuropathol. (Berl.)* **17**:248–264.

Vanegas, H., and Ebbesson, S. O. E., 1976, Telencephalic projections in two teleost species, *J. Comp. Neurol.* **165**:181–196.

Varon, S., Skaper, S. D., and Manthorpe, M., 1981, Trophic activities for dorsal root and sympathetic ganglionic neurons in media conditioned by Schwann and other peripheral cells, *Dev. Brain Res.* **1**:73–87.

Watson, W. E., 1970, Some metabolic responses of axotomized neurones to contact between their axons and denervated muscle, *J. Physiol. (Lond.)* **210**:321–344.

Watson, W. E., 1973, Some responses of dorsal root ganglia to axotomy, *J. Physiol. (Lond.)* **231**:41P–42P.

Weeks, D. P., Collis, P. S., and Gealt, M. A., 1977, Control of induction of tubulin synthesis in *Chlamydomonas reinhardi, Nature* **268**:667–668.

Wells, M. R., and Bernstein, J. J., 1978, Amino acid incorporation into rat spinal cord and brain after simultaneous and interval sciatic nerve lesions, *Brain Res.* **139**:249–262.

Weinberg, E. L., and Spencer, P. S., 1979, Studies on the contol of myelinogenesis. 3. Signalling of oligodendrocyte myelination by regenerating peripheral axons, *Brain Res.* **162**:273–277.

Weiss, P., and Taylor, A. C., 1944, Further evidence against 'neurotropism' in nerve regeneration, *J. Exp. Zool.* **99**:233–257.

Whitnall, M. H. and Grafstein, B., 1982, Perikaryal routing of newly synthesized proteins in regenerating neurons: Quantitative electron microscopic autoradiography, *Brain Res.* **239**:41–56.

Whitnall, M. H., Currie, J. R., and Grafstein, B., 1982, Bidirectional transport of glycoproteins in goldfish optic nerve, *Exp. Neurol.* **75**:191–207.

Williams, L. R., and Agranoff, B. W., 1983, Retrograde transport of goldfish optic nerve proteins labeled by *N*-succinimidyl (³H)propionate, *Brain Res.* **259**:207–216.

Young, J. Z., and Medawar, P. B., 1940, Fibrin suture of peripheral nerves, Measurement of the rate of regeneration, *Lancet* **2**:126–128.

Zelena, J., 1972, Ribosomes in myelinated axons of dorsal root ganglia, *Z. Zellforsch.* **124**:217–229.

CHAPTER 13

THE RELATIONSHIP OF SLOW AXONAL FLOW TO NERVE ELONGATION AND DEGENERATION

PAUL CANCALON

1. INTRODUCTION

After an axon is injured, the segment distal to the lesion degenerates. The fate of the proximal segment containing the cell bodies is more complex; depending on various factors, the injury can induce cell death or promote axonal regeneration. The succession of events leading to either death or survival remains obscure, and their relative importance has been questioned. Recent investigations appear to downplay the chromatolytic reaction of the perikaryon as a necessary step for regeneration or at least for sprouting (Carlsen *et al.*, 1982; Grafstein, 1983) and suggest that changes taking place in the axon itself might have a major influence on the regenerative as well as distal degenerative processes (Lanners and Grafstein, 1980; Lasek, 1981; Morris and Lasek, 1982; Lasek and Morris, 1982; McQuarrie, 1983).

PAUL CANCALON ● *Department of Biological Science, Florida State University, Tallahassee, Florida 32306*

Numerous attempts have been made to correlate the various events occurring in the nerve after an axonal lesion with the rapid and slow phases of axonal transport. The degeneration of the nerve segment severed from its cell bodies has been extensively studied; however, it has not been possible so far to determine with an absolute certainty if the degenerative process appears simultaneously over the entire nerve stump or spreads progressively over the isolated segment. The involvement of axonal transport has been suggested by Schlaepfer and Bunge (1973) and Joseph (1973). Attempts have also been made to correlate axonal transport with the regenerative mechanism (for review see McQuarrie, 1983). In most cases, however, the rate of slow flow is significantly greater than the velocity of axonal elongation (see below).

Analysis of the kinetics of slow flow in the garfish olfactory nerve has revealed an identical acceleration of the transport process in developing and regenerating neurons as well as in nerve stumps isolated from their cell bodies (Cancalon, 1982*b*, 1983*a–d*). This might reflect a similar posttraumatic alteration of the axoplasm over the entire length of the axon proximally and distally to the injury. A possible explanation (Lasek and Morris, 1982) might be that developing and regenerating axons are characterized by a less rigid cytoskeletal organization with few neurofilaments and a high concentration of soluble microfilament and microtubule polymers. An alteration of the cytoskeletal matrix of developing, regenerating, and degenerating neurons may result in a more fluid axoplasm and/or a reorganization of the transport mechanism that will induce faster flow rates. Accelerated flow, in turn, might be responsible for a quick loss of components essential to survival in axons detached from their perikarya or a rapid delivery of molecules to the growing area, promoting a fast extension of the elongating axons.

Axonal transport, nerve degeneration, and regeneration have all been shown to be temperature dependent. Therefore, by analyzing their kinetics over a wide range of temperature, we hoped to reveal some of the links between intraaxonal transport and the degenerative and regenerative processes. Prior to summarizing these studies, I review some of the previous work on the effect of temperature on the various mechanisms occurring in intact and damaged neurons.

2. INFLUENCE OF TEMPERATURE ON MECHANISMS INVOLVED IN NEURONAL MAINTENANCE AND REGENERATION

2.1. Rapid Axonal Transport

In several studies, an exponential or at least a nonlinear increase of the fast axonal transport rate with temperature has been reported. Grafstein *et al.*

(1972) estimated a Q_{10} of at least 2.6 between 9 and 20.5°C in the goldfish visual system for the transport of labeled proteins. A similar Q_{10} (2.5) was determined by Elam and Agranoff (1971) for the transport of glycosamino-glycans in the same preparation. In the frog sciatic nerve, a nonlinear increase of transport rate with temperature was noted by Edstrom and Hanson (1973) between 5.5 and 28°C, with the Q_{10} decreasing from 3.4 to 2.3. The authors determined that below 15°C an increase in transport rate occurs if the animals are acclimated to the temperature for 2 weeks. By direct detection of radio-activity in the bullfrog sciatic nerve, the rate of fast transport was found to be an exponential function of temperature between 5 and 24°C (Q_{10} = 2.5) (Tak-enaka *et al.*, 1978). In the mussel *Anondata,* fast transport increases exponen-tially with temperature between 4 and 15°C (Heslop and Howes, 1972). An exponential relationship between fast transport and temperature between 13 and 38°C has been characterized by Bisby and Jones (1978) in hibernating and nonhibernating ground squirrel, with a Q_{10} ranging from 2.6 to 3.2. Below 13°C, transport is totally inhibited. A linear relationship between fast trans-port and temperature has been demonstrated by Gross and Beidler (1975) in the garfish olfactory nerve between 10 and 28°C with a $Q_{10}{}_{21}^{31}$ of 2.2. In exper-iments performed at 37°C (Cancalon, 1982a) in the same preparation, a rate of 389 $\pm$ 10 mm/day was measured. The value is similar to that obtained for peripheral nerves in warm-blooded animals such as the cat (Ochs and Smith, 1975). Similar values were recorded at 15 and 19°C in the pike by Gross and Kreutzberg (1978). In preliminary studies (Cancalon, 1982a), slightly lower rates were measured in the garfish optic nerve with a $Q_{10}{}_{21}^{31}$ of 1.69.

2.2. Retrograde Axonal Transport

Optical techniques have been used to measure the retrograde rate of trans-port of microscopically visible organelles. Forman *et al.* (1977) determined that in bullfrog sciatic nerve the velocity of retrogradely moving particles is less than half the rate of fast transport but increases exponentially with tem-perature between 8 and 37°C with a Q_{10} of 2.5 to 3.5 but stops entirely at about 5°C. An exponential influence of temperature on retrograde axonal transport has also been measured between 5 and 35°C in the sciatic nerve of the toad *Xenopus* with a Q_{10} of 3 between 15 and 25°C (Smith and Cooper, 1981).

2.3. Slow Axonal Flow

Contradictory results have been obtained regarding the effect of temper-ature on slow axonal flow. Biondi *et al.* (1972) suggested that slow flow is tem-perature independent. A similar conclusion was drawn by Grafstein *et al.* (1972) and Alpert *et al.* (1980) for the goldfish optic system. A very low Q_{10}

(1.3) was measured by Ochs *et al.* (1962) in mammalian peripheral nerves. In contrast, Fernandez *et al.* (1970) showed that in the crayfish ventral nerve cord, the slow flow rate increases linearly with temperature between 5 and 20°C but stops at 3°C. A linear function between rate and temperature has also been determined in the garfish olfactory nerve at temperatures ranging from 14 to 35°C with a $Q_{10} {}_{21}^{31}$ of 2.08 (Cancalon, 1979a, 1982a). Extrapolation indicates that slow flow should stop around 10.3°C; however, a movement of radioactivity was still noted at 10°C. Recently (Cancalon, 1982a), an increase in the rate of slow flow in the garfish optic nerve was observed between 21 and 31°C, corresponding to a $Q_{10} {}_{21}^{31}$ of 1.68.

It should be emphasized that most of these experiments indicate that every phase of axonal transport (fast, slow, or retrograde) stops at a temperature between 5 and 10°C.

The discrepancy between the exponential and linear changes in transport rates as a function of temperature noted among several preparations has never been resolved. It has been suggested that the linear functions were in fact exponential but with a very low coefficient. However, a slight deviation from linearity of the rate of slow flow in intact garfish olfactory nerves at high temperatures (above 30°C) was not found to be statistically significant (Cancalon, 1983d).

2.4. Protein Synthesis

A marked influence of temperature on the rate of protein synthesis in the nervous system has been determined by several groups. In chloropromazine-treated animals, a decrease in protein synthesis has been correlated with decrements in body temperature (Shuster and Hannan, 1964). A 35% decrease in the incorporation of leucine into brain proteins of newborn rats was noted by Schain and Watanabe (1971) when the ambient temperature was reduced from 35 to 22°C. However, no such difference was found in newborn guinea pigs, which, in contrast to newborn rats, are able to regulate their body temperature. A similar result was obtained by Lajtha and Dunlop (1974). More recently, Sershen *et al.* (1981) measured a decrease of 8% in protein synthesis in adult mouse brain for each degree of reduction in body temperature. Lathja and Dunlop (1981) estimated that the absolute rate of synthesis in 2- to 3-day-old rat brain increases linearly with temperature at about 6%/°C. The authors determined that the rate of protein synthesis in young rat brain is maximal between 37 and 39°C but declines rapidly above 40°C. Both hypothermia (Raghupathy *et al.*, 1981) and hyperthermia (Murdock *et al.*, 1978; Millan *et al.*, 1979) were shown to decrease protein synthesis in rat brain by inducing disaggregation of the polyribosomes.

Similar studies have also been performed on poikilotherms. In the goldfish brain, Lajtha and Sershen (1975) measured the rate of incorporation of tyrosine into proteins at 10, 22, and 34°C. Care was taken by the authors to take into account the influence of amino acid transport. The values, ranging from 0.026%/hr at 10°C to 0.52%/hr at 34°C, show a 20-fold increase between the two extreme temperatures. If extrapolated to 37°C, the rate is similar to that found in rat brain. No sign of temperature adaptation was noted when fish were maintained up to 4 weeks at the experimental temperatures. Davison *et al.* (1971) showed that nearly all visual signals disappear within 14 days if goldfish are maintained at 5°C. The authors concluded that at low temperature the retinal cells are unable to keep pace with the requirement for new outer segment protein when retinal illumination remained high. Slow recovery was achieved within 52 days after return to room temperature.

2.5. Regeneration

Rates of nerve regeneration have been studied on a large variety of animals and fibers (for review, see Lubinska, 1964, 1975; Grafstein and McQuarrie, 1978; Grafstein and Forman, 1980). Velocities varying between 2 and 6 mm/day are usually determined for mammals. In cold-blooded animals, however, rates of only a fraction of a millimeter to 1 mm/day are usually measured at temperatures ranging from 8 to 25°C.

The effect of temperature on the regeneration velocity of damaged nerves has been known for a long time. Deinaka (1908) showed that in the rabbit sciatic nerve a similar degree of regeneration is obtained in 5 days at 30°C as in 12 days at 12–14°C. The regeneration of the central caudal nerve of rats maintained at 2–2.5°C, 18–21°C, and 37–38°C has been followed by Gamble (1957, 1958): no nerve regeneration occurs in animals maintained at coldest temperatures, and regeneration at the highest temperatures starts 10 days earlier than in animals kept at 18–21°C. Similar results were obtained by Jha *et al.* (1959) for regenerating rat sural nerve, but the authors did not see any changes in regeneration velocity for the genitofemoral nerve, which is protected from the external temperatures by its position in the peritoneal cavity. Lubinska and Olekiewicz (1950) showed that in the sciatic nerve of toads the rate of regeneration increases from 0.6 mm/day at 12.1°C to 1.4 mm/day at 25.8°C and in the frog from 0.6 mm/day at 12.5°C to 2.2 mm/day at 25.9°C. In these preparations, regeneration stops below 8–9°C (Lubinska, 1952). Niemierko and Zawadzka (as quoted by Lubinska, 1964) showed that regeneration stops at 8°C, although axoplasmic streaming is only slightly reduced compared to its 25°C value. An increase in the rate of regeneration of the goldfish optic nerve between 20 and 30°C was also reported by Springer and Agranoff (1977). The authors noted, however, that higher temperature (35°C) does not lead to a faster recovery of function than that at 30°C. More recently, Carlsen *et al.* (1982) have show that at 15°C frog spinal neurons regenerate at 0.5 mm/day compared to 2.4 mm/day at 25°C. Information was also provided by *in vitro* studies of neurite growth of chick embryo. Levi (1934) measured an elongation rate of 23.5 mm/hr at 38°C, whereas a rate of 33 mm/hr at 39°C was recorded by Mossa (1926). The latter study also showed that elongation stops below 26°C.

These studies indicate that axonal transport, protein synthesis, and axonal regeneration are affected relatively similarly by temperature. This relationship might be an indication that protein synthesis and axonal transport may be linked with the axonal elongation process.

3. CHANGES IN AXONAL TRANSPORT DURING DEVELOPMENT AND REGENERATION

3.1. Changes in Amounts, Rates, and Molecular Composition

Alterations of the amount, the composition, and the rates of transported molecules have been reported in developing and regenerating nerves (for review see Lubinska, 1964, 1975; Grafstein and McQuarrie, 1978; Grafstein and Forman, 1980; Carbonetto and Muller, 1982; Forman, 1983). The results are very often contradictory and reflect the complexity of the events occurring in the axon and in the perikarya during the regenerative process. Some generalizations can nevertheless be made. (1) Higher rates and amounts of transported material are usually noted in developing neurons and in very young animals, a decrease occurring when maturation is achieved (Black and Lasek, 1979; Komiya, 1980, 1981*a,b*). (2) Increases in the rates and amounts of transported material have also been noted during regeneration. Most studies indicate that the rate of fast transport is not affected but that the amount of moving proteins increases (for review, see Grafstein and Forman, 1980). More recent studies have focused on the quantitative and qualitative alteration of specific polypeptides (see Willard and Skene, 1982; D. L. Wilson, L. I. Benowitz, and M. Willard *et al.,* Chapters 9–11, this volume). Changes in the composition of slow flow have also been reported and are often characterized by an increase in both the rate and the amount of material flowing in the nerve. The rise in transported radioactivity appears to be mainly concentrated in a few polypeptides such as tubulin and actin (see S. T. Brady, B. W. Agranoff and T. S. Ford-Holevinski, P. N. Hoffman *et al.,* Chapters 2, 5, 14, this volume). (3) A further increase over regenerative values has also been reported to follow a second conditioning lesion applied to a nerve within a few days to a few weeks after an initial injury (see I. G. McQuarrie, Chapter 12, this volume).

3.2. Correlation between Transport Rates and Elongation

Weiss and Hiscoe (1948) originally suggested that the proximodistal movement of the column of transported material was responsible for the axonal elongation occurring during nerve regeneration. Since that time, the discovery of several phases of axonally transported molecules moving at rates from less than 1 mm/day to more than 400 mm/day has complicated the original hypothesis.

An attempt to correlate fast transport and axonal elongation was made by Lubinska (1975). She pointed out a similar temperature dependence between the rate of fast transport measured by Heslop and Howes (1972) in the mussel *Anondata* and the elongation velocity of regenerating fibers in sciatic nerves of frogs and toads (Lubinska and Olekiewicz, 1950), although a tenfold difference existed between the rates of transport and elongation. More recently, Lasek and Hoffman (1976) observed that the velocity of elongation of rat motor axons is equal to the rate of SCb, the fastest of the two slow peaks identified in this preparation. Identical rates of transport of SCb and axonal elongation were meaured by McQuarrie *et al.* (1980, 1981) in rat spinal nerves. A correlation between the velocity of SCb and regeneration has also been determined by Wujek and Lasek (1982) in each branch of the rat dorsal root ganglion.

Several studies, however, have shown that the rate of slow flow is significantly faster than the regeneration velocity (see S. Ochs, Chapter 1, this volume). In the rabbit vagus nerve, Frizell and Sjostrand (1974) measured an elongation velocity of 3 to 4 mm/day but a rate of slow flow of 20–25 mm/day. However, a much closer correspondence was found in the hypoglossal nerve, with a slow flow rate of 4–5 mm/day and a regeneration velocity of 4 mm/day. In goldfish optic axons, Edwards *et al.* (1981) determined a maximal elongation velocity of 0.74 mm/day after a conditioning lesion, but McQuarrie and Grafstein (1982b) estimated the rate of slow flow to be in excess of 1.5 mm/day under similar conditions. Similar discrepancies were noted by Komiya (1981b). However, he was able to demonstrate that a linear relationship exists between the transport rates of actin, tubulin, and neurofilament proteins in intact rat sensory nerves and axonal regeneration velocities.

4. REGENERATION OF THE GARFISH OLFACTORY NERVE

The elongation velocities of regenerating garfish olfactory nerves have been compared with the rates of axonal transport at temperatures ranging from

10 to 35°C. The methods have been described in detail elsewhere (Cancalon, 1982*b*, 1983*b–d.*).

4.1. Velocities of Axonal Elongation

Previous studies of the olfactory nerve, mainly in higher vertebrates, have indicated that even in mature nerves, the olfactory neurons are constantly turning over (Graziadei and Monto-Graziadei, 1978). Axonal injury causes total degeneration of the mature neurons followed by replacement with new neuronal cells arising from undifferentiated mucosal stem cells. It should therefore be emphasized that the regeneration of an olfactory nerve damaged near the mucosa involves the *de novo* genesis and development of new neurons rather than the regeneration of the distal axonal segments of mature nerve cells (Monti-Graziadei and Graziadei, 1979). Regeneration of the nerve, crushed 1.5 cm from the cell bodies (Cancalon and Elam, 1980*a*), was found to produce three distinct populations of developing fibers depending on their stage of differentiation at the time of injury (Figure 1). At 21°C, the first population (phase I), which appears to originate from already growing nerve cells, progresses along the nerve at a rate of 5.8 ± 0.3 mm/day for the leading fibers of the group. The second group of fibers (phase II), which is thought to correspond to mucosal basal cells in their final stage of differentiation, advances at a rate of 2.1 ± 0.1 mm/day for the leading fibers. The leading fibers in the third group of regenerating axons (phase III), which originate from the mass of the quiescent basal cells, advance at a rate of 0.8 ± 0.2 mm/day. The first two phases of regenerating axons each represent between 3 and 5% of the original axonal population, and the third phase of fibers between 50 and 70%.

Morphological differences among the axons of the three subpopulations were revealed by electron microscopy. Early during regeneration, phase I axons appear very immature: they have a small diameter (0.1 to 0.15 μm), and no structure can be characterized in the axoplasm except for one to two microtubes. By contrast, the slowly growing phase III axons appear much more similar to mature fibers (Figure 2).

The elongation velocities of the three phases of developing axons were examined at temperatures ranging from 10 to 35°C (Cancalon, 1983*c*). The growth rate of phase I fibers increases linearly with temperature (Figure 3) from 1.6 mm/day at 14°C to 10.2 mm/day at 31°C at a rate of 0.52 ± 0.02 mm/day per °C. Between 14 and 31°C, the rate of elongation of phase II and III fibers increases exponentially with temperature, and the rate of phase II fibers remains essentially twice that of phase III axons. In this range of temperature, these rates are significantly smaller than phase I elongation velocities.

Since the elongation velocities of phase II and III increases exponentially, by extrapolation it can be estimated that they should become greater than

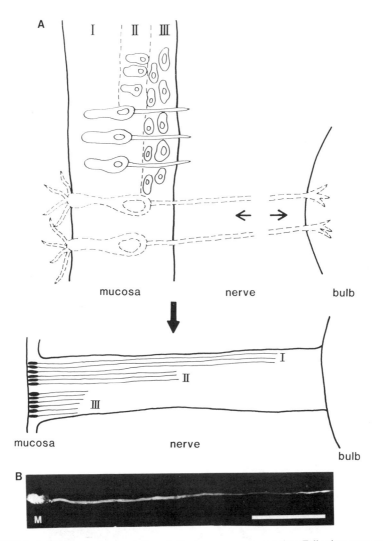

FIGURE 1. A: Schematic representation of olfactory nerve regeneration. Following nerve crush near the cell body, all mature neurons degenerate completely, and three populations of regenerating axons successively invade the olfactory nerve. It has been hypothesized that phase I axons originate from immature nerve cells that were growing at the time of injury, phase II axons from mucosal basal cells in their final stage of differentiation, and phase III fibers from stem cells quiescent at the time of injury. B: The successive arrival of the three phases of growing axons is apparent in a regenerating nerve (170 days p.o. at 21 °C). The proximal area is significantly thicker than the distal segment. (M, mucosa; bar, 5 cm.) (From Cancalon, 1983*d*.)

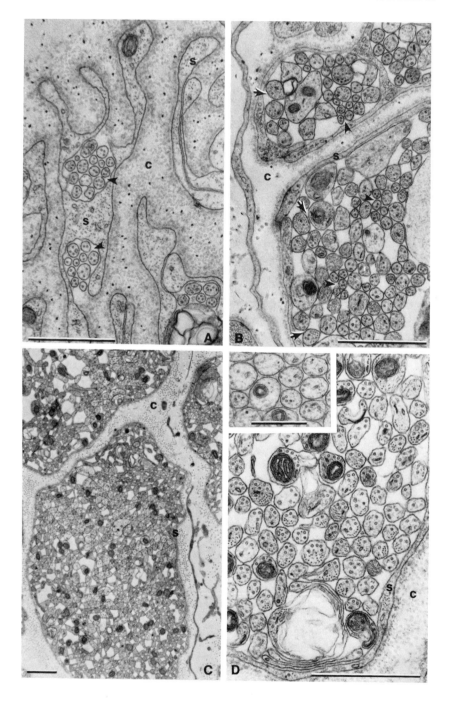

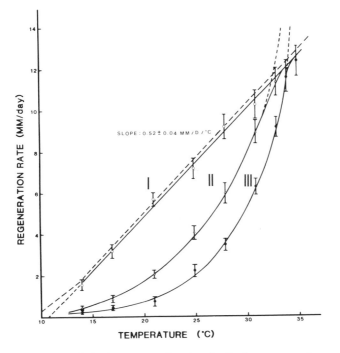

FIGURE 3. Elongation velocity/temperature functions for the three regenerating axonal populations (———). Extrapolation of the exponential functions determined between 14 and 31°C (---). Rate/temperature function for slow intraaxonal flow in regenerating axons (— —). The elongation velocities of phase I and the rates of slow flow are superimposed. Above 31°C, the three axonal phases fuse, and the elongation velocity of this new axonal population is identical to the rate of slow flow. (From Cancalon, 1983*d*.)

FIGURE 2. A: Transmission electron micrographs (TEM) of the three phases of regenerating axons. Phase I fibers (21°C at 5 cm from the mucosa, 20 days p.o.). The nerve is mostly filled with collagen (C). Thick Schwann cell processes (s) surround small fascicles of immature axons (arrows). They have a diameter of 0.1 to 0.15 μm and contain few microtubules and no mitochondria. Bar = 1 μm. B: Transmission EM of a nerve 170 days p.o. at 24 cm from the mucosa (21°C). Only phase I and II axons have penetrated this area. The small-diameter fibers (black arrows) might represent recently arrived phase II axons, and the larger fibers (black-and-white arrows) the matured phase I axons, which invaded the area about 4 months previously. Bar, 1 μm. C: Transmission EM of a nerve area containing phase III fibers (25°C at 4.5 cm from the mucosa, 62 days p.o.). Large domain surrounded by a thin Schwann cell process (s) are filled by numerous fibers. The amount of collagen (c) is greatly reduced. Bar, 1 μm. D: Transmission EM of phase III fibers (25°C at 4.5 cm from the mucosa 62 days p.o.). Bar, 1 μm. Their aspect is similar to that of the intact axons shown in the inset. Bar, 0.5 μm. (From Cancalon, 1983*d*.)

phase I velocities at temperatures above 33°C. To assess this possibility, rates of regeneration were measured at 33, 34, and 35°C. At 34 and 35°C, only one population of regenerating fibers was found, and velocities never reach the very high values that can be predicted by the phase II and III equations. No elongation rate was found to be faster than the rate that can be calculated from the linear equation determined for phase I. Phase II and III elongation velocities increase exponentially with temperature until the rates catch up with phase I velocities; then, above 33°C, their elongation rates increase linearly with temperature.

Attempts were made to have nerves regenerate at 10°C. This was performed on animals (1) acclimated and maintained at 10°C during the entire experiments, (2) kept at 10°C only after surgery, (3) kept at 21°C for 2 weeks post-operative to allow the perikarya to develop and then maintained at 10°C for the remainder of the experiments. Electron micrographs taken up to 150 days post-operative indicate that no intact fibers could be seen in the nerve segment proximal to the crush, although radioactivity is still transported at fast and slow rates in regenerating nerves subjected to temperature shift to 10°C.

4.2. Rates of Axonal Transport in Growing Fibers

4.2.1. Rapid Transport

The rate of rapid transport is not altered during the regeneration process since, at 21°C, the velocities measured in phase I and III axons (Cancalon and Elam, 1980*b;* Cancalon, 1982*a*) are identical to those recorded previously in intact nerves (Cancalon, 1979*a*, 1982*a*). At 21°C, the amount of radioactivity transported with the rapid phase, in contrast, is greatly increased in regenerating nerves (Table 1), and each phase I fiber contains about twice as much label as a phase III axon.

4.2.2. Slow Flow

The rate of slow flow was measured between 10 and 35°C in the three populations of developing axons (Cancalon, 1983*d*). In both intact and regenerating nerves, slow flow is determined as a broad peak of radioactivity.

In intact nerve, the velocity of the front edge of the peak of slow flow increases linearly from 0.54 ± 0.02 mm/day at 14°C to 4.10 ± 0.06 mm/day at 35°C (Figure 4). Slow flow rates were also determined in the three populations of regenerating fibers. The velocity of the peak front edge also increases linearly from 1.6 ± 0.2 mm/day at 14°C to 12.7 ± 0.7 mm/day at 35°C (Figure 4). No statistically signficant differences were determined in phase I fibers alone or in a mixture of phase I and II axons or in phase III fibers. In all cases, the average velocity of slow flow in the regenerating fibers

TABLE 1. Relative Amounts of Radioactivity Moving in a Single Axon at 21 °C

	Intact axon	Phase I regenerating axon	Phase III regenerating axon
Relative amount of rapidly transported radioactivity	1	6–16	3–8
Relative amount of slow radioactivity	1	3.2–5.4	2.3–3.2
Percent of normal axonal population	100	3–5	50–70

is 3.3 times faster than the rate measured in intact nerve at the same temperature. The mechanism responsible for this acceleration of the transport rate has not been clarified. However analysis of the transport rate of individual slowly moving polypeptides in intact nerves has revealed that traces of tubulin and actin are moving at the accelerated velocity. It can be hypothesized that the velocity changes during regeneration might be the result of a shift in the amount of material transported at preexisting rates. At 10 °C, a similar rate of slow flow (0.3 ± 0.1 mm/day) was determined in intact nerves or in nerves allowed to regenerate at higher temperature before their transfer to 10 °C (Figure 4).

Recent studies have pointed out the relationship between axonal elongation and protein synthesis. McQuarrie and Grafstein (1982a,b) have shown that in conditioning experiments, the enhanced outgrowth occurring after the second lesion is correlated with an increase in the amount of rapidly and slowly transported proteins synthesized in the cell bodies in response to an initial stimulus, which might be a lesion (see I. G. McQuarrie, Chapter 12, this volume) or even the initial outgrowth of an embryonic neuron (Collins and Lee, 1982). Phase I fibers represent the population of neurons that, at the time of injury, were growing in the nerve segment proximal to the crush and might therefore be conditioned by the crush. We have, indeed, seen that they contain significantly more rapidly and slowly transported radioactivity (Table 1) than other regenerating olfactory neurons.

Phase II and III fibers differentiate into neurons during or after the lesion. As a consequence, they might be less conditioned, and their cell bodies will produce less axonal component as reflected by the lower amount of fast and slow moving radioactivity measured in phase III fibers (Table 1).

4.2.3. Slow Flow Rate and Axonal Elongation Velocity

The rates of slow flow measured in this study correspond to the movement of the front of the peak of slowly moving radioactivity. Preliminary studies (P. Cancalon, S. T. Brady, and R. J. Lasek, unpublished data) indicate that in the garfish olfactory nerve the molecules corresponding to the subcomponents SCa

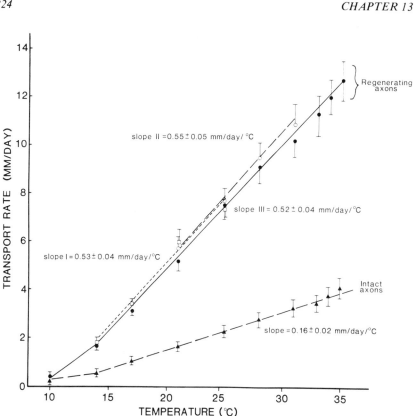

FIGURE 4. Rate of slow versus temperature in intact and regenerating axons: ▲, intact fibers; □, phase I axons; O, phase I and II axons; ●, phase III axons. No significant difference was found among the rates of slow flow in the three populations of regenerating fibers. Rates are 3.3 times faster than the velocities measured in intact nerves except at 10°C. (From Cancalon, 1983c.)

and SCb move as a single peak. Therefore, the front of the slow peak corresponds to the SCb material. Such overlap of the two slow subcomponents might be characteristic of nerve having a very good regenerating ability (McQuarrie *et al.* 1980). Furthermore, as shown previously (Cancalon *et al.,* 1976), tubulin is by far the main polypeptide of the garfish olfactory axon (Cancalon, 1979b). The presence of large amounts of actin and few neurofilament proteins is also characteristic of nerves with a good regenerative potential (Lasek and Morris, 1982).

These results indicate that slow flow or, more specifically, the SCb component is transported at a similar rate in the three populations of regenerating fibers (Cancalon, 1983d), although up to a sevenfold difference exists in the corresponding elongation velocities (Cancalon, 1983c). The rate–temperature functions for slow flow and axonal elongation are completely superimposed for phase I axons. On the contrary, for phase II and III, below 31 °C the elongation velocity is always slower than the rate of flow. Above 31 °C, the three populations of regenerating axons fuse as a single phase whose elongation velocity increases linearly with temperature according to the function defined for slow flow. It can be concluded that the SCb subcomponent constitutes the upper limit of the regeneration velocity.

The role of fast and slow transport in providing axonal components necessary to axonal elongation has been proven by several groups (Grafstein, 1971; Pfenninger, 1980; Pfenninger and Maylie-Pfenninger, 1981; Hoffman *et al.,* 1980, 1981; Griffin *et al.,* 1981). A lack of even a few molecules, such as specific enzymes or membranous or cytoskeletal polypeptides, may act as a growth-limiting factor. The failure of elongation velocity to keep pace with slow flow in some axons can be the result of the inability of the perikarya to provide sufficient amounts of molecules essential to the constitution of an axon. Therefore, a rate of elongation will be set when the rate of incorporation of new rapidly and slowly transported molecules in the axon and the growth cone equals the rate of synthesis of these molecules in the cell body. However, this process might be further complicated by the intraaxonal reutilization of components. As the temperature increases, a significant rise in the level of protein synthesis can be expected in the olfactory perikarya (see above). Since protein synthesis is already high in phase I neurons because of the conditioning effect, the influence of temperature might be more drastic on phase II and III nerve cells. If more proteins are delivered to the axons and the growing tips by the perikarya, the elongation velocity will increase until it reaches the maximal value set by the rate of slow flow. Similarly McQuarrie (Chapter 12, this volume) has postulated that the axonal elongation velocity is determined by a combination of both the amount and the rate of transport of the slow moving material. Concomitantly with the changes in elongation velocities, the lag period between the time of crush and the beginning of axonal elongation decreases as the temperature increases and becomes similar for the three axonal populations. As a result, at high temperature, the neurons seem to appear simultaneously and progress at the same rate along the nerve.

The effect of temperature on the regenerative ability of the axons may also, to some extent, reflect temperature-induced changes in the plasticity of the fiber. Lowering the temperature has been shown to result in an increase in the number of neurofilaments (Matheson *et al.,* 1980). A high neurofilament content will increase the stability of the cytoskeleton and lower the regenerative potential of the fiber. This might explain the lack of regeneration occurring at low temperatures when axonal transport has not yet stopped. Conversely, at high temperature a decrease in the ratio of neurofilaments/microtubules (NF/MT) in phase II and III fibers might allow these axons to reach a level of plasticity equivalent to that of the conditioned phase I fibers.

These results may contribute to the reconciliation of the discrepancies that have been revealed when slow flow and elongation rates have been compared. If the velocity of SCb is only the upper limit that can be reached by the rate of elongation of a fiber, it can be expected that regenerative rates will be either smaller or equal to the rate of transport of slow flow.

5. AXONAL DEGENERATION

Axonal degeneration has been extensively studied in a large variety of preparations by use of anatomic and electrophysiological methods (for review, see Fuxe *et al.,* 1973; Lubinska, 1964, 1975; Donat and Wisniewski, 1973). The conflicting results have not answered the question whether the degeneration invades the entire nerve stump simultaneously (Huber, 1900; May, 1925; Cajal, 1928) or spreads centrifugally from the site of injury toward the periphery.

Joseph (1973) hypothesized that degeneration of the isolated nerve stump was the direct result of the interruption of the delivery to the fiber of essential factors synthesized by the cell body and that therefore degeneration should progress from the site of injury towards the nerve endings. A few studies have revealed a proximodistal degenerative wave progressing at a slow rate. In various regions of the toad CNS, Joseph and Whitlock (1972) demonstrated a somatofugal degeneration ranging from 0.07 to 2 mm/day at 20°C and 0.33 to 6 mm/day at 30°C with an average Q_{10} of 3.5. Matsumoto and Scalia (1979, 1981) showed that after destruction of the frog's retina, the myelinated fibers have disappeared after 6 weeks, but 12% of the unmyelinated fibers persist for more than 12 weeks. They also observed a more rapid degeneration of the optic nerve than of the tract, which indicates that the process might be spreading from the site of injury toward the terminals.

Much higher rates of proximodistal degeneration, usually of the order of several millimeters per day, have been measured in several preparations. Following transection of the frog sciatic nerve (Parker, 1933), the fibers remain normal for 16 days but degenerate proximodistally in 4 days. Parker and Paine (1934) measured a centrifugal degeneration rate of 20–30 mm/day in the catfish lateral line. Lubinska (1977) estimated that in the rat phrenic nerve, degeneration spreads at 46 to 250 mm/day. More recently, Lubinska (1982) has shown that in the rat phrenic nerve, Wallerian degeneration of the distal stump progresses centrifugally by jumping from one internode to another; she suggested that a trophic factor transported in intact axons keeps the Schwann cells in a quiescent state. Following axotomy, the factor no longer being provided, the Schwann cells hypertrophy and induce the destruction of the axon. Donat and Wisniewski (1973) studied the spatiotemporal pattern of degeneration in the sciatic nerve of cats and rabbits between 12 and 144 hr after transection at 0.5 and 20 cm from the lesion. The authors determined that the histological change is a function of the distance from the injury. The nerve area close to the lesion is characterized by an accumulation of organelles. In the distal area, on the contrary, the process consists of the loss of microtubules and filaments and appears to occur simultaneously over the entire nerve segment. However, Donat and Wisniewski did not measure the rate at which the proximal zone was spreading along the nerve. Their results can be interpreted by assuming that two degenerating processes successively invade the nerve (see below), a rapid wave affecting mainly the cytoskeletal elements and a slow wave acting on the other axonal components.

5.1. Influence of Temperature on Degeneration

The accelerating effect of higher temperatures on degeneration has been known for a very long time. The gradient of temperature that exists in the limb of warm-blooded animals has been postulated by Gamble and Jha (1958) to be responsible for the proximodistal movement of degeneration. The proximal area, being warmer, will be destroyed more rapidly than the cooler distal segment.

As early as 1899, Monckeberg and Bethe studied the influence of temperature in nerve degeneration in frogs. Similar studies were performed by Merzbacker (1903) on hibernating bats and by Armstrong (1950, 1951) on *Lacerta vivipara*. Gamble *et al.* (1957) determined that in poikilotherms similar degeneration was obtained after 21 days at 13°C or 3 days at 20°C but that no intact fibers could be found after 5 days at 35°C. The authors also noted that degeneration and regeneration are affected to the same extent by temperature. Similar results were obtained by Gamble and Jha (1958) on the rat ventral caudal nerve. As mentioned previously, Joseph and Whitlock (1972) measured a Q_{10} of 3.5 for the proximodistal degeneration of CNS toad nerves at 20 or 30°C. A faster centrifugal degeneration was also observed by Matsumoto and Scalia (1981) in the frog visual system at 35 than at 20°C.

5.2. Axonal Transport in Nerve Segments Isolated from in the Cell Bodies

5.2.1. Fast Transport

Numerous data indicate that fast transport can proceed unaltered after removal of the cell body. Ochs and Ranish (1969) demonstrated that the rapid peak of radioactivity moves at the same rate in cat sciatic nerve with or without cell bodies. Similar results were obtained by Heslop and Howes (1972) on the mussel *(Anondata)*. Recently, Matsumoto and Scalia (1981) showed that unmyelinated frog optic nerves were able to transport horseradish peroxidase rapidly 69 days after destruction of the retina. Identical rates of rapid transport were also measured by Gross and Beidler (1975) in garfish olfactory nerve before and after severing of the olfactory mucosa. The only difference observed by these authors was a decrease in the material remaining in the nerve behind the moving peak; furthermore, a similar composition of fast transport in intact and isolated garfish nerve was also determined (Cancalon and Beidler, 1975). Several studies (Ranish *et al.,* 1978, 1980; Oakley *et al.,* 1980, 1981) have shown that various enzymes and trophic factors are delivered to the nerve endings until depletion of the amount present in the nerve at the time of cell body removal. These studies showed that the time during which the material is delivered depends on the length of the stump.

5.2.2. Slow Flow

Much less is known of the fate of the slow flow in isolated nerve stumps. Frizell *et al.* (1975) hve shown that in the rabbit vagus nerve a phase of transported moleucules moving at 25 mm/day stops immediately after axotomy. However, this velocity is so high that it might be difficult to associate this material unequivocally with slow flow, and the composition of the material transported at this rate might be somewhat different from that of slow flow (McLean *et al.,* 1983). A persistence of slow flow in the goldfish visual system for at least 24 hr after injury has been reported by Alpert *et al.* (1980). It is possible that a rapid degeneration of the myelinated fibers (see below) induces an early stop in the slow movement of molecules. Indirect evidence from the growth of transected neurites by Hughes (1953) and Shaw and Bray (1977) also indicates that slow flow may persist for some time in isolated fibers.

5.3. Degeneration of the Olfactory Nerve

5.3.1. Slow Flow in Axons Detached from Their Perikarya

Slow flow was investigated in the garfish olfactory nerve after removal of the mucosa containing the nerve cell bodies at 14, 21, and 31°C (Cancalon, 1982*b*). The right olfactory mucosa was removed when a peak of labeled slowly transported proteins had been established along the axon. Profiles determined by slowly moving radioactivity were followed in these detached axons up to a month after surgery.

From the distance–time functions, slow flow rates of 1.6 ± 0.2 mm/day, 5.1 ± 0.5 mm/day, and 10.5 ± 0.7 mm/day were measured in isolated stumps at 14, 21, and 31°C, respectively (Figure 5). These accelerated velocities are

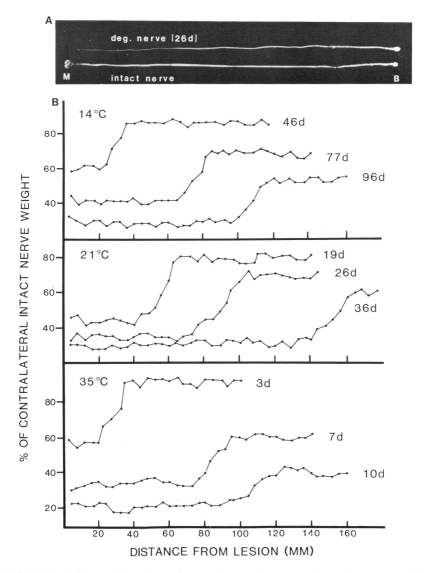

FIGURE 5. A: Degenerating and intact nerves 26 days after removal of the right mucosa (M, mucosa; b, olfactory bulb). The proximal area is significantly thinner than the distal area. B: Proximodistal degeneration as measured by the weight decrease of successive 3-mm nerve segments at 14, 21, and 35 °C. (From Cancalon, 1983*b*.)

identical to the rates of slow flow measured in axons regenerating after crushing of the olfactory nerve 1.5 cm from the mucosa. In both cases, accelerated velocities are 3.3 times faster than the rates of slow flow characteristic of intact nerves. A transient increase in the slow flow rate was also measured in the intact contralateral nerve.

The nature of the labeled material present in the moving peak was assessed by gel electrophoresis 15 days after removal of the right mucosa. In the degenerating ipsilateral and in the intact contralateral nerve, the polypeptide distribution of slowly moving radioactivity was similar to that determined previously in olfactory nerves of noninjured fish (Cancalon, 1979b). However, the level of resolution of these gels was too low to allow a precise comparison.

Not only does slow flow not stop in the isolated distal stump but, on the contrary, it accelerates to a value characteristic of regenerating nerves (Cancalon, 1983d). A more detailed analysis of the polypeptide composition of the material moving in isolated axons should help to determine whether that material corresponds to all or only part of the molecules slowly transported in intact nerve cells. A similar two- to threefold increase in the rate of slow flow of neurofilaments and several other polypeptides has been reported in nerves displaying giant axonal neuropathy following 2,5-hexadione (2,5-HD) intoxication (Monaco et al., 1983). Such nerves are characterized by a two-fold reduction in the NF/MT ratio. The mechanism responsible for this acceleration remains to be determined, but the injury or the chemical may induce an alteration of the NF–MT network, resulting, as proposed by Lasek and Morris (1982), in a more fluid axoplasm in which a large proportion of polymers are transported as subunits. Such a mechanism for the regulation of slow flow velocity has been postulated by M. Willard et al. (Chapter 11, this volume). According to this hypothesis, the rate of transport depends on the amount of high-molecular-weight neurofilament polypeptides responsible for the cross linkage of the cytoskeletal neurofilaments.

A transient acceleration of the rate of slow flow also occurs in the intact nerve contralateral to the injured nerve. It is possible that a factor maintaining slow flow at an accelerated velocity, for example, by preventing the polymerization of cytoskeletal subunits, is repressed in intact neurons but is released into the bloodstream after injury. Such a phenomenon may be a general response of the nervous system to an injury: an increase in the rate of fast transport in the goldfish optic nerve has been reported by McQuarrie and Grafstein (1982a) not only after a lesion of the contralateral nerve but also as a result of the removal of the cerebral hemispheres.

The presence of a soluble factor inducing changes in the rate of slow flow has recently been indirectly corroborated by a study of neurites from chicken embryo ciliary ganglion. Collins and Dawson (1982) extracted two factors from chicken heart embryos. The first factor supports a rapid and extensive neurite outgrowth. The second factor is unable by itself to support neurite outgrowth but increases the rate of neurite elongation threefold. It appears likely that this latter factor interacts with the mechanism of axonal flow.

5.3.2. Proximodistal Degeneration of Unmyelinated Olfactory Axons Detached from Their Perikarya

The degeneration of the olfactory nerve was followed by measuring changes in the weight of successive 3-mm nerve segments (Figure 5) at various times after removal of the cell bodies and at temperatures ranging from 10 to 35°C (Cancalon, 1983b). At each temperature, degeneration progresses from the site of injury toward the olfactory bulb at constant velocity. The degeneration rates increase linearly with temperature from 1.6 mm/day at 14°C to 13 mm/day at 35°C (Figure 6). A degeneration velocity of 0.3 ± 0.1 mm/day was measured in injured nerves maintained at 10°C. These values are identical to the accelerated rates of slow flow measured in regenerating and degenerating axons.

Further analysis performed by electron micrography (Figure 7) indicates that during degeneration four different areas of the nerve can be distinguished: (1) the dengerated zone—in this area proximal to the degenerative wave, no intact axons can be seen; (2) the intermediate zone—in this area of the nerve, corresponding to the drop in nerve weight, degenerating axons can be seen. Their diameter is one-third to one-fourth that of a normal axon, and no internal structure can be recognized. These abnormal fibers might represent the last form of the degenerating axons once most of the components provided by slow flow have moved away; (3) the distal zone—in this area a large number of axons appear morphologically intact; (4) the preterminal zone, corresponding to the last few millimeters of nerve near the olfactory bulb. In this area, degeneration is much more advanced than in the distal zone. A rapid degeneration of nerve preterminal segments has been reported by various groups (Weddell and Glies, 1941; Miledi and Slater, 1970). This might be the result of more active proteolylic activity near the synapses (Lasek and Black, 1977) or of a decrease in the delivery of transported molecules (Munoz-Martinez, 1981).

5.3.3. Mechanism of Slow Proximodistal Degeneration

In the studies of garfish olfactory nerve, the slow proximodistal degeneration of the detached fibers moves along the nerve at a velocity equivalent to that of SCb and is therefore temporally correlated with the depletion of the slowly moving components. Following cell body removal, new axonal elements are no longer provided. Since slow flow keeps moving in the detached stump (Cancalon, 1982b), the proximal area of the severed axons becomes depleted

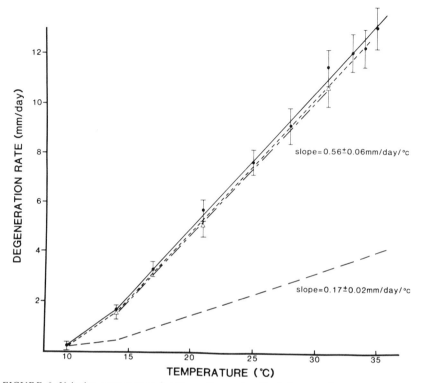

FIGURE 6. Velocity–temperature functions: ●, proximodistal degeneration; △, slow flow in axons detached from their cell bodies; – – –, slow flow in regenerating nerves; ——, slow flow in intact nerves. The velocity of proximodistal degeneration is identical to the rate of slow flow in degenerating and regenerating nerves and 3.3 times faster than the rate of slow flow measured in intact nerves. (From Cancalon, 1983*b*.)

of its matrix elements, and, finally, the disappearance of the cytoskeleton brings about the collapse of the neuronal architecture, leaving only the axolemmal ghost as seen in the intermediate zone (Figure 7). The collapse of the axons progresses toward the nerve endings at a rate corresponding to the velocity of withdrawal of the cytoskeleton and therefore at the rate of slow flow in detached nerves. Finally, the axolemmal ghosts are decomposed very rapidly into membranous fragments.

5.3.4. Rapid Degeneration of Olfactory Axons

Although a well-defined somatofugal slow degeneration has been characterized at all temperatures investigated, a significant degeneration also occurs in the distal zone before the arrival of the slow wave. This distal degeneration can be demonstrated by a decrease in nerve weight and diameter. These changes most probably represent the compounded effects of numerous events occurring in the isolated stump, but they are mainly related to a decrease in the number of axons, although a slight decrease in axonal diameter has also been noted. The decrease in the axonal population is highly temperature dependent and varies from only 30% after 78 days at 10°C to 80% after 10 days at 35°C.

Rapid changes in detached unmyelinated axons have been reported by various groups. A reaction of the distal segment of the rabbit olfactory nerve characterized by the swelling and vacuolization of numerous axons has been observed as early as 8 hr after lesion of the nerve (Berger, 1971). Matsumoto and Scalia (1981) estimated that in frogs maintained in 20°C, more than half of the unmyelinated optic axons have disappeared in the first 10 days after injury, but that 12% remains after 10 weeks.

An explanation for the rapid degeneration of isolated axons has been provided by Schlaepfer (Schlaepfer and Bunge, 1973; Schlaepfer, 1974; W. W.

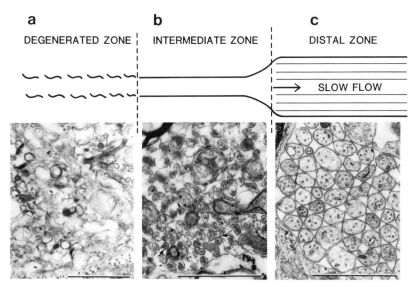

FIGURE 7. Schematic of slow proximodistal degeneration. The proximal area of the axon becomes depleted of cytoskeletal elements, no longer provided by the cell body, as slow flow moves centrifugally. As a result, the axon collapses and is rapidly decomposed. B: Electron micrographs of degenerating olfactory nerves at 10°C 78 days post-operative. (a) Section 5 mm from the site of injury; degenerated zone (×28,000). This area does not contain any intact axons but is filled with membranous material. (b) Section at 15 mm; intermediate zone (×38,000). Only shrunken axons (arrows) about one-third to one-fourth of their normal size can be found. (c) At 120 mm, distal zone (×38,000). The area contains numerous apparently intact axons. Bar, 1 μm. (From Cancalon, 1983b.)

Schlaepfer and U-J. P. Zimmerman, Chapter 15, this volume), who demonstrated that this type of degeneration is induced by calcium-dependent proteases affecting neurofilaments (Figure 8). The author postulated that the increase in proteolytic activity might be triggered by an influx of calcium into the axon as a result of increased permeability of the axolemma. The changes in the membranous properties in turn seem to arise from a lack of membrane components delivered by fast axonal transport.

Such rapid degenerative mechanisms might explain the observation that degeneration occurs simultaneously over the entire nerve (Huber, 1900; May, 1925; Ramon y Cajal, 1928). In myelinated fibers, the intraaxonal degenerative process might be limited to this rapid phase because of the phagocytic activity of the myelin sheath, as proposed by Lubinska (1982).

It remains to be determined why certain fibers are rapidly affected while others remain intact for extended periods of time (Figure 8). A constant turnover of the olfactory neurons has been demonstrated (Graziadei and Monti-Graziadei, 1978), and several studies (Kiyohara and Tucker, 1978; Small and Pfenninger, 1980; Schrichartz *et al.*, 1980; Cancalon and Elam, 1980b, Tessler *et al.*, 1980) have indicated that young axons might lack axolemmal protein components. Such fibers, which already have an immature membrane, might

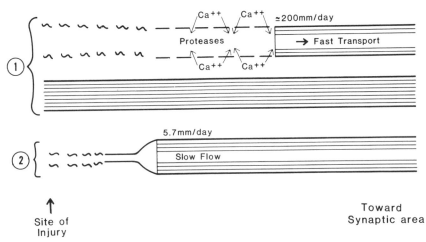

FIGURE 8. Schematic representation of the hypothesis explaining olfactory nerve degeneration. (1) In the unmyelinated olfactory nerve, some fibers, which might be immature, degenerate rapidly. The lack of rapidly transported material may alter the axolemma and allow an influx of calcium. A higher intraaxonal calcium level in turn activates proteases and induces axonal decomposition (see Chapter 15, this volume). (2) Other fibers degenerate only with the withdrawal of the cytoskeletal elements no longer provided to the axon but still moving with slow flow.

be less resistant to an influx of calcium and eventually to degeneration than older axons having a fully developed membrane.

6. CONCLUSIONS

Rates of slow flow have been followed in developing neurons during axonal elongation. An identical rate of flow, 3.3 times faster than the velocity characteristic of an intact nerve, was measured in both preparations. The reasons for this change in slow flow velocity have not been clarified. It can be postulated that following injury the cytoskeletal architecture of the axon is affected and reverts to an embryonic form characteristic of developing neurons. A more fluid organization of the axon may result in an easier displacement of the microtrabecular system according to the mechanism described by Lasek (1980) or a decrease in the amount of time during which the slowly transported molecules are not moving, as proposed by Ochs (1974).

By comparing the rates of slow flow and the elongation velocities in the three populations of regenerating axons, it can be determined that the rate of slow flow or, more precisely, of SCb represents the upper limit of axonal growth. However, other factors may limit the regenerative ability of a neuron, and only nerve cells growing under the most favorable conditions are able to reach the optimal elongation velocity.

An acceleration of slow flow, which might also be induced by a posttraumatic alteration of the cytoskeletal organization, has been recorded in degenerating axons isolated from their cell bodies. The proximodistal movement of this slowly moving material has been shown to be associated with axonal degeneration, which may be the result of the disappearance of the cytoskeleton.

ACKNOWLEDGMENT

The support of NIH grant 17198 is acknowledged.

7. REFERENCES

Alpert, R. M., Grafstein, B., and Edwards, D. L., 1980, Slow axonal transport in goldfish optic axons, *Soc. Neurosci. Abstr.* **6**:83.

Armstrong, J. A., 1950, An experimental study of the visual pathways in a reptile *(Laceria vivipara)*, *J. Anat. (Lond.)* **84**:146–147.

Armstrong, J. A., 1951, An experimental study of the visual pathways in a snake *(Natrix natrix)*, *J. Anat. (Lond.)* **85**:275–288.

Berger, B., 1971, Etude ultrastructurale de la degenerescence Wallerienne experimentale d'un nerf entierment amyelinique: Le nerf olfactif, *J. Ultrastruct. Res.* **37**:105–118.

Biondi. R. J., Levy, M. J., and Weiss, P. A., 1972, An engineering study of the peristaltic drive of axonal flow, *Proc. Natl. Acad. Sci. U.S.A.* **69:**1732–1736.

Bisby, M. A., and Jones, D. L., 1978, Temperature sensitivity of axonal transport in hibernating and non-hibernating rodents, *Exp. Neurol.* **61:**74–83.

Black, M. M., and Lasek, R. J., 1979, Slowing of the rate of axonal regeneration during growth and maturation, *Exp. Neurol.* **63:**108–119.

Cancalon, P., 1979*a,* Influence of temperature on the velocity and on the isotope profile of slowly transported labeled proteins, *J. Neurochem.* **32:**997–1007.

Cancalon, P., 1979*b,* Subcellular and polypeptide distributions of slowly transported proteins in the garfish olfactory nerve, *Brain Res.* **161:**115–130.

Cancalon, P., 1982*a,* Some characteristics of slow flow in the olfactory and optic nerves of the garfish, in: *Axoplasmiç Transport* (D. Weiss, ed.), pp. 218–225, Springer-Verlag, Berlin, Heidelberg, New York.

Cancalon, P., 1982*b,* Slow flow in axons detached from their perikarya, *J. Cell Biol.* **95:**989–992.

Cancalon, P., 1983*a,* Slow flow in regenerating C-fibers, *Dev. Brain Res.* **6:**197–201.

Cancalon, P., 1983*b,* Proximodistal degeneration of C-fibers detached from their perikarya, *J. Cell Biol.* **97:**6–14.

Cancalon, P., 1983*c,* Regeneration of three populations of olfactory axons as a function of temperature, *Dev. Brain Res.* **9:**265–278.

Cancalon, P., 1983*d,* Influence of temperature on slow flow in populations of regenerating axons with different elongation velocities, *Dev. Brain Res.* **9:**279–289.

Cancalon, P., and Beidler, L. M., 1975, Distribution along the axon and into various subcellular fractions of molecules labeled with ^{3}H leucine and rapidly transported in the garfish olfactory nerve, *Brain Res.* **89:**225–244.

Cancalon, P., and Elam, J. S., 1980*a,* Study of regeneration in the garfish olfactory nerve, *J. Cell Biol.* **84:**779–794.

Cancalon, P., and Elam, J. S., 1980*b,* Rate and composition of rapidly transported proteins in regenerating olfactory nerves, *J. Neurochem.* **35:**(4):889–897.

Cancalon, P., Elam, J. S., and Beidler, L. M., 1976, SDS gel electrophoresis of rapidly transported proteins in garfish olfactory nerve, *J. Neurochem.* **27:**687–693.

Cancalon, P., Cole, G. J., and Elam, J. S., 1982, The role of axonal transport in the growth of the olfactory nerve axons, in: *Axoplasmic Transport in Physiology and Pathology* (D. Weiss, and A. Gorio, eds), pp. 62–69, Springer-Verlag, Berlin, Heidelberg, New York.

Carbonetto, S., and Muller, K. J., 1982, Nerve fiber growth and the cellular response to axotomy, *Curr. Topics Dev. Biol.* **17:**33–76.

Carlsen, R. C., Kiff, J., and Ryugo, K., 1982, Suppression of the cell body response in axotomized frog spinal neurons does not prevent initiation of nerve regeneration, *Brain Res.* **234:**11–25.

Collins, F., and Dawson, A., 1982, Conditioned medium increases the rate of neurite elongation: Reparation of the activity from the substratum-bound inducer of neurite outgrowth, *J. Neurosci.* **2:**1005–1010.

Collins, F., and Lee, M. R., 1982, A reversible developmental change in the ability of ciliary ganglion neurons to extend neurites in culture, *J. Neurosci.* **2:**424–430.

Davison, W. W., Hope, G. M., and Bernstein, J. J., 1971, Goldfish retinal structure and function in extended cold, *Exp. Neurol.* **31:**368–382.

Deineka, D., 1908, L'influence de la temperature ambiante sur la regeneration des fibres nerveuses, *Fol. Neurobiol.* **2:**13–24.

Donat, J. R., and Wisniewski, H. M., 1973, the spatio-temporal course of Wallerian degeneration in mammalian peripheral nerves, *Brain Res.* **53:**41–53.

Edstrom, A., and Hanson, M., 1973, Temperature effects on fast axonal transport of proteins *in vitro* in frog sciatic nerves, *Brain Res.* **58:**345–354.

Edwards, D. L., Alpert, R. M., and Grafstein, B., 1981, Recovery of vision in regeneration of goldfish optic axons: Enhancement of axonal outgrowth by a conditioning lesion, *Exp. Neurol.* **72**:672–686.

Elam, J. S., and Agranoff, B. W., 1971, Rapid transport of protein in the optic system of the goldfish, *J. Neurochem.* **18**:375–387.

Fernandez, H. L., Huneeus, F. C., and Davison, P. F., 1970, Studies on the mechanism of axoplasmic transport in the crayfish cord, *J. Neurobiol.* **1**:395–409.

Forman, D. S., 1983, Axonal transport and nerve regeneration: A review, in: *Spinal Cord Reconstruction* (C. C. Kao and R. P. Bunge, eds.), Raven Press, New York, pp. 75–86.

Forman, D. S., Padjen, A. L., and Siggins, G. R., 1977, Effect of temperature on the rapid retrograde transport of microscopically visible intra-axonal organelles, *Brain Res.* **136**:215–226.

Frizell, M., and Sjostrand, J., 1974, The axonal transport of slowly migrating [^{3}H]leucine labeled proteins and the regeneration rate in regenerating hypoglossal and vagus nerves of the rabbit, *Brain Res.* **81**:267–283.

Frizell, M., McLean, W. G., and Sjostrand, J., 1975, Slow axonal transport of proteins blockade by interruption of contact between cell body and axon, *Brain Res.* **86**:67–73.

Fuxe, K., Olsson, L., and Zotterman, Y., 1973, *Dynamics of Degeneration and Growth in Neurons,* Pergamon Press, Oxford.

Gamble, H. J., 1957, Temperature effects in mammalian nerve regeneration, *Nature* **180**:146–147.

Gamble, H. J., 1958, Effect of a raised environmental temperature upon the rate of regeneration in a mammalian peripheral nerve, *Nature* **181**:287.

Gamble, H. J., and Jha, B. D., 1958, Some effects of temperature upon the rate and progress of Wallerian degeneration in mammalian nerve fibres, *J. Anat. (Lond.)* **92**:171–177.

Gamble, H. J., Goldby, F., and Smith, G. M. R., 1957, Effect of temperature on the degeneration of nerve fibres, *Nature* **179**:527.

Grafstein, B., 1971, Role of slow axonal transport in nerve regeneration, *Acta Neuropathol.* [*Suppl.*] **5**:144–152.

Grafstein, B., 1983, Chromatolysis reconsidered—a new view of the reaction of the nerve cell body to axonal injury, in: *Nerve, Organ and Tissue Regeneration: Research Perspectives* (F. J. Seil, ed.), pp. 37–50, Academic Press, New York.

Grafstein, B., and Forman, D. S., 1980, Intracellular transport in neurons, *Physiol. Rev.* **60**:1167–1283.

Grafstein, B., and McQuarrie, I. G., 1978, The role of the nerve cell body in axon regeneration, in: *Neuronal Plasticity* (C. Cotman, ed.), pp. 155–195, Raven Press, New York.

Grafstein, B., Forman, D. S., and McEwen, B. S., 1972, Effects of temperature on axonal transport and turnover of protein in goldfish optic system. *Exp. Neurol.* **34**:158–170.

Graziadei, P. P. C., and Monto-Graziadei, G. A., 1978, Continuous nerve cell renewal in the olfactory system, in: *Handbook of Sensory Physiology,* Volume 9 (M. Jacobson, ed.) pp. 55–83, Springer-Verlag, Berlin, Heidelberg, New York.

Griffin, J. W., Price, D. L., Drachman, D. B., and Morris, J., 1981, Incorporation of axonally transported glycoproteins into axolemma during nerve regeneration, *J. Cell Biol.* **88**:205–214.

Gross, G. W., and Beidler, L. M., 1975, A quantitative analysis of isotope concentration profiles and rapid transport velocities in the C-fibers of the garfish olfactory nerve, *J. Neurobiol.* **6**:213–232.

Gross, G. W., and Kreutzberg, G. W., 1978, Rapid axoplasmic transport in the olfactory nerve of the pike. I. Basic parameters for proteins and amino acids, *Brain Res.* **139**:65–76.

Heslop, J. P., and Howes, E. A., 1972, Temperature and inhibitor effects of fast axonal transport in molluscan nerve, *J. Neurochem.* **19**:1709–1716.

Hoffman, P. N., and Lasek, R. J., 1975, The slow component of axonal transport. Identification of major structural polypeptides of the axon and their generality among mammalian neurons, *J. Cell Biol.* **66**:351–366.

Hoffman, P. N., Griffin, J. W., and Price, D. L., 1980, The role of slow component a (SCa) in determining axon caliber: Changes during regeneration, *Soc. Neurosci. Abstr.* **6**:93.

Hoffman, P. N., Griffin, J. W., and Price D. L., 1981, Changes in the axonal transport of the cytoskelton during development, aging, and regeneration, *Soc. Neurosci Abstr.* **7**:743.

Huber, G. C., 1900, Observations on the degeneration and regeneration of motor and sensory nerve endings in voluntary muscle, *Am. J. Physiol.* **3**:339–344.

Hughes, A., 1953, The growth of embryonic neurites, *J. Anat. (Lond.)* **87**:150–62.

Jha, B. D., Goldby, F., and Gamble, H. J., 1959, The effect of temperature on the maturation of regenerating peripheral nerves in the rat, *J. Anat. (Lond.)* **93**:436–447.

Joseph, B. S., 1973, Somatofugal events in Wallerian degeneration: A conceptual overview, *Brain Res.* **59**:1–18.

Joseph, B. S., and Whitlock, D. G., 1972, The spatio–temporal course of Wallerian degeneration within CNS of toads *(Bufo marinus)* as defined by the Nauta silver method, *Brain Behav. Evol.* **5**:1–17.

Kiyohara, S., and Tucker, D., 1978, Activity of new receptors after transection of the primary olfactory nerve in pigeons, *Physiol. Behav.* **21**:997–994.

Komiya, Y., 1980, Slowing with age of the rate of slow axonal flow in bifurcating axons of rat dorsal root ganglion cells, *Brain Res.* **183**:477–480.

Komiya, Y., 1981*a,* Axonal regeneration in bifurcating axons of rat dorsal root ganglion cells, *Exp. Neurol.* **73**:824–826.

Komiya, Y., 1981*b,* Growth, aging and regeneration of axons and slow axonal flow, in: *New Approaches to Nerve and Muscle Disorders. Basic and Applied Contributions* (A. D. Kidman, J. K. Tomkins, and R. A. Westerman, eds.), pp. 173–182, Excerpta Medica, Amsterdam.

Lajtha, A., and Dunlop, D. S., 1974, Alterations of protein metabolism during development of the brain, in: *Drugs and the Developing Brain* (A. Vernadakis and N. Weiner, eds.), pp. 215–229, Plenum Press, New York.

Lajtha, A., and Dunlop, D., 1981, Turnover of protein in the nervous system, *Life Sci.* **29**:755–767.

Lajtha, A., and Sershen, H., 1975, Changes in the rates of protein synthesis in the brain of goldfish at various temperatures, *Life Sci.* **17**:1861–1868.

Lanners, H. N., and Grafstein, B., 1980, Early stages of axonal regeneration in the goldfish optic tract: An electron microscopic study, *J. Neurocytol.* **9**:733–751.

Lasek, R. J., 1980, Axonal transport: A dynamic view of neuronal structures, *Trends Neurosci.* **3**:87–91.

Lasek, R. J., 1981, The dynamic ordering of neuronal cytoskeletons, *Neurosci. Res. Prog. Bull.* **19**:125–135.

Lasek, R. J., and Black, M. M., 1977, How do axons stop growing? Some clues from the metabolism of the proteins in the slow component of axonal transport, in: *Mechanisms, Regulation and Special Functions of Protein Synthesis in the Brain* (S. Roberts, A. Lajtha, and W. H. Gispen, eds.), pp. 161–169, Elsevier, Amsterdam.

Lasek, R. J., and Hoffman, P. M., 1976, The neuronal cytoskeleton, axonal transport and axonal growth, in: *Cell Mobility,* Volume 3 (R. Goldman, T. Pollard, and J. Rosenbaum, eds.), pp. 1021–1049, Cold Spring Harbor Laboratory, Cold Spring Harbor, New York.

Lasek, R. J., and Morris, J. R., 1982, The microtubule–neurofilament network: The balance between plasticity and stability in the nervous system, in: *Biological Functions of Microtubules and Related Structures* (H. Sakai, H. Mohri, and G. Borisy, eds.), pp. 329–342, Academic Press, New York.

Levi, G., 1934, Explanation, besonders die Struktur and die biologischen Eigenschaften der *in vitro* gezuchteten Zellen and Gewebe, *Z. Ges. Anat. Ergeb. Entwinkt. Gesch.* **31**:125–707.

Lubinska, L., 1952, On the arrest of regeneration of frog peripheral nerves at low temperatures, *Acta Biol. Exp. (Warsaw)* **16**:55–71.

Lubinska, L., 1964, Axoplasmic streaming in regeneration and in normal nerve fibers, in: *Mechanisms of Neural Regeneration, Progress in Brain Research,* Volume 13, (M. Singer and J. P. Schade, eds.), pp. 1–66, Elsevier, Amsterdam.

Lubinska, L., 1975, On axoplasmic flow, *Int. Rev. Neurobiol.* **17**:241–296.

Lubinska, L., 1977, Early course of Wallerian degeneration in myelinated fibers of the rat phrenic nerve, *Brain Res.* **130**:47–63.

Lubinska, L., 1982, Patterns of Wallerian degeneration of myelinated fibers in short and long peripheral stumps and in isolated segments of rat phrenic nerves. Interpretation of the role of axoplasmic flow of the trophic factor, *Brain Res.* **233**:227–240.

Lubinska, L., and Olekiewicz, M., 1950, The rate of regeneration of amphibian peripheral nerves at different temperatures, *Acta Biol Exp. (Warsaw)* **15**:125–45.

Matheson, D. F., Diocee, M. S., and Roots, B. I., 1980, Distribution of neurofilaments in myelinated axons of the optic nerve of goldfish *(Carrassius auratus L.), J. Neurol. Sci.* **48**:233–242.

Matsumoto, D. E., and Scalia, F., 1979, Long term survival of centrally projecting optic nerve axons following enucleation in the frog *(R. pipiens), Anat. Rec.* **193**:615–616.

Matsumoto, D. E., and Scalia, F., 1981, Log-term survival of centrally projecting axons in the optic nerve of the frog following destruction of the retina, *J. Comp. Neurol.* **202**:135–155.

May, R. M., 1925, The relation of nerves to degenerating and regenerating taste buds, *J. Exp. Zool.* **42**:371–410.

McLean, W. G., McKay, A. L., and Sjostrand, J., 1983, Electrophoretic analysis of axonally transported proteins in rabbit vagus nerve, *J. Neurobiol.* **14**:227–236.

McQuarrie, I. G., 1983, Role of the axonal cytoskeleton in the regenerating nervous system, in: *Nerve, Organ and Tissue Regeneration: Research Perspectives* (F. J. Seil, ed.), pp. 51–88, Academic Press, New York.

McQuarrie, I. G., and Grafstein, B., 1982a, Protein synthesis and fast axonal transport in regenerating goldfish retinal ganglion cells, *Brain Res.* **235**:213–223.

McQuarrie, I. G., and Grafstein, B., 1982b, Protein synthesis and axonal transport in goldfish retinal ganglion cells during regeneration accelerated by a conditioning lesion, *Brain Res.* **251**:25–37.

McQuarrie, I. G., Brady, S. T., and Lasek, R. J., 1980, Polypeptide composition and kinetics of Sca and Scb in nerve motor axons and optic axons of the rat, *Soc. Neurosci. Abstr.* **6**:501.

McQuarrie, I. G., King, M., and Lasek, R. J., 1981, Transport of cytoskeletal proteins in newly formed axons of regenerating rat sciatic nerve motor neurons, *Soc. Neurosci. Abstr.* **7**:38.

Merzbacker, L., 1903, Untersuchungen an Winterschlafenden Fledermausen. II. Mitteilung. Die Nervendegeneration wahrend des Winterschlafes. Die Beziehungen zwischen Temperatur und Winterschlaf. *Pfluegers Arch.* **100**:568–85.

Miledi, R., and Slater, C. R., 1970, On the degeneration of rat neuromuscular junctions after nerve section, *J. Physiol. (Lond.)* **207**:507–328.

Millan, N., Murdock, L. L., Bleier, R., and Siegel, F. L., 1979, Effects of acture hyperthermia on polyribosomes, *in vivo* protein synthesis and ornithine decarboxylase activity in the neonatal rat brain, *J. Neurochem.* **32**:311–317.

Monaco, S., Autilio-Bambetti, L., Crane, R., and Gambetti, P., 1983, Transport of neurofilaments polypeptides is accelerated in giant axonal neuropathy, *Soc. Neurosci. Abstr.* **9**:1191.

Monckeberg, G., and Bethe, A., 1899, Die Degeneration der markhaltigen Nervenfasern der Wirbelthiere unter hauptsachlicher Berucksichtigung des Verhaltens der Primitivfibrillen, *Arch. Mikrosk. Anat.* **54**:135–83.

Monti-Graziadei, G. A., and Graziadei, P. P. C., 1979, Neurogenesis and neuron regeneration in the olfactory systems of mammals. II. Degeneration and reconstruction of the olfactory sensory neurons after axotomy, *J. Neurocytol.* **8:**197–213.

Morris, J. R., and Lasek, R. J., 1982, Stable polymers of the axonal cytoskeleton: The axoplasmic ghost, *J. Cell Biol.* **92:**192–198.

Mossa, S., 1926, La vitesse d'accroisement des fibres nerveuses cultivees *in vitro* en function de la temperature, *C.R. Assoc. Anat.* **21:**403–407.

Munoz-Martinez, E. J., Nunez, R., and Sanderson, A., 1981, Axonal transport: A quantitative study of retained and transformed protein fractions in the cat, *J. Neurobiol.* **12:**15–26.

Murdock, L. L. Berlow, S., Colwell, R. E., and Siegel, F. L., 1978, The effects of hyperthermia on polyribosomes and amino acid levels in rat brain, *Neuroscience* **3:**349–357.

Oakley, B., Jones, L. B., and Hosley, M. A., 1980, The effect of nerve stump length upon mammalian taste responses, *Brain Res.* **194:**213–218.

Oakley, B., Chu, J. S., and Jones, L. B., 1981, Axonal transport maintains taste responses, *Brain Res.* **221:**289–298.

Ochs, S., 1974, A unitary concept of axoplasmic transport based on the transport filament hypothesis, *Proceedings of the 3rd International Congress on Muscle Disease, Exerpta Medica Int. Cong. Ser.* **360:**189–194.

Ochs, S., and Ranish, N., 1969, Characteristics of the fast transport system in mammalian nerve fibers, *J. Neurobiol.* **1:**247–261.

Ochs, S., and Smith, C. B., 1975, Low temperature slowing and cold-block of fast axoplasmic transport in mammalian nerves *in vitro, J. Neurobiol.* **6:**85–102.

Ochs, S., Dalrymple, D., and Richards, G., 1962, Axoplasmic transport in ventral root nerve fibers of the cat, *Exp. Neurol.* **5:**349–363.

Parker, G. H., 1933, The progressive degeneration of frog nerve, *Amer. J. Physiol.* **106:**398–403.

Parker, G. H., and Paine, V. L., 1934, Progressive nerve degeneration and its rate in the lateral line nerve of the catfish, *Am. J. Anat.* **54:**1–46.

Pfenninger, K. H., 1980, Mechanism of membrane expansion in the growing neuron, *Soc. Neurosci. Abstr.* **6:**661.

Pfenninger, K. H., and Maylie-Pfenninger, M. F., 1981, Lectin labeling of sprouting neurons. II. Relative movement and appearance of glyconjugates during plasmalemma expansion, *J. Cell Biol.* **89:**547–559.

Raghupathy, E., Patterson, N. A., and Ko, G. K. W., 1971, Formation of ribosome dimers in the brains of hypothermic rats, *Biochem. Biophys. Res. Commun.* **43:**1223–1231.

Ramon y Cajal, S., 1928, *Degeneration and Regeneration of the Nervous System* (R. M. May, trans.), Oxford University Press, Oxford.

Ranish, N. A., and Dettbarn, W. D., 1978, Nerve stump length and cholinesterase activity in muscle and nerve, *Exp. Neurol.* **58:**377–386.

Ranish, N. A., Dettbarn, W. D., and Wecker, L., 1980, Nerve stump length dependent loss of acetylcholinesterase activity in endplate regions of rat diaphragm, *Brain Res.* **191:**379–386.

Schain, R. J., and Watanabe, K., 1971, Postnatal changes in protein metabolism of brain. II. Effects of alteration of ambient temperature and gaseous composition of inspired air. *Pediatr. Res.* **5:**173–180.

Schlaepfer, W. W., 1974, Calcium-induced degeneration of axoplasm in isolated segments of rat peripheral nerve, *Brain Res.* **69:**203–215.

Schlaepfer, W. W., and Bunge, R. P., 1973, Effects of calcium ion concentration on the degeneration of amputated axons in tissue culture, *J. Cell Biol.* **59:**456–470.

Sershen, H., Reith, M. E. A., Lajtha, A., and Gennaro, J., 1981, Effect of cigarette smoke on protein synthesis in brain and liver, *Neuropharmacology* **20:**451–456.

Shaw, G., and Bray, D., 1977, Movement and extension of isolated growth cones, *Exp. Cell Res.* **104**:55–62.

Shuster, L., and Hannan, R. V., 1964, The indirect inhibition of protein synthesis *in vivo* by chlorpromazine, *J. Biol. Chem.* **239**:3401–3406.

Small, R., and Pfenninger, K. H., 1980, Properties and maturation of axolemma in growing neurons, *Soc. Neurosci. Abstr.* **6**:661.

Smith, R. S., and Cooper, P. D., 1981, Variability and temperature dependence of the velocity of retrograde particle transport in myelinated axons, *Can. J. Physiol. Pharmacol.* **59**:857–863.

Springer, A. D., and Agranoff, B. W., 1977, Effect of temperature on rate of goldfish optic nerve regeneration: A radioautographic and behavioral study, *Brain Res.* **128**:405–415.

Strichartz, G., Small, R., Nicholson, C., Pfenninger, K. H., and Llinas, R., 1980, Ionic mechanisms for impulse propagation in growing nonmyelinated axons: saxitoxin binding and electrophysiology, *Soc. Neurosci. Abstr.* **6**:660.

Takenaka, R., Horie, H., and Sugita, T., 1978, New technique for mesuring dynamic axonal transport and its application to temperature effects, *J. Neurobiol.* **9**:317–324.

Tessler, A., Autilio-Gambetti, L., and Gambetti, P. L., 1980, Axonal growth during regeneration: A quantitative autoradiographic study, *J. Cell Biol.* **87**:197–203.

Weddell, G., and Glees, P., 1941, The early stages in the degeneration of cutaneous nerve fibers. *J. Anat. (Lond.)* **76**:65–93.

Weiss, P., and Hiscoe, H. B., 1948, Experiments on the mechanism of nerve growth, *J. Exp. Zool.* **107**:315–395.

Willard, M., and Skene, J. H. P., 1982, Molecular events in axonal regeneration, in: *Repair and Regeneration of the Nervous System* (J. G. Nichols, ed), pp. 71–89, Springer-Verlag, Berlin, Heidelberg, New York.

Wujek, J. R., and Lasek, R. J., 1983, Correlation of axonal regeneration and slow flow component b in two branches of a single axon, *J. Neurosci.* **3**:243–251.

CHAPTER 14

NEUROFILAMENT TRANSPORT IN AXONAL REGENERATION
Implications for the Control of Axonal Caliber

PAUL N. HOFFMAN, JOHN W. GRIFFIN, and DONALD L. PRICE

1. INTRODUCTION

Regenerating axons have been intensively studied with regard to the mechanisms and determinants of elongation, and several lines of evidence suggest that the delivery of cytoskeletal proteins (tubulin and actin, in particular) are correlates of outgrowth and may be rate limiting (see Lasek and Hoffman, 1976;

PAUL N. HOFFMAN • Department of Ophthalmology, The Johns Hopkins University School of Medicine, Baltimore, Maryland 21205   JOHN W. GRIFFIN • Departments of Neurology and Neuroscience, The Johns Hopkins University School of Medicine, Baltimore, Maryland 21205   DONALD L. PRICE • Departments of Pathology, Neurology, and Neuroscience, The Johns Hopkins University School of Medicine, Baltimore, Maryland 21205

Wujek and Lasek, 1983). In addition to changes in axonal length, regeneration involves marked changes in axonal caliber and in cytoskeletal composition. The regenerating axon provides the best available system in which to test critically the hypotheses underlying several of our recent studies. These hypotheses are that neurofilament content is the major correlate of axonal caliber and that axonal neurofilament content is, in turn, determined, in large part, by neurofilament delivery via slow axonal transport. This review will first summarize the general problem of the determinants of axonal caliber and then focus on recent data from regenerating nerves. These data can be considered in terms of three regions of the regenerating axon—the proximal stump, the maturing sprouts, and the distal sprouts.

2. CYTOSKELETAL COMPOSITION IN NORMAL NERVES

Axons in the peripheral nervous system (PNS) of mature animals range from about 0.1 to 10 μm in diameter; in other words, cross-sectional areas vary by a factor of 10^4. Electron microscopy reveals that the cytoskeletal organelles and the surrounding domains occupy > 98% of the cross-sectional area of large fibers; particulate organelles occupy the remaining area (Hoffman et al., 1984). Routine electron micrographs demonstrate two types of longitudinally oriented cytoskeletal organelles, microtubules and neurofilaments. Microtubules are composed primarily of tubulin. The composition of neurofilaments, now known to contain three distinct polypeptides with molecular masses of 68, 145, and 200 kilodaltons (kd), was first deduced on the basis of isotopic pulse-labeling studies of slow axonal transport, which demonstrated the constitutive migration of these proteins (Hoffman and Lasek, 1975). This composition has been abundantly confirmed by direct biochemical and immunologic approaches (Liem et al., 1978; Schlaepfer, 1978; Schlaepfer and Freeman, 1978).

There is a large normal range of both absolute and relative numbers of microtubules and neurofilaments. Three lines of evidence indicate that neurofilament content is the primary correlate of axonal caliber: morphometry of cytoskeletal composition among fibers of different calibers; morphometry of differing regions along the course of individual axons; and examination of normal developing axons. The first approach was used by Friede and Samorajski (1970), who compared quantitatively the cytoskeletal composition among axons of different calibers. Small axons had a high proportion of microtubules with relatively few neurofilaments. Among larger fibers, neurofilament number was the major correlate of axonal caliber. Although both neurofilament and microtubule numbers were directly correlated with caliber, neurofilaments greatly outnumbered microtubules in large-caliber axons (by as much as 10:1). Hoffman et al. (1984) similarly found a linear relationship between neurofilament number and axonal cross-sectional area; microtubule numbers were related in a nonlinear fashion with little increase in microtubule number in axons with cross-sectional areas $> 30 \ \mu m^2$.

The second approach, assessment of cytoskeletal composition along different regions of single axons, provides a dramatic illustration of the relationship between neurofilament number and axonal diameter. Large myelinated fibers in the PNS have periodic variations in axonal caliber: in the region around the node of Ranvier, there is a segment of reduced caliber. This constricted segment, composed of myelin sheath attachment sites in the paranodes and node of Ranvier, is as little as one-tenth the cross-sectional area of the adjacent internodes (Figure 1). The constricted segments, which are evenly spaced along the fiber at distances ranging from 200 to 2000 μm, divide the myelinated axon into a series of contiguous internodal segments of equal length. Berthold (1978) used skip-serial electron micrographs of individual large myelinated fibers from the cat to assess neurofilament numbers and densities as well as microtubule numbers and densities in internodes and in constricted segments. He found that the number of neurofilaments/μm^2 was similar in nodal and internodal regions (Figure 2). In other words, neurofilament number was markedly reduced in regions of smaller caliber, and this reduction directly correlated with axonal area. In contrast, microtubule number was comparable in internodal regions and in constricted segments; the density was, thereby, greatly increased in the constricted segments (Figure 2). Consequently, the ratio of neurofilaments to microtubules was much greater in internodes than in nodes.

The third line of evidence relating neurofilament content to caliber comes from studies of normal axonal development. Immature axons in the PNS and central nervous system (CNS) are composed largely of microtubules, with relatively few neurofilaments (Peters and Vaughn, 1967). Growth in caliber is associated with an increase in the neurofilament content of the axon. Microtubule numbers also increase as the axon grows in caliber, but they do so at a much slower rate than neurofilament numbers.

Neurofilament density in fibers of a wide range of calibers is about 100/μm^2 (Hoffman et al., 1984). The relatively regular spacing between neurofilaments (Weiss and Mayr, 1971; Yamada et al., 1971) apparently reflects the presence of interfilament cross links (Ellisman and Porter, 1980; Hirokawa, 1982; Tsukita et al., 1982). Recent evidence indicates that the 200-kd neurofilament protein is associated with these cross links (Willard and Simon. 1981; Hirokawa et al., 1984). Thus, cross-link formation may be an intrinsic property of neurofilaments that regulates their spacing and thereby determines the volume they occupy. Similarly, the cross links between microtubules and intermediate filaments, of which the neurofilament is an example, may be mediated by microtubule-associated protein 2 (MAP-2) (Bloom and Vallee, 1983). Although antibody staining for MAP-2 is less intense in axons than in den-

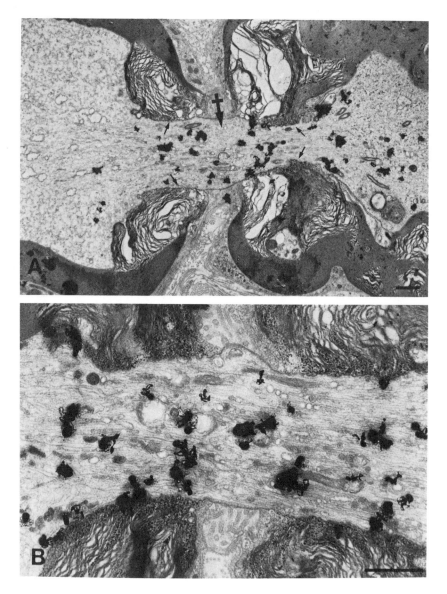

FIGURE 1. Electron microscopic autoradiograms showing the discrepancy in caliber between the internode and the constricted segment of a large myelinated rat sciatic nerve fiber. In A, note that this segment contains the paranodal myelin sheath attachment sites (arrows) and the node of Ranvier (barred arrow). These electron microscopic autoradiograms show the passage of [³H]fucose-labeled material carried by fast axonal transport. The increase in silver grain density within the constricted segment is, in part, a reflection of reduced caliber. In B, a longitudinal section through the node of Ranvier is shown at higher magnification; note the prominence of microtubules within the constricted segment as well as the density of rapidly transported organelles. Bars, 1 μm.

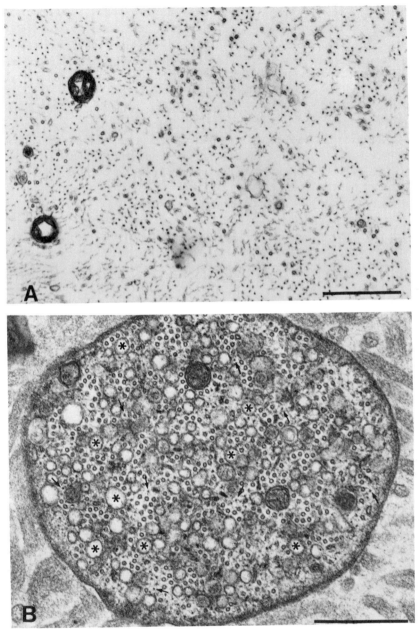

FIGURE 2. Electron micrographs illustrating transverse sections through axoplasm of a large internode (A) and through the node of Ranvier (B) in a rat sciatic nerve fiber. Note, in A, the prominence of neurofilaments as compared to microtubules. Note also the relative paucity of particulate organelles. In B, particulate organelles are numerous (asterisks identify smooth membrane-bound vesicles), and the cytoskeleton is composed primarily of microtubules. Neurofilaments (arrows) are much reduced in number compared to internodes. Bars, 0.5 μm.

drites (Matus *et al.* 1981), recent evidence suggests that MAP-2 is present in the axon (Papasozomenos *et al.,* 1983). Furthermore, the protein kinase assocaited with MAP-2 (Vallee *et al.,* 1981) appears to preferentially phosphorylate the 145-kd neurofilament protein (Leterrier *et al.,* 1981).

The principal cytoskeletal proteins of the axon, which include the neurofilament proteins, tubulin, and actin, are made in the cell body and conveyed along the axon by slow axonal transport (Hoffman and Lasek, 1975). The transport of MAP-2 has not yet been firmly established. Although Takenaka and Inomata (1981) claim to have demonstrated its transport in spinal sensory neurons of the rat, Tytell and Lasek (1978) were unable to demonstrate its transport in retinal ganglion cell neurons of guinea pigs.

In their original description of neurofilament transport, Hoffman and Lasek (1975) proposed that, at the time of their synthesis in the cell body, neurofilament proteins are immediately added onto the ends of existing neurofilaments that extend into the axon and that, as a result of this, all the neurofilament protein in the axon is in the form of polymerized neurofilaments rather than unassembled subunits. This was originally deduced on the basis of the coherent migration of pulse-labeled neurofilament proteins (Hoffman and Lasek, 1975); it was later confirmed by observations that these proteins are assembled almost immediately after synthesis (M. M. Black, personal communication) and that essentially all the neurofilament protein in the axon is in the polymeric (filamentous) form (Morris and Lasek, 1982). Lasek and Hoffman (1976) also proposed that neurofilaments remain intact as they are transported along the axon and are normally disassembled as they enter axon terminals, possibly through the action of a calcium-activated protease. Pulselabeling studies confirmed that there is negligible degradation of neurofilament protein as it is transported along the axon and that it disappears shortly after entering axon terminals (Lasek and Black, 1977). The role of a calcium-activated protease in the degradation of neurofilaments at the terminal is supported by the recent observation that leupeptin, a relatively specific inhibitor of this protease, leads to the accumulation of neurofilament-filled loops at the axon terminals (Roots, 1983).

Taken together, previous morphometric and axonal transport studies make a circumstantial case for the hypothesis that neurofilament transport is a determinant of axonal caliber. Two pathological systems add to this body of evidence. A role for neurofilaments in the control of caliber is apparent in studies using the toxin β, β'-iminodipropionitrile (IDPN). Morphological studies demonstrate that intoxication with this agent leads to the formation of giant neurofilament-filled swellings in the most proximal region of the axon (Chou and Hartmann, 1965) as well as arrested growth in caliber and atrophy of the distal axon (Clark *et al.,* 1980). These changes in caliber appear to result from the selective impairment of neurofilament transport by this agent (Griffin *et al.,* 1978). Pulse-labeling studies indicated that neurofilament proteins enter these swellings from the cell body but are severely retarded in their subsequent transport along the axon. The transport of actin and tubulin, two other major cytoskeletal proteins of the axon, is relatively unaffected, and the rates of rapid axonal transport in both the anterograde and retrograde directions are unaffected. These studies demonstrated that the local accumulation of neurofilaments, i.e., in the proximal axon, leads to a marked increase in axonal caliber and that impaired delivery of neurofilament proteins to the distal axon is associated with a reduction in axonal caliber.

Additional evidence for the role of neurofilaments in the control of caliber comes from the study of hypoplastic axons produced in chronically constricted sciatic nerves of 10- to 14-day-old rats (Duncan, 1948; Friede, 1971). With subsequent nerve growth, progessive compression developed at the constriction and led to the arrest of growth in caliber distal to the ligature. These hypoplastic nerve fibers had a profound paucity of neurofilaments; the cytoskeleton consisted largely of microtubules. In contrast, caliber increased in a normal manner proximal to the ligature; the neurofilament content of this region was indistinguishable from that of control axons in age-matched animals. Thus, the relative absence of neurofilaments distal to the constriction was associated with an arrest of radial growth. This observation provides additional support for the concept that the normal proximal-to-distal transport of neurofilaments along the axon plays a major role in growth in caliber.

None of these systems, however, provides a critical test of the association between neurofilament transport and axonal caliber; either quantitative studies of axonal transport are difficult (as in the hypoplastic axonal preparation) or transport of other cytoskeletal elements is altered in the same direction as alterations in neurofilament transport. For example, in the IDPN model, there are modest reductions in the transport of all slow-component proteins, with neurofilaments being the most severely affected (Griffin *et al.,* 1978, 1983*a*). In addition, IDPN administration reduces interfilament spacing and increases neurofilament density. This factor complicates the comparison with normal systems. For these reasons, the regenerating system provides an important model for critically testing the relationship between fiber caliber and neurofilament transport.

3. NEUROFILAMENT TRANSPORT AND AXONAL CALIBER IN REGENERATING AXONS

3.1. Changes in the Proximal Stump

Recent observations demonstrated a direct correlation between the axonal transport of neurofilaments and the regulation of axonal caliber in the regenerating system. A number of investigators, using both classical morphology and electrophysiological approaches, have previously demonstrated that axonal caliber is reduced in the proximal stump of regenerating axons, i.e., the portion proximal to the site of injury (Greenman, 1913; Gutmann and Sanders, 1943; Cragg and Thomas, 1961; Aitkin and Thomas, 1962; Kreutzberg and Schubert, 1971a,b; Kuno et al., 1974a,b) (Figure 3). Previous studies by Hoffman and Lasek (1980) demonstrated that the amount of labeled neurofilament protein transported in regenerating axons is selectively reduced in relation to tubulin and actin. Thus, given the relationship between axonal caliber and neurofilament number suggested above, it seemed reasonable to presume that these reductions in caliber of the proximal stump resulted from the transport of a decreased number of neurofilaments into these axons. According to this hypothesis, reductions in caliber resulting from this alteration in neurofilament transport should spread in a proximal-to-distal direction along the axon at a rate equal to the velocity of neurofilament transport, i.e., 1–2 mm/day. In addition, reductions in axonal area should be associated with a proportional decrease in the number of neurofilament cross sections per axon.

These predictions were tested morphometrically by studying the spatial and temporal evolution of changes in the caliber of motor axons in the L5 ventral root following injury of the rat sciatic nerve and by correlating these changes with alterations in the number of neurofilament cross sections per

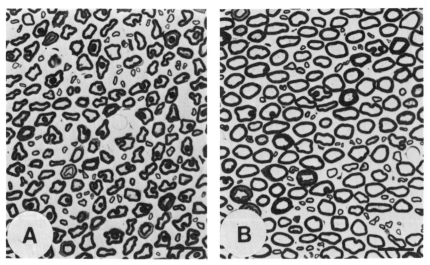

FIGURE 3. Light micrographs comparing caliber in regenerating (A) and control (B) motor axons in the rat L5 ventral root (proximal level) 3 weeks after crushing the sciatic nerve. Reductions in caliber are associated with a loss of circularity and the presence of inappropriately thick myelin sheaths in regenerating fibers (A). Bars, 25 μm.

axon. Our experimental observations confirmed these predictions. Following injury to the rat sciatic nerve, reductions in caliber spread along motor axons in a proximal-to-distal direction at a rate equal to the velocity of neurofilament transport in these neurons, i.e., 1.7 mm/day (Figure 4). Reductions in the area of these regenerating axons were associated with a proportional decrease in the number of neurofilaments but not of microtubules. This latter finding is consistent with the observation that labeling of the transported neurofilament protein was reduced in relation to tubulin (Hoffman and Lasek, 1980). Thus, these observations demonstrated that alterations in the amount of neurofilament protein transported into the axon are associated with changes in axonal caliber.

Observations in the regenerating neuron also suggest that neuron–target cell interactions may influence the level of neurofilament transport and possibly synthesis. Disconnecting the neuron and its target by axotomy leads to a decrease in neurofilament transport (Hoffman and Lasek, 1980) that appears to be responsible for atrophy of the proximal stump (Hoffman *et al.,* 1984). Failure of regeneration and/or reconnection with targets results in persistent

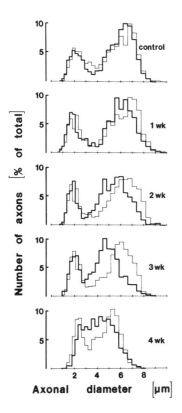

FIGURE 4. Histograms comparing axonal caliber at the proximal (bold lines) and distal levels (thin lines) of the L5 ventral root between 1 and 4 weeks after crushing of the sciatic nerves of 7-week-old rats. Unoperated control animals were killed at 8 weeks of age (upper profile). The mean number of axons in each size class is plotted as a function of axonal diameter (n = three roots in each case). In the control roots, axons fall into two size classes (large and small), which account for two-thirds and one-third of the total number of axons, respectively (also see Figure 3). Between 1 and 3 weeks after crush, reductions in the caliber of large axons are present at the proximal level but not distally. At 4 weeks, reductions are nearly equal at both levels. This demonstrates a proximal-to-distal progression of reductions in caliber along regenerating fibers.

atrophy (Kuno *et al.,* 1974*a*), whereas recovery of caliber coincides with reconnection (Kuno *et al.,* 1974*b*). Recently, we found that recovery correlates with
the return of neurofilament transport to normal levels (P. N. Hoffman and G.
W. Thompson, unpublished observations).

3.2. Regenerating Sprouts

Following crush of peripheral nerve (rat sciatic nerve), outgrowth proceeds at a rate up to 4.5 mm/day in young animals (Gutmann *et al.,* 1942;
Black and Lasek, 1979). Cytoskeletal composition of the distal (elongating)
region of sprouts is simple and monotonous; microtubules are the predominant
organelle with relatively few neurofilaments, and neurofilaments that are present are often segregated into discrete fascicles (Figures 5, 6). Even as the grow-

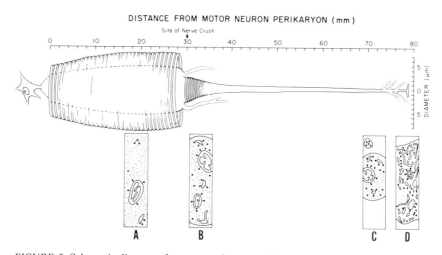

FIGURE 5. Schematic diagram of a regenerating rat sciatic motor fiber 2 weeks after nerve
crush. To emphasize the differences in caliber among the regions of this regenerating nerve, this
idealized fiber is diagrammed with the diameter scale (in micrometers) magnified 1000-fold in
relation to the length scale (in millimeters). The growth cones of the most rapidly elongating
sprouts have reached 50 mm from the site of transection, correlating with a growth rate greater
than 4 mm/day. The growth cone itself (D) contains abundant particulate organelles including
smooth membrane-bound vesicular and tubular structures as well as bundles of microfilaments.
The distal (immature) sprout region (C) contains cytoskeleton composed predominantly of
microtubules with relatively few neurofilaments. In the maturing region of the sprout (B), myelination has already commenced, and the cross-sectional area of the sprout is more than ten times
greater than that of the distal, immature sprouts. The cytoskeleton contains an increased proportion of neurofilaments in relation to microtubules. The parent axon proximal to the crush (A)
shows a reduction in caliber in the most proximal regions, reflecting an intermediate phase in the
development of proximal stump atrophy and reflecting the proximal-to-distal spread of atrophy
from the cell body. The cytoskeleton contains the high ratio of neurofilaments to microtubules
characteristic of large myelinated fibers. (Note that the cell body is not drawn to scale.)

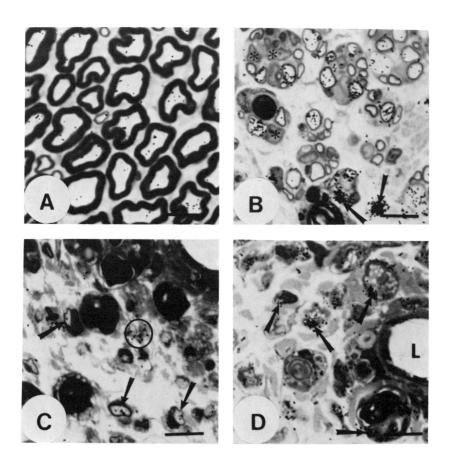

FIGURE 6. Cross sections of rat sciatic nerve 2 weeks after nerve crush. Sections A–D were taken from levels of the nerve containing fibers in the stages of growth labeled A–D in Figure 5. These light microscopic autoradiograms illustrate the localization of [³H]leucine-labeled rapidly transported proteins. A shows the appearance of large myelinated fibers in the proximal stump. In B, a few millimeters distal to the crush, there are clusters of regenerating axons that are already myelinating. The very densely labeled regions (arrows) represent growth cones. Numerous Schwann cell nuclei (*) and dark spheroidal bodies representing Wallerian degeneration of the distal stump are present. In C, a few myelinated fibers are apparent (arrows), and other grains are associated with axonal sprouts not well resolved at the light microscopic level (within circles). In D, the axonal sprouts are often very small and are seen on the basis of dense collections of silver grains associated with the growth cone regions (arrows). L, blood vessel lumen. Bars, 10 μm. (Reprinted with permission from Griffin et al., 1976.)

ing tip elongates, more proximal regions begin to mature; i.e., there is an increase in caliber, and myelination begins. This increase in caliber is associated with increasing neurofilament content, as previously suggested in developing systems.

4. MODELS FOR THE CONTROL OF AXONAL CALIBER BY NEUROFILAMENT TRANSPORT

Any model for the control of caliber in myelinated fibers must account for the reduced neurofilament content of the nodes. We will consider three models that account for this finding with varying degrees of success. Implicit in each of them is the assumption that alterations in cross-sectional area result directly from changes in the neurofilament content of the axon.

The first model, which was proposed by Hoffman and Lasek (1975) in their original description of neurofilament transport, postulates that the relative positions of neurofilaments and microtubules in the cytoskeleton are maintained throughout the course of their movement within the axon. Although several features of this model concerning the synthesis and degradation of neurofilaments are applicable to large myelinated fibers (as discussed previously), it does not account for the reduced neurofilament content of the nodes. Instead, it predicts that neurofilament density should increase markedly (in proportion to reductions in area).

The second model that we consider postulates that the axon contains two populations of neurofilaments—one undergoing transport and a second that is stationary. Stationary neurofilaments result from the retention of a relatively small fraction of the moving population within each internodal segment. Over time, this could lead to the accumulation of a substantial population of stationary neurofilaments. In this model, the nodal neurofilaments would be comprised exclusively of the moving population, whereas the internodes would contain both moving and stationary neurofilaments.

The major deficiency of this model is that it would require axonal caliber to be substantially greater proximally than distally; i.e., the axon would have to be tapered. This reflects a progessive decrease in the neurofilament content (and cross-sectional area) of the transported fraction with increasing distance along the axon as neurofilaments are transferred to the stationary population. For example, in order for the area of large motor axons in the rat L5 ventral root to increase at the observed rate of 1.5 μm^2/week during growth (Hoffman *et al.*, 1984), the transported fraction would have to occupy a cross-sectional area of 32.1 μm^2 in the proximal axon. (This calculation assumes that growth occurs at this rate along the entire length of these axons, that these axons are 100 mm long, that the mobile phase has a conical distribution along the axon, and that the rate of neurofilament transport is 2 mm/day.) Yet, since the mean cross-sectional area of these axons in 8-week-old animals is only 31 μm^2 (Hoffman *et al.,* 1984), essentially all the neurofilaments in the proximal axon would be moving; i.e., there would be no stationary population in the proximal axon. Therefore, this model is untenable.

We now propose a third model that is consistent with our current understanding of neurofilament metabolism and axonal structure. As we have already discussed, evidence indicates that neurofilament assembly does not occur locally within the axon and that there is negligible degradation of neurofilaments along the axon. Therefore, axonal transport appears to represent the only mechanism for neurofilaments to enter or leave any nonterminal region of the axon.

In this model, we assume that neurofilaments are either continuous structures extending from the cell body to the axon terminal or that neurofilaments are joined to form uninterrupted chains that extend the entire length of the axon. This assumption is compatible with the observation that pulse-labeled neurofilament protein is transported within the axon as a coherent wave (Hoffman and Lasek, 1975). In the nodes, these chains are aligned parallel to the longitudinal axis of the fiber and move unidirectionally proximal to distal. In contrast, in the internodes, they are folded so that an individual chain may be seen several times in a single cross-sectional view (Figure 7). This accounts for the lower neurofilament content of the nodes, since folding occurs exclusively in the internodes. Since interfilament distance and, therefore, density is maintained during this folding, the cross-sectional area of an internode is proportional to the total length of the neurofilament chains within that segment.

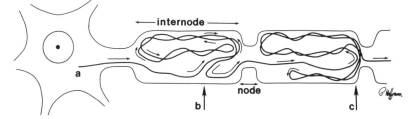

FIGURE 7. Schematic representation of proposed model for the control of axonal caliber. In this model, neurofilaments are linked to form a discrete number of continuous chains, which extend from the cell body, where neurofilaments are assembled, to the axon terminals, where they presumably are degraded. In the nodes, these chains are aligned parallel to the longitudinal axis of the fiber and move unidirectionally proximal to distal. In the internodes, portions of these chains are folded so that an individual chain may be seen several times in a single cross-sectional view. This accounts for the reduced neurofilament content and caliber of the nodes. Radial growth results from increasing the total length of the neurofilament chains in each internode. In order for this to occur, there must be a decrease in the velocity of these chains across each internodal segment. Hypothetical sites for this slowing are indicated by arrows at b and c.

This model has several implications for radial growth of the axon. If, for the sake of clarity, we assume that internodal length remains constant, then increasing the total length of the neurofilament chains in each internode will result in radial growth (of the internodal segments). In order for this to occur, the rate at which these chains enter the internode must be faster than the rate at which they leave, i.e., there must be a decrease in the velocity of these chains across each internodal segment (Figure 7). This would allow caliber to increase without changing the total number of neurofilament chains in the axon.

One correlate of this model is that the net velocity of neurofilament transport within an internode should decrease as internodal caliber increases. The net velocity is the rate at which radioactive neurofilament proteins move distally along the axon in pulse-labeling studies. Since these proteins are transported along a circuitous path (through regions of folding) in internodal segments, the distance they actually travel while crossing an internode may be substantially greater than the internodal length (measured along the fiber). Consequently, as folding becomes more extensive (and internodal caliber increases), the net velocity should decrease proportionately. This is consistent with our observation that the net velocity of neurofilament transport decreases in motor axons of the rat sciatic nerve as they grow in caliber during development (Hoffman *et al.*, 1983).

Another correlate of this model is that there should be a sequential decrement in the velocity of neurofilament transport from internode to internode along axons undergoing radial growth. In our model, neurofilament chains simultaneously undergo folding in successive internodal segments along the length of the axon. As we have previously mentioned, since radial growth is associated with a decrease in the velocity of these chains across each internodal segment, there should be a sequential decrement in velocity at successive internodes along the fiber, i.e., a sequential decrement in velocity with increasing distance along the axon. Conversely, once growth has stopped (after the axon has reached its mature caliber), the length of the chains and the extent of their folding within the internodes should remain constant. Consequently, velocity should remain constant along nongrowing axons.

We can only speculate as to how the velocity of neurofilament transport could undergo decrements in successive internodes during growth. If we assume that transport involves interactions between neurofilaments and other axonal structures, e.g., microtubules (Griffin *et al.*, 1983*b*) or the axolemma (Hoffman and Lasek, 1975), then it is conceivable that the velocity of transport is proportional to the frequency of these interactions. In theory, the frequency of these interactions could be regulated by allosteric modification of proteins associated with the neurofilaments. In this regard, it is particularly intriguing that the 200- and 145-kd neurofilament proteins contain an exceptionally large number of phosphorylated sites (Pant *et al.*, 1978; Jones and Williams, 1982), since phosphorylation is a known mechanism for altering the functional properties of proteins (for review, see Ingebritsen and Cohen, 1983). Thus, one possibility is that stepwise alterations in the level of phosphorylation of these proteins at successive internodal segments could be responsible for reductions in the velocity of neurofilament transport along growing axons.

Recent observations indicate that the velocity of transport does, in fact, decrease as labeled neurofilaments are carried distally along axons undergoing radial growth, i.e., in lumbar motor axons of 3- and 12-week-old rats (P. N. Hoffman, J. W. Griffin, and D. L. Price, unpublished observations). There is a lack of slowing, i.e., no change in velocity, of neurofilament proteins along motor axons in phrenic nerves of adult guinea pigs (Lasek and Black, 1977). Since axons in the phrenic nerve complete their radial growth very early during postnatal development (Nystrom, 1968), it is likely that these axons in adult guinea pigs are no longer growing, and the absence of any change in neurofilament velocity is consistent with our model.

This model also has implications for the growth of regenerating sprouts. Radial growth should begin as neurofilament chains enter the sprouts from the proximal stump. This growth, which results from folding of these chains, should proceed along the sprouts in a proximal-to-distal direction, and the sprouts should be tapered within the region containing these neurofilaments (Figure 5). Since folding begins as chains enter the sprouts, the extent to which each chain is folded should be much greater in the proximal stump than in the sprouts, particularly at early times after axotomy. Therefore, we would expect the net transport velocity to increase as labeled neurofilament proteins enter the sprouts from the proximal stump. Studies currently underway are designed to test this prediction.

5. CONCLUSION

The regenerating neuron provides an ideal system in which to explore the role of the cytoskeleton in the control of cellular volume. Evidence derived from these studies indicates that neurofilaments (neuronal intermediate filaments) are a primary intrinsic determinant of axonal caliber and that the axonal transport of neurofilaments plays an important role in the control of caliber. This role has major physiological significance for the neuron, since caliber is the principal determinant of impulse conduction velocity along the axon (Hursh, 1939). In a more general sense, these studies suggest that intermediate filaments play an important role in the control of cellular volume.

ACKNOWLEDGMENTS

Dr. Hoffman is a John A. and George L. Hartford Foundation Fellow and an Alfred P. Sloan Foundation Research Fellow. This work was supported by grants from the U.S. Public Health Service (NIH EY 03791, NS 10580, and NS 15721). Dr. Griffin is the recipient of a Research Career Development Award (NIH NS 00450). The authors thank Mrs. Carla Jordon and Ms. Adelaine Stocks for their careful assistance during preparation of the manuscript.

6. REFERENCES

Aitkin, J. T., and Thomas, P. K., 1962, Retrograde changes in fibre size following nerve section, *J. Anat.* **96**:121–129.

Berthold, C. H., 1978, Morphology of normal peripheral axons, in: *Physiology and Pathobiology of Axons* (S. G. Waxman, ed.), pp. 3–63, Raven Press, New York.

Black, M. M., and Lasek, R. J., 1979, Slowing of the rate of axonal regeneration during growth and maturation, *Exp. Neurol.* **63**:108–119.

Bloom, G. S., and Vallee, R. B., 1983, Association of microtubule-associated protein 2 (MAP 2) with microtubules and intermediate filaments in cultured brain cells, *J. Cell Biol.* **96**:1523–1531.

Chou, S.-M., and Hartmann, H. A., 1965, Electron microscopy of focal neuroaxonal lesions produced by β, β'-iminodipropionitrile (IDPN) in rats, *Acta Neuropathol. (Berl.)* **4**:590–603.

Clark, A. W., Griffin, J. W., and Price, D. L., 1980, The axonal pathology in chronic IDPN intoxication, *J. Neuropathol. Exp. Neurol.* **39**:42–55.

Cragg, B. G., and Thomas, P. K., 1961, Changes in conduction velocity and fibre size proximal to peripheral nerve lesions, *J. Physiol. (Lond.)* **157**:315–327.

Duncan, D., 1948, Alterations in the structure of nerves caused by restricting their growth with ligatures, *J. Neuropathol. Exp. Neurol.* **7**:261–273.

Ellisman, M. H., and Porter, K. R., 1980, Microtrabecular structure of the axoplasmic matrix: Visualization of cross-linking structures and their distribution, *J. Cell Biol.* **87**:464–479.

Friede, R. L., 1971, Changes in microtubules and neurofilaments in constricted, hypoplastic nerve fibers, *Acta Neuropathol. (Berl.)* [*Suppl.*] **5**:216–225.

Friede, R. L., and Samorajski, T., 1970, Axon caliber related to neurofilaments and microtubules in sciatic nerve fibers of rats and mice, *Anat. Rec.* **167**:379–388.

Greenman, M. J., 1913, Studies on the regeneration of the peroneal nerve of the albino rat: Number and sectional areas of fibers: Area relation of axis to sheath, *J. Comp. Neurol.* **23**:479–513.

Griffin, J. W., Drachman, D. B., and Price, B. L., 1976, Fast axonal transport in motor nerve regeneration, *J. Neurobiol.* **7**:355–370.

Griffin, J. W., Hoffman, P. N., Clark, A. W., Carroll, P. T., and Price, D. L., 1978, Slow axonal transport of neurofilament proteins: Impairment by β, β'-iminodipropionitrile administration, *Science* **202**:633–635.

Griffin, J. W., Fahnestock, K. E., Price, D. L., and Hoffman, P. N., 1983, Microtubule–neurofilament segregation produced by β, β'-iminodipropionitrile: Evidence for the association of fast axonal transport with microtubules, *J. Neurosci.* **3**:557–566.

Griffin, J. W., Anthony, D. C., Fahnestock, K., Hoffman, P. N., and Graham, D. G., 1984, 3,4-Dimethyl-2,5-hexanedione impairs axonal transport of neurofilament proteins, *J Neurosci.* **4**:1516–1526.

Gutmann, E., and Sanders, F. K., 1943, Recovery of fibre numbers and diameters in the regeneration of peripheral nerves, *J. Physiol. (Lond.)* **101**:489–518.

Gutmann, E., Gutmann, L., Medawar, P. B., and Young, J. Z., 1942, The rate of regeneration of nerve, *J. Exp. Biol.* **19**:14–44.

Hirokawa, N., 1982, Cross-linker system between neurofilaments, microtubules, and membranous organelles in frog axons revealed by the quick-freeze, deep-etching method, *J. Cell Biol.* **94**:129–142.

Hirokawa, N., Glicksman, M. A., and Willard, M., 1984, Organization of mammalian neurofilament polypeptides within the neuronal cytoskeleton, *J. Cell Biol.* **98**:1523–1536.

Hoffman, P. N., and Lasek, R. J., 1975, The slow component of axonal transport. Identification of major structural polypeptides of the axon and their generality among mammalian neurons, *J. Cell Biol.* **66**:351–366.,

Hoffman, P. N., and Lasek, R. J., 1980, Axonal transport of the cytoskeleton in regenerating motor neurons: Constancy and change, *Brain Res.* **202**:317–333.

Hoffman, P. N., Lasek, R. J., Griffin, J. W., and Price, D. L., 1983, Slowing of the axonal transport of neurofilament protein during development, *J. Neurosci.* **3**:1694–1700.

Hoffman, P. N., Griffin, J. W., and Price, D. L., 1984, Control of axonal caliber by neurofilament transport *J. Cell Biol.* (in press).

Hursh, J. B., 1939, Conduction velocity and diameter of nerve fibers, *Am J. Physiol.* **127**:131–139.

Ingebritsen, T. S., and Cohen, P., 1983, Protein phosphatases: Properties and role in cellular regulation, *Science* **221**:333–338.

Jones, S. M., and Williams, R. C., Jr., 1982, Phosphate content of the polypeptides of mammalian neurofilaments, *J. Cell Biol.* **95**:227a.

Kreutzberg, G. W., and Schubert, P., 1971*a,* Volume changes in the axon during regeneration, *Acta Neuropathol. (Berl.)* **17**:220–226.

Kreutzberg, G. W., and Schubert, P., 1971*b,* Changes in axonal flow during regeneration of mammalian motor nerves, *Acta Neuropathol. (Berl.)* [*Suppl.*] **5**:70–75.

Kuno, M., Miyata, Y., and Munoz-Martinez, E. J., 1974*a,* Differential reactions of fast and slow α-motoneurones to axotomy, *J. Physiol. (Lond.)* **240**:725–739.

Kuno, M., Miyata, Y., and Munoz-Martinez, E. J., 1974*b,* Properties of fast and slow alpha motoneurones following motor reinnervation, *J. Physiol. (Lond.)* **242**:273–288.

Lasek, R. J., and Black, M. M., 1977, How do axons stop growing? Some clues from the metabolism of the proteins in the slow component of axonal transport, in: *Mechanisms, Regulation and Special Functions of Protein Synthesis in the Brain* (S. Roberts, A. Lajtha, and W. H. Gispen, eds.), pp. 161–169, Elsevier/North Holland Biomedical Press, Amsterdam.

Lasek, R. J., and Hoffman, P. N., 1976, The neuronal cytoskeleton, axonal transport and axonal growth, *Cold Spring Harbor Conf. Cell Prolif.* **3**:1021–1049.

Leterrier, J.-F., Liem, R. K. H., and Shelanski, M. L., 1981, Preferential phosphorylation of the 150,000 molecular weight component of neurofilaments by a cyclic AMP-dependent, microtubule-associated protein kinase, *J. Cell Biol.* **90**:755–760.

Liem, R. K. H., Yen, S-H., Salomon, G. D., and Shelanski, M. L., 1978, Intermediate filaments in nervous tissues, *J. Cell Biol.* **79**:637–645.

Matus, A., Bernhardt, R., and Hugh-Jones, T., 1981, High molecular weight microtubule-associated proteins are preferentially associated with dendritic microtubules in brain, *Proc. Natl. Acad. Sci. U.S.A.* **78**:3010–3014.

Morris, J. R., and Lasek, R. J., 1982, Stable polymers of the axonal cytoskeleton: The axoplasmic ghost, *J. Cell Biol.* **92**:192–198.

Nystrom, B., 1968, Fibre diameter increase in nerves to "slow-red" and "fast-white" cat muscles during postnatal development, *Acta Neurol. Scand.* **44**:265–294.

Pant, H. C., Shecket, G., Gainer, H., and Lasek, R. J., 1978, Neurofilament protein is phosphorylated in the squid giant axon, *J. Cell Biol.* **78**:R23–R27.

Papasozomenos, S. Ch., Binder, L. I., Bender, P. K., and Payne, M. R., 1983, The axonal cytoskeleton in the β,β'-iminodipropionitrile (IDPN) model, *J. Neuropathol. Exp. Neurol.* **42**:310.

Peters, A., and Vaughn, J. E., 1967, Microtubules and filaments in the axons and astrocytes of early postnatal rat optic nerves, *J. Cell Biol.* **32**:113–119.

Roots, B. I., 1983, Neurofilament accumulation induced in synapses by leupeptin, *Science* **221**:971–972.

Schlaepfer, W. W., 1978, Observations on the disassembly of isolated mammalian neurofilaments, *J. Cell Biol.* **76**:50–56.

Schlaepfer, W. W., and Freeman, L. A., 1978, Neurofilament proteins of rat peripheral nerve and spinal cord, *J. Cell Biol.* **78**:653–662.

Takenaka, T., and Inomata, K., 1981, Axoplasmic transport of microtubule-associated proteins in the rat sciatic nerve, *J. Neurobiol.* **12**:479–486.

Tsukita, S., Usukura, J., Tsukita, S., and Ishikawa, H., 1982, The cytoskeleton in myelinated axons: A freeze-etch replica study, *Neuroscience* **7**:2135–2147.

Tytell, M., and Lasek, R. J., 1978, Axonal transport in guinea pig optic neurons: Each component consists of a distinct pattern of proteins, *Neurosci. Abstr.* **6**:37.

Vallee, R. B., DiBartolomeis, M. J., and Theurkauf, W. E., 1981, A protein kinase bound to the projection portion of MAP 2 (microtubule-associated protein 2), *J. Cell Biol.* **90**:568–576.

Weiss, P. A., and Mayr, R., 1971, Organelles in neuroplasmic ("axonal") flow: Neurofilaments, *Proc. Natl. Acad. Sci. U.S.A.* **68**:846–850.

Willard, M., and Simon, C., 1981, Antibody decoration of neurofilaments, *J. Cell Biol.* **89**:198–205.

Wujek, J. R., and Lasek, R. J., 1983, Correlation of axonal regeneration and slow component *b* in two branches of a single axon, *J. Neurosci.* **3**:243–251.

Yamada, K. M., Spooner, B. S., and Wessells, N. K., 1971, Ultrastructure and function of growth cones and axons of cultured nerve cells, *J. Cell Biol.* **49**:614–635.

CHAPTER 15

CALCIUM-ACTIVATED PROTEASE AND THE REGULATION OF THE AXONAL CYTOSKELETON

WILLIAM W. SCHLAEPFER and UN-JIN P. ZIMMERMAN

1. INTRODUCTION

The synthesis, assembly, and intracellular dissemination of a prominent and elaborate cytoskeleton are basic properties of neurons that enable these cells to establish and maintain a highly asymmetric cell form. Variations in size and shape among different neurons are determined by the quantity and quality of their cytoskeletal components. A complex interplay among cytoskeletal elements undoubtedly underlies the formation of growth cones and their transformation into neurites as well as the subsequent maintenance of established neuritic processes. Similar interactions of cytoskeletal components are probably

WILLIAM W. SCHLAEPFER and UN-JIN P. ZIMMERMAN ● *Division of Neuropathology, Department of Pathology and Lab Medicine, University of Pennsylvania Medical School, Philadelphia, Pennsylvania 19104*

also reponsible for the regeneration of cell processes that occurs following injury to the axonal extension of the cell.

Homeostasis of the cytoskeleton requires that the synthesis and assembly of cytoskeletal components be balanced by a concomitant breakdown and turnover of these elements. It would seem reasonable to assume that a major portion of this cytoskeletal degradation occurs in the distal ends of neurites after the cytoskeleton has traversed the full expanse of its extension across the cell. It may well be expected that the turnover of cytoskeletal components is geared primarily to maintain the anatomic continuities of neuritic processes. Furthermore, it would be advantageous if the turnover of cytoskeletal proteins were regulated so that synthesis and assembly of cytoskeletal components are coordinated with changing rates and/or patterns of degradation.

Very limited information is presently available on the turnover of neuronal cytoskeletal proteins. Nevertheless, an interesting study by Lasek and Black (1977) indicates that labeled cytoskeletal proteins are rapidly turned over on reaching axonal terminals. They concluded that synaptic endings are active sites of cytoskeletal degradation and speculated that cytoskeletal breakdown may be regulated by activation of proteases as a result of local increases in calcium concentration. Experimental data in support of this hypothesis are reviewed in this chapter.

2. CALCIUM-DEPENDENT BREAKDOWN OF THE AXONAL CYTOSKELETON

The adverse effects of calcium on axoplasm were initially noted by physiologists while studying the relative calcium impermeability of the axolemma surrounding the squid giant axon. Immersion of intact giant axons in artificial sea water resulted in very limited penetration of ^{45}Ca (Hodgkin and Keynes, 1957). Damaged regions of axonal membrane were sites of increased calcium permeability, causing a visible cloudy alteration in the underlying axoplasm (Fluckiger and Keynes, 1957). Similar opacification as well as liquefaction of axoplasm occurred following microinjection of calcium into axoplasm (Hodgkin and Keynes, 1956). Identical changes were reproduced by local application of calcium to extruded axoplasm (Hodgkin and Katz, 1949).

Susceptibility of mammalian axoplasm to calcium-induced alterations was noted in studies of minced segments of rat peripheral nerve that were placed in solutions of different composition before fixation and examination by electron microscopy (Schlaepfer, 1971). These studies showed that brief exposure to calcium led to a granular disintegration of the axoplasmic cytoskeleton (Figures 1, 2), a change that could be prevented by chelation of calcium. Similar changes did not occur during parallel incubation with high levels of mag-

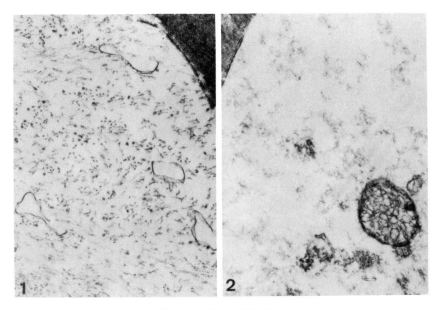

FIGURE 1. Transverse section of large myelinated fiber from rat sciatic nerve showing intact neurofilaments and microtubules after 3-day incubation in 0.1 M phosphate buffer, pH 7.0 ×32,000. (From Schlaepfer, 1979.)

FIGURE 2. Transverse section of large myelinated fiber from rat sciatic nerve showing granular disintegration of neurofilaments and microtubules after 1-hr incubation in Ringer's solution. ×32,000. (From Schlaepfer, 1979.)

nesium or during incubations with aluminum or lead. The same granular disintegration of axonal neurofilaments and microtubules occurred in long excised segments of rat peripheral nerves provided that they were incubated in solutions containing free calcium (Schlaepfer, 1974a). The rate of calcium-induced disintegration was accelerated by increased calcium concentrations and, especially, by permeabilizing the axolemma by including detergents or calcium ionophores in the incubation media (Schlaepfer, 1978). Degradative changes were also hastened by the use of cyanide or dinitrophenol to facilitate the influx of calcium into the axoplasm (Schlaepfer, 1974b). It is noteworthy that the disintegration of the axoplasmic cytoskeleton by calcium was associated with collapse and fragmentation of myelin, suggesting that the morphological changes were accompanied by liquefaction of axoplasm in myelinated nerve fibers.

Experimental calcium influxes into the axoplasm of peripheral nerve segments also led to selective breakdown and/or loss of cytoskeletal proteins when the total protein content of these nerves was examined by SDS gel electrophoresis (Schlaepfer and Micko, 1979). Loss of neurofilament triplet proteins (M_r = 200,000, 150,000, and 68,000) and some tubulin occurred in parallel with the calcium-induced morphological disintegration of the axonal cytoskeleton (Figure 3). The same biochemical alterations of neurofilament proteins occurred when different methods were used to induce calcium influxes, including permeabilization by addition of the calcium ionophore A23187 or triton X-100 to the incubation media.

Calcium-dependent granular disintegration of the axonal cytoskeleton occurs not only in excised nerve segments subjected to experimental influxes of

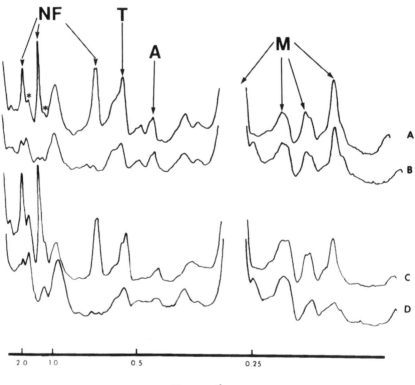

MW x 10⁻⁵

FIGURE 3. Densitometric tracing of nerve proteins in acrylamide gels from excised nerve segments incubated for 2 hr with ionophore A23187 (A and B) or detergent Triton X-100 (C and D) in the presence (B and D) or absence (A and C) of calcium. Calcium caused the selective loss of neurofilament (NF) proteins and some loss of tubulin (T) but no significant alterations of actin (A) or myelin (M) proteins. Metachromatic proteins (asterisks) of collagen served as internal marker proteins in acrylamide gels. Molecular weight (MW) scale constructed from protein standards. (From Schlaepfer, 1979.)

calcium but also in transected nerves left to degenerate *in situ*. The granular axoplasmic disintegration in transected neurites can be prevented if calcium is removed from the incubation medium of cultured rat dorsal root ganglia (Schlaepfer and Bunge, 1973). Replacement of calcium in these cultures brings about a resumption of the granular disintegration of axoplasm. The same granular degeneration of axoplasm occurs in transected rat peripheral nerves *in vivo* (Schlaepfer, 1974a) and is accompanied by a loss of neurofilament triplet proteins when the proteins of transected nerves are examined by SDS gel electrophoresis (Schlaepfer and Micko, 1978; Soifer *et al.*, 1981). The biochemical changes in cytoskeletal proteins in transected nerves are identical to those that can be simulated by experimental calcium influxes into excised and isolated nerves (Schlaepfer and Micko, 1979).

3. CALCIUM-ACTIVATED PROTEOLYSIS OF AXONAL CYTOSKELETAL PROTEINS

The nature of the calcium-mediated disruption of the axonal cytoskeleton has been elucidated in studies on isolated preparations of rat neurofilaments. Neurofilaments are readily obtained from the supernatants of spinal cord homogenates and can be seen and monitored by negative staining techniques (Schlaepfer, 1977). Addition of calcium to these neurofilament preparations causes a granular disruption of the isolated filaments (Schlaepfer and Freeman, 1980). At the same time, there is a rapid and extensive loss of neurofilament triplet proteins when neurofilament preparations are examined by SDS gel electrophoresis. The progression of calcium-dependent loss of neurofilament triplet proteins is identical to that that occurs *in situ* following experimental influx of calcium into rat peripheral nerve.

A major advance in our understanding of calcium-mediated disruption of neurofilaments was provided by the observation that washed neurofilaments are not susceptible to calcium degradation (lSchlaepfer and Freeman, 1980). Washed neurofilaments in these experiments represented neurofilaments that had been pelleted and resuspended in fresh buffer, whereas unwashed neurofilaments were admixed with many proteins that coexisted in the crude supernatant from rat spinal cord homogenates. Parallel incubations of washed and unwashed neurofilaments of the same preparation showed that only the latter were degraded by calcium (Figures 4, 5). Susceptibility to calcium degradation could be restored to washed neurofilaments by addition of soluble proteins from the crude supernatant. Accordingly, it was shown that calcium does not act directly to disrupt neurofilaments. Instead, the crude supernatant contained soluble factor(s) that mediated the calcium-dependent disruption of neurofilaments. These soluble factor(s) were identified as calcium-activated neutral

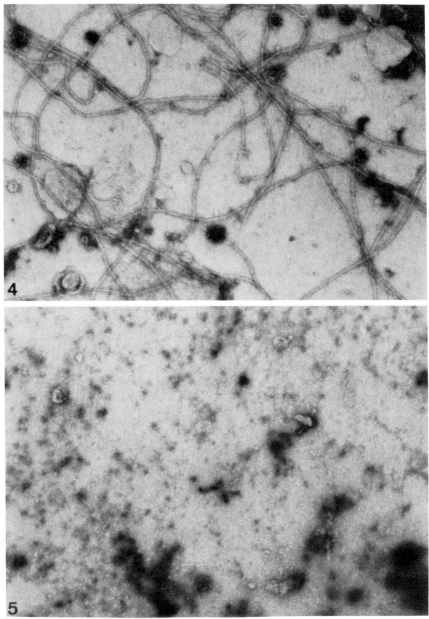

FIGURE 4. Intact neurofilaments from saline-washed neurofilament preparation after 2-hr incubation with 4 mM calcium. Susceptibility to calcium-induced disruption of neurofilaments was restored by additions (20% v/v) of saline wash. ×65,000. (From Schlaepfer, 1979.)

thiol protease(s), since they were inactivated by heat, could be recovered from ammonium sulfate precipitates, were active between pH 6.0 and 9.0, and were selectively susceptible to the thiol group of enzyme inhibitors.

Disruptive morphological features were used to localize degradative reactions in nerve that corresponded to the activity of a calcium-activated, neutral thiol protease. The calcium-dependent granular disintegration of axoplasm was found to fit with characteristics of such a reaction. For example, calcium-induced axoplasmic changes occur in the neutral and alkaline pH range and are totally prevented by thiol reagents (Schlaepfer and Hasler, 1979a). Furthermore, these studies showed that preincubation of frozen sections in calcium-free media progressively diminished the capacity of axoplasm to undergo granular disintegration, a finding interpreted as indicating that the latter reaction is mediated by a soluble factor that could diffuse out of the axoplasm. Finally, it is noteworthy that the same pattern of calcium-dependent disintegration of axoplasm occurred universally among myelinated and unmyelinated fibers of peripheral nerve, in the optic tract, and in spinal cord white matter of tissues incubated in calcium (Schlaepfer and Zimmerman, 1981). Other studies have suggested that calcium-activated protease(s) occur in the distal but not in the proximal regions of mouse optic nerve (Nixon *et al.,* 1982).

4. ISOLATION OF CALCIUM-ACTIVATED PROTEASE FROM NEURAL TISSUES

Calcium-activated protease has been successfully isolated from rat brain and spinal cord (Zimmerman and Schlaepfer, 1982). The isolated enzyme degrades neurofilament triplet proteins very rapidly with apparent K_m values of 3.9×10^{-8}, 4.4×10^{-8}, and 8.2×10^{-8} M for the M_r 68,000, 150,000, and 200,000 neurofilament proteins, respectively. Proteolytic activity is dependent on calcium concentration, with threshold and saturation values of about 10^{-6} and 10^{-4} M, respectively. Similar calcium levels cause enzyme inactivation by autoproteolysis. The enzyme is sensitive to thiol protease inhibitors, is activated by Sr^{2+}, Ba^{2+}, Mn^{2+}, and La^{3+} at 1–10 mM, and has an optimal pH range of 7.4–8.0. These features of the isolated enzyme are identical to the biochemical characteristics of calcium-activated proteolysis that occurs in rat peripheral nerve *in situ* (Schlaepfer *et al.,* 1981).

These findings suggest that there is a relative homogeneity among calcium-activated proteases in rat neural tissues, including the calcium-activated

---

FIGURE 5. Granular debris from unwashed neurofilament preparation after 2-hr incubation with 4 mM calcium. Calcium-induced breakdown of neurofilaments was prevented by addition of 1 mM PCMB. ×65,000. (From Schlaepfer, 1979.)

protease that is believed to occur in astroglial cells (Schlaepfer and Zimmerman, 1981). Further evidence of the homogeneity of calcium-activated proteases is provided by the similarities in the patterns of neurofilament protein degradation by different preparations of rat brain and spinal cord, including crude brain supernatant, different column fractions during enzyme purification, and purified calcium-activated protease. In each case, the neurofilament triplet proteins show the same relative susceptibility to calcium-activated proteolysis, which is roughly inversely proportional to their molecular sizes. Furthermore, similar-sized intermediate breakdown fragments appear during neurofilament protein breakdown. Evidence for selective proteolysis of individual neurofilament proteins, as seen by Nixon *et al.* (1982), was not encountered. Finally, conditions that decreased or abolished enzymatic activity had uniform effects on all three neurofilament proteins.

More recent studies on the calcium-activated protease from rat brain indicate that some heterogeneity in enzymatic activity arises from multiple forms of enzyme that share the same catalytic subunit (Zimmerman and Schlaepfer, 1984). At least two forms of enzyme can be eluted separately from DEAE-cellulose chromatography. A protease that is activated by micromolar concentrations of calcium elutes from DEAE-cellulose at 0.07–0.1 *M* NaCl. This enzyme, with high affinity for calcium (i.e., high-affinity enzyme), has optimal activity at pH 7.0–7.5 and is not susceptible to inactivation during incubations with micro- or millimolar levels of calcium. A second enzyme form with low affinity for calcium (i.e., low-affinity enzyme) elutes from DEAE-cellulose at 0.27–0.3 *M* NaCl. The low-affinity enzyme is a highly active form of the enzyme but requires near-millimolar levels of calcium for activation. It is readily inactivated by autocatalysis during incubation with millimolar calcium. It can also be inactivated by the high-affinity enzyme at micromolar levels of calcium. The pH optimum (7.5–8.5) of the low-affinity enzyme is slightly more alkaline than that of the high-affinity enzyme form. Most enzyme preparations contain admixtures of low- and high-affinity enzyme forms. The proteolytic activity profiles of admixed enzyme preparations are dominated by the much higher activity of the low-affinity enzyme when calcium-mediated activity is monitored using millimolar concentrations of calcium.

Both high- and low-affinity forms of calcium-activated protease degrade neurofilament proteins in the same manner. Autoradiographs of radioiodinated neurofilament triplet proteins during their degradation show identical patterns and sequences of change by high- and low-affinity enzyme forms. These findings strongly support the view that the high- and low-affinity forms of calcium-activated protease share the same catalytic subunit.

Substrate affinity chromatography has been used to purify and further characterize the high- and low-affinity forms of calcium-activated protease. With either neurofilament proteins or casein as substrate, the high-affinity enzyme selectively binds the affinity column when enzyme and column have been equilibrated at 10^{-5} M calcium. Enzyme forms with lower affinity for calcium do not bind to the substate and can be washed away. Purified high-affinity enzyme can then be separated by lowering the calcium concentration to 10^{-7} M in the eluting Ca/EGTA buffer. The purified high-affinity enzyme from rat brain and spinal cord reveals a M_r of 96,000 when monitored by SDS acrylamide electrophoresis.

Separation of the low-affinity enzyme by substrate affinity chromatography is complicated by the autocatalysis of enzyme when activated by calcium. Nevertheless, the enzyme form is retarded during passage through the affinity column at 10^{-3} M calcium and is markedly enriched in fractions eluted with 10^{-5} M calcium. The eluted low-affinity enzyme is very active enzymatically and appears as a single band at M_r 76,000 by SDS gel electrophoresis. This protein band is degraded into progressively smaller fragments during calcium inactivation of the enzyme.

Western immunoblot studies using rabbit antisera to low-affinity protease reveals extensive if not total immunologic cross reactivity between the high- and low-affinity forms of calcium-activated protease from rat brain. These antibody probes also indicate that calcium-activated protease may well exist in a larger molecular mass complex *in vivo*. For example, fresh brain tissues that are rapidly solubilized in SDS contain prominent antiprotease binding sites in electrophoretic protein bands at M_r 96,000 and 160,000. The M_r 96,000 protein corresponds to the high-affinity protease, which elutes from DEAE-cellulose at 0.07–0.1 M NaCl. The M_r 160,000 protein corresponds to an additional high-affinity protease, which elutes from DEAE-cellulose at 0.07–0.1 M NaCl and can be separated from the M_r 96,000 protease by gel filtration. Further characterization of the larger high-affinity enzyme form is complicated by its instability as well as its coisolation with endogenous enzyme inhibitors.

5. TURNOVER OF NEUROFILAMENT PROTEINS AND THE REGULATION OF THE AXONAL CYTOSKELETON

There is very little direct information on the fate of neurofilament and other cytoskeletal proteins that form the bulk of slow axonal transport. Only a single study has examined the turnover of cytoskeletal proteins in distal neurites (Lasek and Black, 1977). This study has shown that there is, indeed, a rapid dispersal of radiolabeled cytoskeleton, especially neurofilament triplet proteins, as they reach synaptic terminals. What exactly happens to neurofilament proteins at this stage, the nature of their transformation by proteolysis, and the fate of degradation products are unknown. Do proteolytic fragments maintain any neurofilament protein characteristics, or are they degraded to small amorphous peptide fragments? Are these products lost or dispersed through exocytosis, or are they retained within the parent neuron? Are they compartmentalized within axonal terminals, and are they subject to translocation via retrograde axonal transport? Finally, is it possible that translocated fragments of neurofilament proteins return to the perikaryon where they influence transcription, translation, and/or assembly of neurofilaments? This hypothetical sequence would imply that breakdown fragments of neurofilament proteolysis function as a feedback control mechanism to regulate the synthesis and delivery of cytoskeletal components in accordance with changing needs and requirements for cytoskeletal proteins in the distal neurites.

The hypothesis that neurofilament synthesis is regulated in part by a feedback mechanism involving products of neurofilament degradation is entirely speculative at this time. The theory requires complex movements and interactions among intermediates of neurofilament metabolism that have not yet been defined and identified. It is therefore unlikely that any single piece of evidence will be forthcoming that will either establish or refute the above hypothesis. Instead, it seems more reasonable to address the validity of the hypothesis by examining some of the premises that underlie the overall theory.

Evidence for the persistence of distinctive neurofilament fragments in tissues following proteolytic degradation of neurofilament proteins *in vivo* is provided by immunoblot studies on transected rat sciatic nerves (Schlaepfer *et al.,* 1984). Breakdown of neurofilament proteins in transected nerves is mediated by endogenous calcium-activated proteolysis and results in the loss of neurofilament triplet proteins from SDS gel electrophoretic profiles (Schlaepfer and Micko, 1978; Bignami *et al.,* 1981; Kamakura *et al.,* 1983). Indeed, the complete loss of neurofilament triplet proteins during the 24- to 60-hr interval following nerve transection is confirmed by immunoblotting the transected nerve proteins and probing the transferred proteins with polyclonal and monoclonal neurofilament antibodies. Many of the immunogenic foci on neurofilament proteins are markedly diminished or lost during the breakdown of axonal proteins in transected nerves. Some antigenic sites, however, are retained and can be used to identify and monitor neurofilament fragments that survive proteolytic degradation. It is of interest that these neurofilament protein fragments retain not only neurofilament antigenicity but also the unusual neurofilament property of insolubility in nonionic detergents such as 1% Triton X-100. The latter property may reflect the tendency of fragments to self-aggregation, possibly because of retention of the α-helical structure of the intermediate filaments (Geisler *et al.,* 1982).

The persistence of neurofilament fragments in transected nerves is not necessarily comparable to that of neurofilament turnover within intact nerves. Neurofilament fragments are part of the axonal debris that probably becomes externalized after disappearance of the axonal compartment in transected nerves (Schlaepfer and Hasler, 1979*b*). Indeed, immunoblot studies indicate that neurofilament fragments of transected nerves remain unaltered during a 3- to 35-day interval following transection. On the other hand, neurofilament fragments from turnover phenomena would presumably be mobilized and disseminated within the intact neurites. Nevertheless, it seems likely that the same enzyme systems would be operative during neurofilament turnover as during neurofilament degradation in transected nerve. In fact, the degree of proteolysis should be more severe under the latter pathological condition. Thus, the survival of neurofilament fragments in transected nerve is a strong indication that similar fragments may be recycled during neurofilament turnover.

Immunoblot studies of normal neural tissues using neurofilament antibodies reveal the presence of multiple immunoreactive fragments in addition to the characteristic neurofilament triplet proteins (Calvert and Anderton, 1982). Some of the immunoreactive bands may represent posttranslational modifications of the neurofilament triplet proteins during anterograde axonal transit. The prominence of some nontriplet bands may also reflect enhanced detectability by the much more sensitive immunoblot methodology. Nevertheless, it is likely that many of the immunoreactive nontriplet neurofilament bands seen in neural tissues represents processing and movement of neurofilament protein fragments that have been degraded and are in the process of being recycled. Evidence that some neurofilament nontriplet bands of intact rat sciatic nerve are proteolytic products of neurofilament degradation is seen in the correspondence of these bands with similar bands from transected nerve. Most prominent neurofilament degradative products seen with immunoblots have M_r of 50,000 to 60,000. The appearance and increasing prominence of neurofilament nontriplet bands during development and maturation of rat brain (Calvert and Anderton, 1982) could also be interpreted as evidence for the turnover and recycling of fragments in neurofilament metabolism.

The presence of proteolytic fragments of neurofilament proteins in neural tissues is a very important observation. Many additional studies, however, will be needed to determine whether these neurofilament fragments have some regulatory role in neurofilament synthesis and assembly or whether they merely reflect the conservation of peptide residues within the confines of a cell. If neurofilament synthesis and, perhaps, other aspects of axonal cytoskeleton elaboration are controlled by feedback mechanisms, then the elucidation of these phenomena will undoubtedly provide crucial insights for our understanding of the basic principles underlying neurite formation during development and during nerve regeneration.

6. REFERENCES

Bignami, A., Dahl, M. D., Nguyen, B. T., and Crosby, C. J., 1981, The fate of axonal debris in Wallerian degeneration of rat optic and sciatic nerves, *J. Neuropathol. Exp. Neurol.* **40**:537–550.

Calvert, R., and Anderton, B. H., 1982, *In vivo* metabolism of mammalian neurofilament poly-peptides in developing and adult rat brain, *FEBS Lett.* **145**:171–175.

Fluckiger, E., and Keynes, R. D., 1957, The calcium permeability of *Loligo* axons, *J. Physiol. (Lond.)* **128**:41–42p.

Geisler, N., Kaufman, E., and Weber, K., 1982, Protein chemical characterization of three struc-turally distinct domains along the protofilament unit of desmin 10 nm filaments, *Cell* **30**:277–286.

Hodgkin, A. L., and Katz, B., 1949, The effect of calcium on the axoplasm of giant nerve fibers, *J. Exp. Biol.* **26**:292–294.

Hodgkin, A. L., and Keynes, R. D., 1956, Experiments on the injection of substances into squid giant axons by means of microsyringe, *J. Physiol. (Lond.)* **131**:592–616.

Hodgkin, A. L., and Keynes, R. D., 1957, Movements of labelled calcium in squid giant axons, *J. Physiol. (Lond.)* **138**:253–281.

Kamakura, K., Ishiura, S., Sugita, H., and Toyokura, Y., 1983, Identification of Ca^{++} activated neutral protease in the peripheral nerve and its effects on neurofilament degeneration, *J. Neurochem.* **40**:908–913.

Lasek, R. J., and Black, M. M., 1977, How do axons stop growing? Some clues from the metab-olism of the proteins in the slow component of axonal transport, in: *Mechanisms, Regulation and Special Functions of Protein Synthesis in the Brain* (S. Roberts, A. Lajtha, and W. H. Gispen, eds.), pp. 161–169, Elsevier/North-Holland Biomedical Press, Amsterdam.

Nixon, R. A., Brown, B. A., and Marotta, C. A., 1982, Posttranslational modification of a neu-rofilament protein during axoplasmic transport: Implications for regional specialization of CNS axons, *J. Cell Biol.* **94**:150–158.

Schlaepfer, W. W., 1971, Experimental alteration of neurofilaments and neurotubules by cal-cium and other ions, *Exp. Cell Res.* **67**:73–80.

Schlaepfer, W. W., 1974a, Calcium-induced degeneration of axoplasm in isolated segments of rat peripheral nerve, *Brain Res.* **69**:203–215.

Schlaepfer, W. W., 1974b, Effects of energy deprivation on Wallerian degeneration in isolated segments of rat peripheral nerve, *Brain Res.* **78**:71–81.

Schlaepfer, W. W., 1977, Studies on the isolation and substructure of mammalian neurofila-ments, *J. Ultrastruct. Res.* **61**:149–157.

Schlaepfer, W. W., 1978, Structural alterations of peripheral nerve induced by the calcium iono-phore, A23187, *Brain Res.* **136**:1–9.

Schlaepfer, W. W., 1979, Nature of mammalian neurofilaments and their breakdown by cal-cium, *Prog. Neuropathol.* **4**:101–123.

Schlaepfer, W. W., and Bunge, R. P., 1973, The effects of calcium ion concentration on the degeneration of amputated axons in tissue culture, *J. Cell Biol.* **59**:456–470.

Schlaepfer, W. W., and Freeman, L. A., 1980, Calcium-dependent degradation of mammalian neurofilaments by soluble tissue factor(s) from rat spinal cord, *Neuroscience* **5**:2305–2314.

Schlaepfer, W. W., and Hasler, M. B., 1979a, The persistence and possible externalization of axonal debris during Wallerian degeneration, *J. Neuropathol. Exp. Neurol.* **38**:242–252.

Schlaepfer, W. W., and Hasler, M. B., 1979b, Characterization of the calcium-induced disrup-tion of neurofilaments in rat peripheral nerve, *Brain Res.* **168**:299–309.

Schlaepfer, W. W., and Micko, S., 1978, Chemical and structural changes of neurofilaments in transected rat sciatic nerve, *J. Cell Biol.* **78**:637–678.

Schlaepfer, W. W., and Micko, S., 1979, Calcium-dependent alterations of neurofilament pro-teins of rat peripheral nerve, *J. Neurochem.* **32**:211–219.

Schlaepfer, W. W., and Zimmerman, U.-J. P., 1981, Calcium-mediated breakdown of glial fil-aments and neurofilaments in rat optic nerve and spinal cord, *Neurochem. Res.* **6**:243–255.

Schlaepfer, W. W., Zimmerman, U.-J. P., and Micko, S., 1981, Neurofilament proteolysis in rat peripheral nerve. Homologies with calcium-activated proteolysis of other tissues, *Cell Calcium* **2**:235–250.

Schlaepfer, W. W., Lee, C., Trojanowski, J. Q., and Lee, V. M.-L., 1984, Persistence of immunoreactive fragments of neurofilament proteins in transected rat sciatic nerve, *J. Neurochem.* (in press).

Soifer, D., Iqbal, K., Czosnek, H., DeMartini, J., Sturman, J. A., and Wisniewski, H. M., 1981, The loss of neuron-specific proteins during the course of Wallerian degeneration of optic and sciatic nerve, *J. Neurosci.* **1**:461–470.

Zimmerman, U.-J. P., and Schlaepfer, W. W., 1982, Characterization of a brain calcium-activated protease that degrades neurofilament proteins, *Biochemistry* **21**:3977–3983.

Zimmerman, U.-J. P., and Schlaepfer, W. W., 1984, Multiple forms of calcium-activated protease from rat brain and muscle, *J. Biol. Chem.* **259**:3210–3218.

INDEX